OXFORD MEDICAL PUBLICATIONS

Head, Neck, and Dental Emergencies

T0202099

**Published and forthcoming titles in
the Emergencies in . . . series:**

Emergencies in Adult Nursing
Edited by Philip Downing

Emergencies in Anaesthesia, Third Edition
Edited by Keith Allman, Andrew McIndoe, and Iain H. Wilson

Emergencies in Children's and Young People's Nursing
Edited by E.A. Glasper, Gill McEwing, and Jim Richardson

Emergencies in Critical Care, Second Edition
Edited by Martin Beed, Richard Sherman, and Ravi Mahajan

Emergencies in Gastroenterology and Hepatology
Marcus Harbord and Daniel Marks

Emergencies in Obstetrics and Gynaecology, Second Edition
Edited by Stergios K. Doumouchtsis and S. Arulkumaran

Emergencies in Paediatrics and Neonatology, Second Edition
Edited by Stuart Crisp and Jo Rainbow

Emergencies in Palliative and Supportive Care
Edited by David Currow and Katherine Clark

Emergencies in Respiratory Medicine
Edited by Robert Parker, Catherine Thomas, and Lesley Bennett

Emergencies in Sports Medicine
Edited by Julian Redhead and Jonathan Gordon

Head, Neck, and Dental Emergencies, Second Edition
Edited by Mike Perry

OXFORD MEDICAL PUBLICATIONS

Head, Neck, and Dental Emergencies

SECOND EDITION

EDITED BY

Mike Perry

Consultant Maxillofacial Surgeon
Regional North West London Craniomaxillofacial Unit,
Northwick Park and St Mary's Major Trauma Service,
Northwick Park Hospital, Harrow, Middlesex, UK

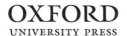
OXFORD
UNIVERSITY PRESS

OXFORD
UNIVERSITY PRESS

Great Clarendon Street, Oxford, OX2 6DP,
United Kingdom

Oxford University Press is a department of the University of Oxford.
It furthers the University's objective of excellence in research, scholarship,
and education by publishing worldwide. Oxford is a registered trade mark of
Oxford University Press in the UK and in certain other countries

© Oxford University Press 2018

The moral rights of the authors have been asserted

First Edition published in 2005
Second Edition published in 2018

Impression: 1

Published in the United States of America by Oxford University Press
198 Madison Avenue, New York, NY 10016, United States of America

British Library Cataloguing in Publication Data
Data available

Library of Congress Control Number: 2017941744

ISBN 978–0–19–877909–4

Printed and bound in China by
C&C Offset Printing Co., Ltd.

Preface

This second edition has been extensively revised to make its contents more practically useful for the user. The aim is to help the reader develop a targeted approach in their assessment and management of those 'emergencies' that occur in the anatomical regions above the collar bones. Such patients may attend an emergency department or general practice clinic, or they may present on the ward. Although this book is part of the 'Emergencies in ...' series of books published by OUP, the strict application of the definition of an emergency to the head and neck (i.e. an immediately life- or sight-threatening condition) would result in just a handful of cases being listed and discussed. Therefore, a more broadly defined remit has been used, that is, to cover urgent and potentially worrying problems which may present to the non-specialist or novice.

How this book works

Generally speaking, patients do not present with a ready-made diagnosis, but rather with either a symptom located to an anatomical region (e.g. toothache, a lump/swelling, or a headache), or an obvious problem (such as a nose bleed or injury). This is the starting point in each of the anatomically based chapters ('Common presentations' and 'Common problems and their causes'). For each symptom a variety of conditions may be the cause and these are listed. These conditions have also been categorized as common or uncommon, although it is accepted that individual clinicians, departments, and specialists will all have differing experiences of their frequency (depending on training and geographical location). We have tried to include the majority of conditions likely to be encountered in non-specialist practice, but clearly it is not possible (nor practical) to include the rare or obscure in view of the aims of this book.

Making a diagnosis

Diagnosis requires a history and examination. As undergraduate students, we are taught this must be all inclusive, with a full detailed history and full examination of the patient. However, the reality of any emergency department setting, busy practice, or assessment of an urgent problem is that a more limited, but targeted approach is required. By necessity the questions and examination are more focused. But at the same time these must not omit those key elements which are required to make an *accurate* diagnosis. In accordance with this, the next section in each chapter ('Useful questions and what to look for') lists relevant and important diagnostic cues, in relation to each presenting symptom. These questions should be regarded as an aide memoire and when appropriate can be tailored accordingly. Some overlap and repetition is inevitable. The aim of this section is therefore to equip the reader with the necessary knowledge to enable them to quickly and accurately triage and diagnose a problem.

The remainder of each chapter is self-evident with details on how to examine each anatomical site, useful investigations (in both the emergency department and outpatient setting), and some notes on the conditions themselves. Management is also covered, based on current evidence, but as guidelines continue to evolve this may change. Where available, local protocols should always be used (e.g. 'clearing' a cervical spine injury).

For the pedants among us, it is accepted that not every known condition is covered. It must also be remembered that some symptoms may be the result of systemic disease (e.g. bleeding gums, halitosis, and headaches), while other head and neck pathologies may present with symptoms outside this site (e.g. cervical rib, overactive thyroid, or secretory pituitary adenoma). Nevertheless, if this book is used as a practical guide, or a manual, we are confident the reader will find it a useful diagnostic aid. Undergraduates may also find it useful when preparing for clinical examinations.

Contents

Contributors to the second edition

Wing Chuen Chan
Consultant Ophthalmologist,
Royal Victoria Hospital,
Belfast, UK
Chapter 10

Ramesh Gurunathan
Consultant Head and
Neck Surgeon, Darlington
Memorial Hospital and James
Cook University Hospital,
Middlesbrough, UK
Chapters 5, 6, and 8

Peter Gordon
Registrar in Oral & Maxillofacial
Surgery, Southern General
Hospital, Glasgow, UK
Chapter 12

John Hanratty
Consultant Oral & Maxillofacial
Surgeon, Ulster Hospital,
Belfast, UK
Chapters 9 and 11

Gina Hooper
Trainee in Emergency Medicine,
Northern Ireland Deanery, UK
Chapter 4

Nida T Ilahi
Medical Student, University of
Glasgow, UK
Chapter 7

Vasuki Gnana Jothi
Consultant Ophthalmologist,
Royal Victoria Hospital,
Belfast, UK
Chapter 10

Kevin Maguire
Consultant in Emergency
Medicine, Ulster Hospital,
Dundonald, UK
Chapter 4

Jonathan Poots
Specialty Registrar, Neurosurgery,
Royal Victoria Hospital, Belfast, UK
Chapter 3

Brian Purcell
Core Surgical Trainee, ENT, Royal
Victoria Hospital, Belfast, UK
Chapter 6

Anna E Raymond
Formerly General Dentist,
TFI Dentistry, Thornlands,
Queensland, Australia
Chapter 13

Henry Neil Simms
Consultant Neurosurgeon,
Training Programme Director,
Neurosurgery, Royal Victoria
Hospital, Belfast, UK
Chapter 3

Gavin Smith
Anaesthetics and ICM Trainee,
Ulster Hospital, Dundonald, UK
Reviewer

Christopher Vinall
Specialist Registrar, Oral &
Maxillofacial Surgery, Peninsula
Deanery, UK
Chapters 1, 2

Contributors to the first edition

Howard Brydon FRCS
Consultant Neurosurgeon,
University Hospital of North
Staffordshire, UK

Anne Dancey MRCS
Specialist Registrar in Plastic
Surgery, West Midlands
Rotation, UK

Nick Grew FRCS, FDS
Consultant Maxillofacial Surgeon,
Wolverhampton, UK

Manoli Heliotis FRCS, FDS
Specialist Registrar in Maxillofacial
Surgery, South Thames
Rotation, UK

Ian Holland FRCS, FDS
Consultant Maxillofacial Surgeon,
West of Scotland, UK

William Kisku FRCS
Staff Grade in Burns and Plastic
Surgery, University Hospital of
North Staffordshire, UK

**Professor Nick Maffulli BSc,
PhD, MBBS, MD, FRCS**
Consultant Orthopaedic Surgeon,
University Hospital of North
Staffordshire, UK

**Kamiar Mireskandari
FRCOpth**
Specialist Registrar in
Ophthalmology, Moorefields Eye
Hospital, London, UK

Jehanzeb Mughal FDS
Maxillofacial Unit, University
Hospital of North
Staffordshire, UK

Mike Perry FRCS, FDS, BSc
Consultant Maxillofacial Surgeon
and Trauma Team Leader,
University Hospital of North
Staffordshire, UK

**Mr Philip Roberts
MBBS, FRCS**
Specialist Registrar Orthopaedic
and Trauma Surgery,
University Hospital of North
Staffordshire, UK

Mr Mike Shelly FRCS, FDS
Specialist Registrar in Maxillofacial
Surgery, South Thames
Rotation, UK

**Richard T Walker RD,
BDS, PhD, MSc, FDS RCS,
FDS, RCPS**
Formerly Centre Director,
International Centre for
Excellence in Dentistry, Eastman
Dental Institute for Oral Health
Sciences, University College
London, UK

**Lt Col. Mike Williams,
FRCS, FDS**
Specialist Registrar in Maxillofacial
Surgery, South Thames
Rotation, UK

Symbols and abbreviations

❢	cross-reference
AACG	acute angle-closure glaucoma
ABG	arterial blood gas
AC	air conduction
ACE	angiotensin-converting enzyme
APD	afferent pupillary defect
ATLS®	Advanced Trauma Life Support®
AVM	arteriovenous malformation
BC	bone conduction
BNBM	nil by mouth
BP	blood pressure
BPPV	benign paroxysmal positional vertigo
BRONJ	bisphosphonate-related osteonecrosis of the jaw
CCS	central cord syndrome
CN	cranial nerve
CNS	central nervous system
COPD	Chronic obstructive pulmonary disease
CPP	cerebral perfusion pressure
CRP	C-reactive protein
CSF	cerebrospinal fluid
CT	computed tomography
CTA	computed tomography angiography
CXR	chest X-ray
DVT	deep vein thrombosis
EAM	external auditory meatus
ECG	electrocardiogram
EMG	electromyography
ENT	ear, nose, and throat
ESR	erythrocyte sedimentation rate
FBC	full blood count
FNA	fine-needle aspiration
GCS	Glasgow Coma Scale
GI	gastrointestinal
GORD	gastroesophageal reflux disease
HDU	high dependency unit
HSV	herpes simplex virus
ICH	intracranial haemorrhage
ICP	intracranial pressure
ICU	intensive care unit
IJV	internal jugular vein
IM	intramuscular
INR	international normalized ratio
IOFB	intraocular foreign body
IOP	intraocular pressure
ITU	intensive therapy unit
IV	intravenous
LFT	liver function test
LMA	laryngeal mask airway
LMN	lower motor neuron
LMW	low molecular weight
LP	lumbar puncture
MRA	magnetic resonance angiography
MRI	magnetic resonance imaging
MS	multiple sclerosis
MVC	motor vehicle collision
NOE	naso-orbitoethmoid
NSAID	non-steroidal anti-inflammatory drug
OCS	orbital compartment syndrome
OM	occipitomental
OPT	orthopantomography
ORN	osteoradionecrosis
OSA	obstructive sleep apnoea
PA	posteroanterior
PCR	polymerase chain reaction
PE	pulmonary embolism
PMH	past medical history
RAPD	relative afferent pupillary defect
RBH	retrobulbar haemorrhage
SCM	sternocleidomastoid

SGS	subglottic stenosis		TMJDS	temporomandibular joint dysfunction syndrome
SJS	Stevens–Johnson syndrome		TON	traumatic optic neuropathy
SLE	systemic lupus erythematosus		U&E	urea and electrolyte
SOF	superior orbital fissure		UMN	upper motor neuron
TB	tuberculosis		UTRI	upper respiratory tract infection
TIA	transient ischaemic attack		VZV	varicella zoster virus
TMJ	temporomandibular joint		WCC	white cell count

Principles of assessment

Taking a history and examining the patient in the emergency department

History taking is the first stage in diagnosis. Even though this can be an arduous task, being repeated every day, one must not lose sight of the fact that for the patient this may be a sensitive or private issue. He or she may be asked questions for which the answers may not be normally shared even with their close contacts (e.g. circumstances resulting in an injury, alcohol/recreational drug usage, and sexual contacts/HIV risk). Therefore be sensitive to this. Introduce yourself and any member of your team who is present. Take time and be clear in the introductions. Try not to interrupt patients when they are talking. Not everyone is able to express themselves clearly in a few words. Know how to contact interpreters if the patient is having problems in communicating or expressing themselves in English. Remain in control.

Setting and privacy

Make sure that you have enough space to be able to create a comfortable environment. For patients accompanied by a carer or member of their family, ask them to join you, as they might be able to provide additional information. However, only include them if the patient consents to this (unless of course the patient is of non-consenting age or deemed mentally unable to give consent).

Sometimes your patient may wish to talk in private. In such a situation, make sure that you take the necessary precautions to safeguard yourself; include a member of staff as a chaperon. If this is not possible, then leave the door or curtains of the consultation area partially open. Document everyone present in the notes.

Documentation and handwriting

This should be clear enough for all future use. Many 'alleged assaults' will result in criminal proceedings and you or your seniors may be called upon to write a report many months later. Be careful what you write. Stick to the facts and what the patient tells you. Avoid speculation. Try to note as much detail as you can of what is told to you—this may avoid the patient having to repeat potentially embarrassing information to another colleague. It may help to highlight important information with a different coloured pen or a sticker, i.e. allergies, HIV, hepatitis C status, and sensitive topics (where the patient does not want others to know).

What is written in the notes is accepted as an accurate account of events, anything more is inadmissible unless a chaperon testifies to it. It is difficult to defend oneself in a court of law on the basis of memory and the law may favour the patient in this regard. Legible writing ensures that colleagues who continue the patient's care can read what you have written.

Photography

Photographs can be very helpful, but can be difficult to take in an emergency department. Make sure that the patient has consented in writing to these if you can. Alternatively, get the consent in retrospect. Nowadays many hospitals are limiting the ability to take photographs so follow your local policies on this.

The presenting complaint

This is best recorded briefly and if possible in the patient's own words. The most common complaint is pain and it is important to be able to differentiate its different origins. This can be difficult in the head and neck. Patients may also present with a whole host of other problems that may or may not be associated with pain. There are of course many other clinical reasons why someone may seek urgent care and the following list gives an idea of the more common ones. These will be covered in more detail in the relevant sections. Some presenting complaints tend to be common in certain age groups, and this becomes more recognizable with experience. However, be warned not to prematurely make a diagnosis without completing the history and examination. It is tempting to do just that and you may miss a rare or unusual condition—these may still be seen in an emergency department.

Some reasons why patients go to an emergency department

Common
- Pain
- Injuries
- Bleeding
- Trismus
- Lumps or swellings
- Rashes and ulcers
- Social-related problems.

Uncommon
- Altered sensation or weakness
- Facial asymmetry
- Stiffness
- Abnormal function (e.g. vision, bite).

History of the presenting complaint

When asking about the presenting symptom, consider the following questions. These are of course just a starting point but will hopefully enable you to identify most problems. Questions can be tailored accordingly and this is discussed in the relevant chapters.

Useful key questions

Pain
- Site of pain—this must be documented with reference to trigger points and/or referred pain. Use a diagram.
- Description of pain—constant, intermittent, dull, aching, throbbing, sharp, burning, or shooting?
- Periodicity—speed of onset, duration, frequency.

- Influences—does anything affect the pain, e.g. movement, heat, or cold?
- Associated symptoms—swelling, dysfunction, numbness or dysaesthesia, pain anywhere else?
- Previous therapies—has anything to date improved the pain?

Assaults/injuries
- Time and place
- Mechanism of injury
- Any loss of consciousness?
- Where did the patient go afterwards (emergency department, home etc.), and how did they get to hospital (walk, ambulance, or other transport)?
- Any other injuries apart from on the head/face?
- Are the police involved? Get consent to speak to them if they arrive later.
- Any previous injuries (the broken nose may be old)?

Bleeding
- How long/often?
- Where from?
- Underlying cause?
- Predisposing history or medication?
- Symptoms of hypovolaemia/shock/anaemia?

Trismus (limitation of mouth opening due to muscle spasm)
- Duration?
- Progression?
- Symptoms of underlying infection or possible tumour?
- Difficulty swallowing?
- Difficulty breathing?

Lumps or swellings
- How long?
- Is it growing?
- Related to mealtimes (salivary obstruction)?
- Is it painful (infected or rapid growth)?
- Any obvious cause/lumps elsewhere?

Rashes and ulcers
- Dermatological history.
- Associated with vesicles/blisters?
- Any ocular/genital/gastrointestinal (GI)/joint symptoms?
- Drug history.

Altered sensation or weakness
- Where (anatomical or diffuse)?
- Any underlying cause?
- Any associated swellings/ulcers (possible tumours)?
- Any other neurological symptoms?

Facial asymmetry
- Localized or generalized?
- Painful/painless?
- Is it static/progressive/speed of swelling?

Stiffness
- Which joint?
- Any preceding cause?
- When is it most stiff (in the morning/evening)?
- Does movement improve the stiffness ('rusty gate')?
- Are other joints affected?
- Is there associated swelling or pain?
- Any neurological symptoms (especially with neck stiffness)?
- Any symptoms to suggest a connective tissue disease?
- Any family history?

Abnormal bite
(See ➡ Chapter 12.)
- When did it change?
- Is it painful?

Infections
- How long?
- Any obvious cause (toothache/viral/injury etc.)?
- Is it getting worse?
- Any signs of systemic upset?
- Has the patient been taking antibiotics?

Other useful information

Systems review
Document the patient's general health. This is important in order to assess the fitness of the patient should surgery be required and to decide on the type of anaesthesia required. It may also modify treatment. There is no real indication to listen to the chest of a medically fit and healthy 18-year-old who complains of pain from a wisdom tooth.

Past medical history, medication, and allergies
Any medication currently in use must be recorded, as well as allergies to medication and any other substances. This will help reduce the risks of a prescription error being made. Anticoagulants are of relevance following

trauma. Knowledge of chronic steroid use is important when dealing with infections. If there is an allergy, is it a true allergy? Or is it drug intolerance (e.g. diarrhoea with penicillin)?

Social history

Occupation, family situation, living conditions, smoking, alcohol consumption, employment, and hobbies. Do they require care? Ask 'On a good day, what is the most active thing you could do?'.

Religious beliefs

Ask about these in certain circumstances. Jehovah's witnesses, for instance, will not accept blood transfusions. This is a potential minefield medico-legally, especially in the unconscious patient (where relatives have been known to be wrong about the patient's beliefs). Seek help in these cases, and preferably find out local protocols before the situation arises.

Remember the possibility of anatomical variations and age-related changes (especially when examining radiographs).

The significance of the past medical, social, and drug history in assessing emergencies and admissions

In all patients requiring admission, or an anaesthetic, a full medical, social, and drug history will eventually be taken. However, when dealing with an emergency this may not be possible in the early stages. This is seen in the management of the seriously injured patient, discussed in Chapter 2. In all sick patients it is essential to rapidly identify those factors which may have an immediate impact on either establishing the diagnosis or managing the clinical problem. These include the following:

Age

Although not a medical condition, the elderly have a decreased physiological reserve and need close monitoring. This is particularly the case following blood loss where prompt fluid replacement is necessary. Care is required not to overload their cardiovascular system. Elderly patients are often taking a variety of medications, each with the potential for problems from withholding, or from drug interactions. Children are also at risk of fluid overload and hyponatraemia. Fluids must be administered with caution (see http://learning.bmj.com/learning/home.html).

Pregnancy

Ask about this in all women of childbearing age. In trauma, the best treatment for the fetus is to treat the mother first. Get the obstetricians involved early. In other emergencies, pregnancy may influence the choice of local anaesthesia and medications. Certain drugs are potentially teratogenic, and affect fetal maturation (closure of ductus arteriosus) or the onset of delivery. If in doubt, refer to medication information sheets or a drug reference book such as the *British National Formulary*. In reality, radiographs (and computed tomography (CT)) of the face carry very little risk to the fetus, but by and large, most units will restrict or minimize these to those regarded as essential.

Ischaemic heart disease

This increases the risks of general anaesthesia and local anaesthesia containing adrenaline (epinephrine). Cardiac pain can occasionally present as discomfort in the neck or mandible or as 'toothache'. It should therefore be considered in the diagnosis. Pain on exertion, relieved by rest or glyceryl trinitrate, is highly suggestive. Nicorandil, a vasodilator prescribed for angina, can cause major solitary ulceration of the oral cavity (and the anus and penis). These ulcers can be confused with malignancy. They typically resolve completely on cessation of the medication within a few weeks.

Hypertension

This increases the risks of general anaesthesia and local anaesthesia. Hypertensive 'crises' (where the blood pressure (BP) is extremely high) can present with headaches and drowsiness.

Rheumatic fever, artificial valves, and endocarditis

Not all abscesses need antibiotics if they are adequately drained (e.g. dental abscess, boils). However, patients with a history of rheumatic fever, prosthetic heart valves, or previous endocarditis are at risk from bacteraemia. In these cases it is important to liaise with the cardiologist and microbiologist. These patients may require a specific antibiotic that covers organisms that cause infective endocarditis (see 'Prophylaxis against infective endocarditis', http://www.nice.org.uk/CG064).

Chronic obstructive pulmonary disease

Do not give oxygen over 28%. The exception to this rule is in the multiply injured patient with life-threatening injuries (see British Thoracic Society guidelines on emergency oxygen, https://www.brit-thoracic.org.uk/guidelines-and-quality-standards/emergency-oxygen-use-in-adult-patients-guideline).

Patients with Chronic obstructive pulmonary disease (COPD) should receive targeted oxygen therapy with the aim of maintaining targeted oxygen saturations. Hypoxia can kill rapidly and is more of a threat than the slower development of hypercapnia. The use of oxygen in respiratory failure is therefore not contraindicated. The vital aspect is that *therapy is adjusted after arterial blood gas (ABG) results are available. Current guidelines suggest these patients are given high priority and that they are not just put on oxygen and then walked away from.*

Asthma

Avoid aspirin and other non-steroidal anti-inflammatory drugs (NSAIDs) if possible. However, not all patients are sensitive to NSAIDs and they are not absolutely contraindicated—they just need to be used with care and the patient reassessed or warned about possible worsening of their asthma. Asthmatics may be taking inhaled steroids which predispose to thrush etc. Rarely, they are taking oral steroids. Get an idea of their asthma control (previous intensive care unit (ICU) admissions, recurrent exacerbations, frequent courses of oral steroids, etc.).

Diabetes

Consider hypoglycaemia in all confused, drowsy, or aggressive head-injured (and non-head-injured) patients, even if they appear to be intoxicated. Patients with diabetes are also at risk of infections, which can spread rapidly (notably dental). Occasionally a severe infection may be the presenting feature of diabetes. All patients with facial abscesses should be screened for this.

Hepatitis

Risks of cross infection. Check liver function tests (LFTs) and clotting.

Epilepsy

Fitting can occur after head injuries, especially in children. It also makes assessment difficult. Status epilepticus aggravates secondary brain injuries (as a result of fluctuations in BP and hypoxia). Intubation, ventilation, and transfer to ICU/intensive therapy unit (ITU) may be required.

Blood dyscrasias

Clotting disorders (haemophilia, platelet disorders, etc.) predispose to the same problems as anticoagulants. Leukaemic patients are also at risk of severe infections. Sickle cell disease requires care with general anaesthesia. It can present acutely with severe pain in the mandible.

Previous injuries

Old facial fractures (e.g. nose, zygoma, or mandible) may make it difficult to decide whether a new injury is a new fracture or just bruising. Acute chest injuries preclude the use of Entonox®, which is particularly helpful in reducing dislocations of the mandibular condyle.

Tetanus status

This is relevant to all lacerations, bites, abrasions, and other penetrating wounds. Wounds can be classified as tetanus prone or non-tetanus prone and depending on the patient's immunization status, a booster, course, or immunoglobulin may be required (see http://www.hpa.org.uk/Topics/InfectiousDiseases/InfectionsAZ/Tetanus/Guidelines).

Drug interactions

Commonly prescribed drugs in the emergency department include opiates, antibiotics, NSAIDs, and sedatives. Each has the potential to interact with commonly prescribed medication that the patient may already be taking. Remember herbal medicines as well (e.g. St John's wort)—they can also interact.

Anticoagulants (e.g. warfarin and aspirin)

Reduced clotting may have an impact following trauma in several ways. Head injuries are at an increased risk of intracranial bleeding and may require admission for observation. Similarly, retrobulbar haemorrhage, and bleeding into easily distensible tissues (floor of mouth, upper airway, and eye), are more likely to occur following trauma to these sites. Panfacial injuries may even require airway protection. Some authorities recommend avoidance of nerve blocks. Bleeding into large body cavities (chest, abdomen, pelvis) around fractures (limbs, retroperitoneum) and externally can rapidly result in haemorrhagic shock. Check clotting and if necessary reverse the anticoagulant. Discuss with haematology.

More recently, new oral anticoagulants (such as apixaban, dabigatran, and rivaroxaban) have become available. These also carry risks of haemorrhage but with these drugs there is no specific reversal agent available (see http://www.mhra.gov.uk/Safetyinformation/DrugSafetyUpdate/CON322347).

Steroids/bisphosphonates

Patients on long-term steroids may require extra steroid cover during infection, trauma, or other periods of stress to prevent adrenal insufficiency. Usually a doubling of their normal dose or conversion to intravenous (IV) is sufficient to ensure reliable administration. Never abruptly stop long-term steroids. The *British National Formulary* has a handy section on this including dose reduction in chronic use. Chronic steroid use also predisposes the patient to the risks of infection, poor wound healing, osteoporosis, and a diabetic potential, each with their own attendant problems. Bisphosphonates may have been prescribed to reduce osteoporosis in the elderly and in patients with metastatic bone disease. These can affect bone healing in the mandible following fracture or dental extractions.

Alcohol intake

Acute alcohol intoxication can result in agitation and unconsciousness, with loss of protective airway reflexes and vomiting. In the head-injured patient, this always makes assessment difficult. Never assume that the drowsy state is simply due to too much 'booze'. Chronic alcoholics are often malnourished and self-neglected and at an increased risk of infection. If it is anticipated that the patient will not be able to drink alcohol for some time, get help in setting up an appropriate withdrawal protocol. They should be given high-potency vitamins B and C, such as Pabrinex®, and require close observation for withdrawal symptoms (see http://publications.nice.org.uk/alcohol-use-disorders-diagnosis-and-clinical-management-of-alcohol-related-physical-complications-cg100; http://www.nice.org.uk/nicemedia/live/12995/49004/49004.pdf).

Home circumstances

One of the criteria for discharge of head-injured patients is appropriate home support. This involves regular observations for at least 24 hours by a responsible adult who can either bring the patient back to casualty or phone for an ambulance if required. If the patient lives in a remote area, it might be better to consider overnight observation.

Allergies

Notably with antibiotics used to treat facial infections.

Family/occupational history

This may sometimes indicate potential risks from anaesthesia and patients should be asked about a history of malignant hyperpyrexia, porphyria, and, if of non-European decent, sickle cell disease.

People in certain occupations may be exposed to hazards that can produce respiratory disease. These include cancers (e.g. asbestos workers), infections (e.g. bird breeders), asthma (e.g. painters), pneumoconiosis (e.g. coal miners), and allergic alveolitis (e.g. farmers). Travel abroad can occasionally result in exotic infections and cervical lymphadenopathy.

Rapid assessment of patients requiring emergency/urgent surgery

Consider the impact of the following in planning management

- Age
- Smoking
- Alcohol abuse
- Ischaemic heart disease
- Respiratory disease (e.g. COPD and asthma)
- Diabetes
- Malnutrition
- Blood disorders (haemophilia, sickle cell anaemia)
- Head/facial injury
- Cervical spine injury.

Management considerations

The initial care of a patient can be considered under several headings. These are applicable to varying extents, but a useful checklist is:
- Treating coexisting medical conditions
- Fluid balance and nutritional support (patient may already be in deficit)
- Deep vein thrombosis (DVT) prophylaxis
- Antibiotic cover
- Steroid cover
- Effective pain relief
- Stress ulcer prophylaxis
- Early involvement of specialists, including physiotherapists and social services.

Whereas patients undergoing elective surgery can be pre-assessed in good time, those requiring emergency surgery cannot and may only be rendered as fit as possible within the time allowed, depending on the degree of urgency. Relatively few emergencies in the head and neck require immediate intervention (such as airway obstruction, extradural haematoma, and retrobulbar haemorrhage) and most can be delayed by at least a few hours, so that the patient's general health can be improved if possible. In selected cases, some patients may benefit from a brief period of intensive management on a high dependency unit (HDU) or ICU. In all cases, early input from an anaesthetist is essential, particularly in those patients with conditions affecting the airway.

Getting patients ready for urgent surgery: medical considerations

Cardiorespiratory assessment

Risk factors for cardiac disease include:
- Smoking
- Diabetes
- Hyperlipidaemia and obesity
- Hypertension
- Male sex
- Family history of cardiac disease.

Thorough assessment of the cardiovascular and respiratory systems is particularly important in patients undergoing surgery. Ischaemic heart disease (myocardial infarction, heart failure, angina), hypertension, asthma, COPD, chest injuries, and chest infections all significantly increase the risks of anaesthesia. Myocardial infarction within the preceding 6 months is a recognized major risk factor in anaesthesia and surgery. There is a 20–50% risk of a further infarction and perioperative death. Patients with a history of ischaemic heart disease should have an up-to-date electrocardiogram (ECG) preoperatively. Patients with a past history of rheumatic fever are predisposed to valvular heart disease, which can lead to heart failure or infective endocarditis. Intraoral procedures, especially those involving the teeth (e.g. removal), are well-recognized risk factors in the development of endocarditis and some patients may require antibiotic cover, depending on the surgical procedure (although not every patient does). Similarly, some types of congenital heart disease and patients with artificial heart valves may require appropriate antibiotic cover.

Chronic obstructive airways disease/tuberculosis

This predisposes to postoperative chest infections and hypoxia. Preoperative measures to reduce postoperative chest infection include:
- Being aware of high-risk patients
- Forbidding smoking for at least a few days before surgery
- Nebulized beta agonists and steroids preoperatively
- Physiotherapy
- Using high dependency or intensive care beds for patients who are particularly at high risk.

Tuberculosis is still seen even in developed countries especially among the homeless and in deprived inner city areas where poverty and overcrowding contribute to its incidence.

Asthma

Lung function in asthmatics can be improved with nebulized beta agonists and steroids preoperatively. Avoid aspirin and other NSAIDs.

Diabetes

Surgical risks in diabetic patients
- Acute hypoglycaemia
- Ketoacidosis
- Ischaemic heart disease
- Hypertension (renal disease)
- Increased risk of infections (chest, urinary, wound)
- Predisposed to pressure sores (spinal injured patients).

Postoperative complications and mortality are more common in diabetic patients. This is partly due to controllable factors such as blood glucose, but also due to established complications such as ischaemic heart disease and infection, both of which are more common in these patients.

The problems with diabetic patients undergoing major surgery are related to the period of starvation (nil by mouth (NBM)) and the metabolic effects secondary to the surgery itself. The main source of nutrition to the brain is glucose, yet persistently high blood sugar predisposes to infections, poor wound healing, and ketoacidosis. The aim of management is therefore to minimize gross variations in blood sugar by ensuring an adequate glucose, calorie, and insulin intake. Blood glucose needs to be within normal limits preoperatively and maintained until normal feeding is resumed following surgery. For many patients, normal feeding may be delayed by many days, especially following major procedures in the head and neck. Preoperative blood glucose control can be determined by urinalysis or preferably, a random blood sugar. Blood urea and electrolyte (U&E) concentrations, creatinine, and estimated glomerular filtration rate should also be checked to exclude renal disease.

Preoperatively determine:
- The type of diabetes
- The adequacy of blood glucose control
- The treatment regimen (diet, oral hypoglycaemic agent, or insulin)
- The presence of any organ impairment (e.g. cardiovascular, renal)
- The likely delay in resumption of oral feeding.

Many regimens exist for stabilizing diabetic patients in the preoperative period.

General principles in diabetic management
- Get expert help—liaise early with the anaesthetist or diabetic specialist.
- Establish good control of blood sugar before surgery if possible.
- Avoid long-acting insulin preparations or oral hypoglycaemic agents 12–24 hours preoperatively, to prevent hypoglycaemia.
- Regularly monitor blood sugar.
- Fast from midnight (if on morning theatre list).
- Place patient first on the list.
- Control blood sugar on the day of surgery using IV short-acting insulin and IV dextrose (many regimens exist).
- Check potassium and supplement if necessary.
- Postoperatively, continue sliding scale until an adequate oral diet is re-established and then restart normal regimen.

All type 1 and type 2 diabetics on insulin should never be left without insulin. They may develop ketoacidosis. Do not withhold insulin because the patient is fasting. Seek advice.

In acute cases, blood glucose may be grossly abnormal secondary to infection, trauma, or reduced oral intake. Patients are often hyper-glycaemic, which can lead to diuresis, dehydration, and ketoacidosis. These patients require IV rehydration, correction of sodium depletion (beware of pseudohyponatraemia), potassium supplementation, and infusion of short-acting soluble insulin. Regular monitoring of blood glucose, sodium, potassium, and acid–base balance is essential. The CO_2 reported with U&E results give an indicator of the acid–base balance. Check ABGs. When rehydration is underway and some correction of acidosis and hyperglycaemia has been achieved, urgent surgery may then be performed while continuing management during and after surgery.

Sliding scales
These involve the continuous infusion (sometimes subcutaneously) of a short-acting insulin, using a syringe pump. The rate of infusion varies according to the patient's blood glucose which is checked regularly (e.g. hourly, depending on its stability). The higher the blood glucose, the more insulin is given. In this way hyperglycaemia can be controlled without risking profound hypoglycaemia. Sliding scales should be reviewed constantly and adjusted to achieve a relatively steady infusion rate. The aim is to establish a steady blood glucose rather than constantly oscillating below low and high infusion rates. Ketoacidosis guidelines include those from the Joint British Diabetes Societies Inpatient Care Group: http://www.diabetes.org.uk/Documents/About%20Us/What%20we%20say/Management-of-DKA-241013.pdf.

Bleeding disorders and anticoagulants
The undiagnosed presence of blood dyscrasias and other causes of delayed clotting should be considered whenever there is prolonged bleeding following apparent minor injury or minor surgery. The com-moner problems include haemophilia A, haemophilia B, von Willebrand disease, liver disease, and patients on anticoagulants. Patients with known or suspected bleeding problems need to be fully assessed by an appropriate specialist. With appropriate prophylactic measures (e.g. local measures, tranexamic acid, DDAVP, factor replacement, or adjustment/reversal of warfarin), urgent surgery can usually be safely performed. Opinions vary considerably as to what is an 'acceptable' international normalized ratio (INR) for surgery, although this depends on the site (superficial vs deep, or within a cavity).

Stopping warfarin: a guide (refer to your local policy)
Patients undergoing low-bleeding-risk procedures (dental extractions, minor skin procedures) do not require alteration of their anticoagulation regimen. In these patients, the procedure can be performed at the ther-apeutic range. Patients undergoing high-bleeding-risk procedures (e.g. abdominal surgery, intracranial or spinal surgery) require discontinua-tion of warfarin preoperatively. If the patient has a metallic heart valve, this should be discussed with their cardiologist. A metallic mitral valve is at higher risk of thrombosis.

After stopping warfarin it takes approximately 2–3 days for the INR to fall below 2, and 4–6 days for the INR to normalize. When the INR is 1.5 or below, most surgery can be performed with relative safety. Patients with the following risk factors may require bridging anticoagulation with either unfractionated or low-molecular-weight (LMW) heparin:

• Prior stroke or systemic embolic event
• Mechanical mitral valve
• Mechanical aortic valve and additional stroke factors
• Atrial fibrillation and multiple stroke risk factors
• Previous thromboembolism during interruption of warfarin therapy.

Bridging anticoagulation with unfractionated heparin may be stopped 4–5 hours before surgery. If LMW heparin has been used, it should be stopped 24 hours before surgery. In some patients, heparin may not be restarted postoperatively until at least 24 hours after major surgery and delayed longer if there is evidence of bleeding. Seek advice on this. Patients at low risk for thrombosis can stop warfarin 5 days preoperatively without the need for bridging anticoagulation. Use other measures (such as antiembolism stockings). Once haemostasis has been achieved, warfarin can be resumed 12–24 hours after surgery.

Stopping dabigatran: a guide (refer to your local policy)
Dabigatran is a thrombin inhibitor approved for use in stroke prevention, atrial fibrillation, and DVT prevention after hip and knee replacement surgery.

Patients with a creatinine clearance >50 mL/minute should stop dabigatran 1–2 days prior to the surgical procedure. If creatinine clearance is <50 mL/minute then stop dabigatran 3–5 days before the procedure. A longer period of time may be required in patients undergoing major surgery. It has been recommended that a normal or near normal activated partial thromboplastin time be documented to ensure that dabigatran has been adequately cleared from the circulation prior to surgery.

In patients undergoing high-bleeding-risk surgery, it is recommended to restart dabigatran 2–3 days post procedure. The rapid offset and onset of dabigatran activity obviates the need for bridging anticoagulation with heparin.

Stopping rivaroxaban and apixaban: a guide (refer to your local policy)
Rivaroxaban and apixaban are direct factor Xa inhibitors. They have a similar onset of action and half-life as dabigatran but are less dependent on renal clearance. The same perioperative management for dabigatran should be used with these anticoagulants.

Deep vein thrombosis

DVT is generally uncommon following head and neck problems or their management. However, it is a potentially life-threatening condition (due to the risk of pulmonary embolism (PE)) and is preventable. Diagnosis is often difficult and it has been estimated that around half of patients with extensive thrombosis have no clinical findings. Such 'silent' thrombi are a particular risk where the condition may remain unrecognized until fatal

PE has occurred. It is therefore important that patients are assessed for risk factors and appropriate preventive measures taken.

Risk factors for DVT
- Previous history of DVT or PE
- Age
- Obesity
- Extensive trauma
- Congestive heart failure
- Malignancy
- Diabetes
- Length and type of operation
- Prolonged immobilization
- Oral contraceptives
- Smoking
- Sex
- Type of anaesthetic
- Pregnancy and the puerperium
- Varicose veins
- Drugs.

DVT prophylaxis
Currently, prevention is directed towards elimination of stasis in the veins, or reducing the tendency to clot in the patient. Measures include
- Full-length antiembolism stockings
- Intermittent pneumatic calf compression
- Low-voltage electrical calf stimulation
- Early mobilization
- Heparin/LMW dextrans, warfarin.

Heparin is currently available as 'fractionated heparin' and 'LMW' which are reported to be more effective but are more expensive. Low-dose subcutaneous heparin significantly reduces the incidence of DVT. LMW heparins may be given once daily, which is more convenient for staff and the patient.

More recently, new oral anticoagulants (such as apixaban, dabigatran, and rivaroxaban) have become available. These also carry risks of haemorrhage but with these drugs there is no specific reversal agent available (see http://www.mhra.gov.uk/Safetyinformation/DrugSafetyUpdate/CON322347).

Steroids in surgery: 'steroid cover'

Patients on long-term or high-dose steroids for whatever reason (asthma, rheumatoid arthritis, inflammatory bowel disease), are at risk of adrenocortical suppression. Following surgery, trauma, and infections, they are unable to mount a normal 'stress response' which can lead to metabolic disturbances and occasionally, collapse. Steroid supplementation may be required in the perioperative period commencing on induction of anaesthesia and continued postoperatively with a reducing dose.

For an 'average' NBM patient, one regimen might be (protocols vary depending on patient and procedure):

• Major surgery: hydrocortisone 100mg intramuscularly (IM) or IV with the premedication and then four times daily for 3 days after which return to previous medication.
• Minor surgery: prepare as for major surgery, except that hydrocortisone is given for 24 hours only.

Stress ulceration

This occurs in patients after prolonged physiological stresses and is classically seen following extensive burns, major trauma, and multiorgan failure. Patients undergoing surgery for head and neck cancer may similarly be 'stressed' postoperatively, particularly if their recovery is complicated. GI ulceration can result in fatal haemorrhage and in such patients prophylaxis is necessary. Current measures include H2 receptor blockade, proton pump inhibitors, sucralfate, and other drugs.

The elderly patient: some specific problems

Urgent preparation of elderly patients can be particularly challenging. Although the principles of assessment in the elderly are no different than in the younger population, some specific points are worth highlighting:

• Chronological age per se is no indication of relative risk and careful assessment is still necessary. Contrary to general belief, most old people are fit. A better indication is the 'biological age', i.e. how old the patient looks.
• Hypertension, ischaemic heart disease, and congestive cardiac failure are all common in the elderly and often undiagnosed.
• Several diseases or problems may coexist.
• Elderly patients are often taking one or more different drugs. These should generally be continued throughout the perioperative period. The potential for drug interactions must always be considered.
• Patients may have impaired metabolism and excretion of drugs.
• One problem (e.g. poor mobility) may have several causes, each requiring attention.
• Complications are relatively common and may present non-specifically, with absence of typical symptoms (e.g. myocardial infarction without chest pain or a urinary tract infection (UTI) without dysuria). Rapid deterioration can occur if these are not recognized and treated.
• Incontinence, instability, immobility, hypothermia, and confusion are common problems in the elderly. However they may be early symptoms of underlying treatable disease (e.g. UTI).
• More time is required for recovery.
• Many elderly people live alone. Early involvement of social services may prevent delayed discharge in patients who go on to become 'social' admissions.

For major surgery, routine preoperative full blood count (FBC), bio-chemistry, blood gases, and chest X-ray (CXR), are useful as a base-line against which postoperative investigations can be compared. This is essential in patients with longstanding medical problems and associated biochemical abnormalities. A preoperative CXR and ECG are manda-tory in all elderly patients, as asymptomatic respiratory or heart disease may be detected.

Physical examination of the head and neck needs to be tailored accord-ing to the individual requirement of the patient.

Examination of the head and neck: an overview

In order to recognize the abnormal, you must first be able to recog-nize what is 'normal'. Practise your examination techniques until you are comfortable with them, this way you will be slick and minimize your chances of missing something. Further details for each anatomical site are given in the appropriate chapters.

If at all possible, document clinical findings (notably injuries) photo-graphically. Not only is this useful from a medico-legal perspective, but wounds etc. can then be dressed and repeated examinations avoided. If photography is unavailable, use diagrams.

Extraoral examination

- Inspection. Standing at a distance from the patient, take a general look at the head and neck. Note any asymmetry, lumps, trauma, discolouration, and muscular neuronal deficit. Remember that hair (and even a hat) can sometime hide problems.
- Function. Check eye movements (blowout fractures), vision (ocular trauma), cranial nerves, swallowing, hearing, and jaw movements where appropriate. Remember the Glasgow Coma Scale (GCS), pupils, and cranial nerves (especially II, V, and VII).
- Palpation of the head and face. Depending on the presenting complaint, a thorough palpation of any visual findings is performed. This includes all surfaces that form the head and neck:
  - Scalp
  - Forehead
  - Supraorbital ridges
  - Zygomaticofrontal sutures (lateral orbital margins)
  - Infraorbital ridges
  - Nasal bridge
  - Maxilla
  - Zygomatic body and arch
  - Temporomandibular joints
  - Mandibular ramus, body, and lower border
  - Mandibular range of movement, i.e. opening and lateral excursions
  - Surface of the neck down to the clavicle, cervical spine, and occiput.
  - Feel for tenderness, fluctuation, steps in bony continuity, and enlarged lymph nodes or swellings in the neck.

- Auscultation and auroscopy. Can be considered for vascularized lumps (e.g. haemangioma, arteriovenous malformation, enlarged thyroid) or following trauma to the neck (surgical emphysema/carotid bruit).

Intraoral examination

- Tongue. Look for any signs of neural weakness, i.e. slurred speech, tingling, or difficulty in swallowing. Trauma, i.e. lacerations or haemorrhage. Change in colour, texture, or size can be due to tumour, fungal infections, anaemia, folate, vitamin B12 deficiency, or acute cyanosis. The condition of the mucosa forming the floor of mouth under the tongue is noted. If this is enlarged it can raise the tongue. This may indicate spread of infection with a potential airway problem, or a sublingual haematoma following mandibular trauma.
- Occlusion (the bite). Note whether this is deranged before asking the patient to open the mouth. If not sure, then ask the patient to close the teeth together and retract the cheeks to see if there is even and balanced contact at the back and front on either side. Ask the patient if the 'bite' feels normal. Be mindful of artificial teeth that can alter the occlusion without underlying bony trauma. There are also natural variations in different bites related to the relative sizes of the jaws.
- Gingival (gums)/oral mucosa overlying the alveolar bone, hard palate, cheeks (buccal mucosa), and soft palate. No intraoral examination is complete without looking at the back of the throat or tonsillar area. The presence of a swelling or discolouration needs to be further examined for size, tenderness, sinus tract, and whether it is associated with a tooth.
- Teeth. Those present in both the upper and lower alveolar ridges are noted. These are 'charted' by assigning numbers to those present in each arch in relation to their position. Following loss of a tooth, its neighbours will drift a little over several years. The more teeth that are lost, the more this occurs. This can make identification difficult.
- Salivary flow. The three paired parotid, submandibular, and sublingual salivary glands secrete into the oral cavity. Parotid glands discharge adjacent to the upper molar teeth through a papilla on the buccal mucosa. Submandibular and sublingual glands discharge though a papilla on either side in the floor of mouth near the lingual frenum. Ductal patency and gland function can be assessed by 'milking' or massaging the glands.
- Palpation. This is just as important inside the mouth as it is on the face. Feel for induration, lumps, swelling, loose teeth, and fracture crepitus.

How the teeth are arranged

For permanent teeth, see Table 1.1 and Figure 1.1. For deciduous teeth, see Table 1.2. Mixed dentition can be any combination of Table 1.1 and Table 1.2.

Table 1.1 Permanent ('adult') teeth

Right	Left
8 7 6 5 4 3 2 1	1 2 3 4 5 6 7 8
8 7 6 5 4 3 2 1	1 2 3 4 5 6 7 8

1 + 2	= incisors
3	= canine
4 + 5	= premolars
6 + 7 + 8	= molars

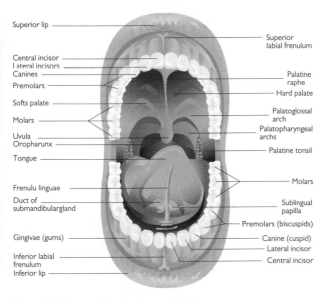

Superior lip

Central incisor
Lateral incisors
Canines
Premolars

Softs palate

Molars

Uvula
Oropharunx
Tongue

Frenulu linguae
Duct of submandibulargland

Gingivae (gums)

Inferior labial frenulum
Inferior lip

Superior labial frenulum

Palatine raphe
Hard palate

Palatoglossal arch
Palatopharyngeal archs
Palatine tonsil

Molars

Sublingual papilla
Premolars (biscuspids)
Canine (cuspid)
Lateral incisor
Central incisor

Figure 1.1 Adult dentition. © stockshopp/123RF.

Table 1.2 Deciduous ('baby') teeth

Right	Left
edcba	abcde
edcba	abcde

a + b	= incisors
c	= canine
d + e	= molars

The injured patient

Initial assessment of the multiply injured patient with facial injuries

Some general points

Injuries to the head, face, and neck in the multiply injured patient need to be prioritized. Injuries resulting in airway compromise, significant and ongoing bleeding, and possible loss of vision are a high priority. But they are uncommon. When multiple coexisting injuries are present, it is important not to be distracted by the obvious facial injuries. A systematic approach beginning with the rapid assessment and management of all life-threatening injuries is required. This is followed by a head-to-toe secondary evaluation and investigations. This will provide information on the full extent of all injuries and help establish priorities. Once airway compromise, significant bleeding, and possible loss of vision have been addressed, all other facial injuries can wait for at least a short while, during which time the entire patient can be assessed. The initial priority is to treat any immediate life-threatening conditions first. The most widely adopted approach is that developed by the American College of Surgeons and known as Advanced Trauma Life Support® or ATLS®. It consists of an initial *rapid primary survey* to identify and treat immediately life-threatening conditions (the ABCDE approach). Once the patient is stable, a more detailed head-to-toe examination (*secondary survey*) can be performed.

Head and neck injuries resulting in life-threatening conditions

- Facial injuries resulting in airway compromise (e.g. panfacial fractures with gross displacement, mobility or swelling, comminuted #s of the mandible, gunshot, foreign bodies, burns).
- Anterior neck injuries resulting in airway compromise (e.g. penetrating injuries, circumferential burns, laryngeal/tracheal injuries) or injuries to the carotid arteries.
- Injuries resulting in profuse blood loss (e.g. penetrating neck, panfacial fractures—rarely).
- Head injuries resulting in intracranial swelling or bleeding.
- Cervical spine injuries with spinal cord injury (hypoventilation, hypotension and other late complications).

Once immediately life-threatening conditions are excluded/managed, specific imaging is undertaken (often a CXR, lateral C-spine and pelvic X-ray CT is now increasingly used to evaluate many injuries). The patient is then reassessed. Only when they are stable can the secondary survey be carried out. This is when attention can be focused on the majority of facial injuries.

The (rapid) primary survey

The initial goal in trauma management is to get adequate oxygen into the blood and then circulate this, notably to the brain. To achieve this, patients need:

- Oxygen.
- A patent airway so that oxygen in the air can get to the lungs.
- Adequate lung ventilation so oxygen can pass into the blood.
- An adequate volume of oxygenated blood to circulate to the vital organs.
- The ability to use oxygen at a cellular level (cf. cyanide poisoning).
- The absence of any intracranial pathology that would irreversibly damage the brain.

These issues are addressed during the primary survey. This is undertaken quickly. The sequence in which the primary survey proceeds is related to those conditions that would lead to loss of life quickest:

- Airway patency (while protecting the cervical spine to prevent neurological damage).
- Breathing (all trauma patients should be given 100% oxygen). They may also need to be ventilated.
- Circulation with control of haemorrhage.
- Disability (brain function).

This sequence ends with 'E'—for Exposure. This must be completed so a full examination front and back can be undertaken. After this, the patient needs to be covered to prevent hypothermia.

The primary survey is preferably performed by a team approach where different team members do the above-listed sequence simultaneously. In such cases, a 'team leader' ensures that each step has been performed. If team numbers are not sufficient for this, an ABCDE sequence is followed. It is also vital to enlist the early help of any speciality not on the receiving team if a problem or is identified (e.g. neurosurgery/maxillofacial surgery).

If a patient is clearly losing a lot of blood from a wound, apply immediate pressure then proceed with the primary survey. This is acceptable practice with massive external haemorrhage, rather than waiting until 'C' in primary survey. The acronym MARCH is sometimes used to describe this: Massive Haemorrhage, Airway, Respiration, Circulation, Hypothermia.

Taking a history in the multiply injured patient

The traditional approach of taking a full history from the patient prior to examination has no place in the preliminary assessment of the multiply injured patient. Instead an 'AMPLE' history is taken at this early stage. If a history of the event cannot be obtained from the patient, prehospital personnel or family members should be consulted regarding the events leading up to the injury. A medical history obtained either from the patient, general practitioner, or hospital notes may help.

History taking in major trauma: the 'AMPLE' history

Certain information may be helpful to understand what injuries may be present, or the effects of any potential treatment. This can be remembered by taking an 'AMPLE' history:

- A: enquire about any allergies related to medications.
- M: any medication that the patient is taking may alert us to potential problems following trauma (e.g. anticoagulants). They may also give us a clue about pre-existing medical problems (e.g. cardiovascular medication). Some medications may alter the response to trauma and need to be taken (e.g. patients taking beta-blockers who are shocked may not exhibit the expected degree of tachycardia). Steroids also affect management. Remember herbal remedies—these can also interact with prescribed drugs.
- P: a brief past medical history (PMH) and pregnancy. MedicAlert® bracelets might provide clues. Some conditions may influence management or alert us to other possible problems (e.g. the patient with known cardiovascular disease may have had a myocardial infarct before the car crashed). Age and reduced physiological reserve may necessitate careful fluid resuscitation.
- L: when the patient last ate (anaesthetic risk of aspiration).
- E: events leading to the trauma and the mechanism of injury.

The mechanism of injury

The mechanism of injury may give clues as to what injuries a patient may have. This may be available from the patient, witnesses, or paramedical personnel attending the patient. Ensure a team member records the information before the people who know it leave the department. As much detail as is known should be recorded.

- If the mechanism involves a single blow, the risk of injuries is localized to some anatomical regions more than others. For example, in the case of a neck stabbing, we need to know how long the blade was, which direction the assault was from (above/below, in front/behind), and whether the blade broke. In this situation, a pelvic, abdominal, and lower limb injury is unlikely, but chest, head, and upper limb trauma are all quite possible. There is also the potential for airway, cervical spine, breathing, and circulatory problems from such a wound.
- Some mechanisms may be more complicated (e.g. a motor vehicle collision (MVC), a fall from a height, or an explosion). In all these cases the details help assess risk. Speed of impact, whether a seat belt was worn, vehicle deformity, and injuries sustained by others (especially any fatalities), are all useful clues following MVCs. If the patient fell, the height and what he/she hit when they landed are clearly important. *Deceleration injuries are particularly worrying*, due to the risk of tearing at vascular pedicles. With explosions, what

exploded, were chemicals involved, and was fire or smoke present? All these and other information help to raise the possibility of injuries over and above the obvious. These need to be actively looked for and treated.

- In circumstances where the details are vague or incomplete, consider what might have happened in addition to what is known. A patient who has been assaulted but is not sure what happened may have obvious facial injuries, but may also have received 'a good kicking' to the chest or abdomen, resulting in potentially life-threatening injuries. These can easily go unnoticed if not specifically looked for.
- The time from injury to help arriving and transfer to hospital is important and should be ascertained, especially following severe burns. Environmental conditions should also be noted—has the patient being exposed to contamination or extreme temperatures, and if so, for how long?

Thorough documentation of both the event and the patient's medical/social history will act as a guide to arriving at the correct diagnosis, and formulating an appropriate management plan (see Figure 2.1).

Some important mechanisms of injury in the head and neck

- A fall from a height of 10 feet or more carries an increased risk of sustaining spinal, pelvic, and long-bone injuries.
- Blunt trauma to the forehead can result in blindness, even in the absence of fractures.
- A blow directly on the chin can result in the well-known 'guardsman's fracture' pattern, or injury to the brainstem.
- Anterior–posterior directed impacts to the face can result in hyperextension injuries to the cervical spine and spinal cord injury (notably in the elderly).
- Successful airbag deployment can result in ocular injury.
- A high-velocity projectile can penetrate both the eye and the brain.
- Strangulation/hanging type injuries can fracture the hyoid/larynx and avulse the trachea.
- Compressed air/blast injuries can result in massive emphysema in the face, neck, and chest. Pneumothorax can occur.
- Rapid deceleration (such as seen in bungee jumping) has resulted in retinal haemorrhages, whiplash, carotid dissection, and stroke.
- Rapid deceleration (as seen in MVCs) can result in subdural haematoma, diffuse axonal injury, whiplash, detached retina, or traumatic optic neuropathy.

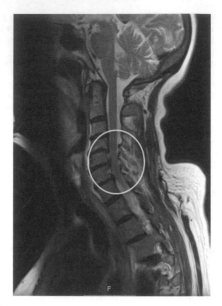

Figure 2.1 MRI showing a cervical cord injury in an elderly patient following hyperextension injury to the neck. The patient tripped and fell forward, striking her face on the ground.

Reproduced from *Atlas of Operative Maxillofacial Trauma Surgery: Primary Repair of Facial Injuries*, 'Initial Considerations: High- vs. Low-Energy Injuries and the Implications of Coexisting Multiple Injuries', 2014, Figure 1.5, eds M. Perry and S. Holmes, Copyright © 2014, Springer-Verlag London. With permission of Springer.

Primary survey: airway

The most important initial step in recognizing a problem with the airway is to talk to the patient. An appropriate verbal response from the patient indicates that the airway is patent and the brain is adequately perfused, although it is no guarantee that it will remain so. *The most common cause of airway compromise is a reduced level of consciousness.* Failure of the patient to appropriately respond to simple questioning signifies an altered level of consciousness indicating a risk of airway compromise. Other common causes of airway compromise include a foreign body, swelling, and bleeding.

In any patient with significant facial injuries, the airway needs to be assessed very carefully. *Even if the patient can talk, this cannot be taken as a guarantee that the airway is free from risk.* Loose teeth, bleeding, or fractures can all be present and yet the patient may still be able to talk to you. In order to assess the airway properly, the patient must therefore be able to open their mouth wide enough for you to look inside. This means that any hard collar will need to be unfastened. You will need an assistant to support the head during this time. This is often a source of anxiety when managing injured patients (due to concerns about cervical spine injury), so be sure you know how to do this safely.

Assessing the airway

The usual steps suggested are to
- Look—for use of accessory muscles of ventilation:
  - Agitation of patient suggesting hypoxia
  - In the mouth—active bleeding, loose teeth, dentures, etc.
- Listen—for abnormal sounds:
  - Noisy breathing indicates partial obstruction.
  - Stridor indicates partial obstruction above the laryngeal inlet.
  - Expiratory wheeze indicates lower airway obstruction.
- Feel—airflow at the mouth:
  - Also check the position of trachea (displacement is a sign of tension pneumothorax).

However, when obvious facial injuries are present, assessment needs to be more thorough. Specifically this requires the following:
- Speak to the patient—if they reply in a clear manner then they have an airway that is patent and have the capacity to use it. A hoarse voice may suggest airway injury. Ask them if they feel any blood trickling down the back of their throat.
- Are there gurgling/stridorous noises indicating partial obstruction? This must be cleared immediately. Common causes are blood/saliva or the base of the tongue falling back into the pharynx. Other causes of obstruction may relate to swelling in the neck from bleeding or direct trauma to the airway (larynx/hyoid).
- High-flow suction should be used and if necessary the mandible manipulated forward to lift the tongue base (chin lift/jaw thrust). To do this requires care and assistance to support the head. Otherwise the neck may be extended. The collar may need to be unfastened so you can suction properly—don't just force the suction tube between the lips and hope for the best. Be very careful, this can precipitate vomiting. If the airway re-obstructs then an oropharyngeal, nasopharyngeal, or a definitive airway will be required. If patients require an oro- or nasopharyngeal airway for more than a short while they probably require a definitive airway—get senior help early.
- If the airway is silent it is either completely occluded or the patient is not breathing. In the former, movement of the chest will be apparent and the patient will be in distress. Immediate relief of obstruction is essential. In severe facial/neck trauma this may require a surgical airway, although this is rarely needed.
- The anterior neck. This is often a forgotten site and requires careful examination. It should be regarded as a watershed between 'Airway' and 'Breathing' during the primary survey. Life-threatening problems arising in both can manifest clinical signs here. Fractures of the larynx and hyoid may lead to substantial glottic swelling. A hoarse voice,

haemoptysis, and crepitus in the neck are highly suggestive of these injuries. Carefully palpate the hyoid and larynx. Again, to assess the front of the neck properly the hard collar will need to be unfastened and the head supported.

Loss of the airway is often due to a combination of factors (more commonly alcohol, head injury, bleeding, and being restrained supine). If the patient is not breathing they require mechanical ventilation. This is usually achieved by orotracheal intubation or with a surgical cricothyroidotomy. Nasotracheal intubation is usually contraindicated in midface trauma or head injuries.

Airway risk factors in facial trauma
- Inability to handle normal secretions
- Foreign bodies
- Altered level of consciousness (this may be secondary to alcohol, drugs, or some medical conditions)
- Uncontrolled haemorrhage
- Surgical emphysema
- Adjacent soft tissue injuries/gross swelling
- Burns
- Hyoid/laryngeal/tracheal injury
- Disrupted mid/lower face anatomy
- A tightly fitting collar when the patient has mandibular fractures.
- Laying supine.

Remember that the unresponsive/comatose patient may also require a definitive airway for protection in the event of vomiting. Remember also the risk to the cervical spine. This must be presumed injured and stabilized using a correctly fitting collar, blocks, and tape. If these are not available, get an assistant to stabilize the head manually.

Some difficult airway-related problems in facial trauma

Sudden vomiting in supine patients

Unexpected vomiting is a difficult problem in all immobilized patients and poses an immediate threat to the airway. In all supine patients vomiting can occur at any time, often after the primary survey has been completed. *Therefore, an experienced nurse escort and suction should be with the patient at all times until they are allowed to sit up.* Early warning signs may include repeated attempts by the patient to try and get up. Restrained supine patients should never be left unattended.

If vomiting occurs in the restrained supine patient, tilting the patient head-down approximately 6–12 inches and clearing the airway using high-flow suction is the safest approach. In the head-down position, vomitus preferentially flows into the oropharynx from the oesophagus reducing the risk of causing obstruction around the laryngeal inlet.

Have an agreed plan of action in the event of unexpected vomiting. When it occurs, there is no time to debate the relative merits of log rolling/sitting up/tilting the table head-down.

Is it safe for the patient to sit up?

See Figure 2.2. A common scenario seen in the emergency department is the intoxicated, aggressive male with apparently isolated facial injuries following an assault or fall. The patient will often sit up with little response to reason. In this situation an unstable cervical spine injury is rare. Allowing the patient to sit up may be the best initial option as it reduces the risk of airway compromise from vomiting or unstable facial fractures. If they will allow you to put a hard collar on them, do so. But never forcibly restrain.

However, in the potentially multiply injured patients with facial injuries a decision needs to be made quickly regarding the relative risks of keeping the patient supine (with potential airway obstruction) against the risks of axially loading a potential spine, torso or pelvic injury, by allowing

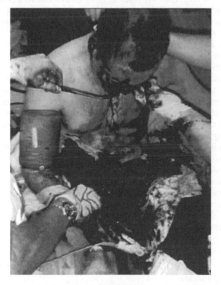

Figure 2.2 A patient with significant, but isolated, facial injuries. In this case, allowing the patient to sit up enabled self-protection of the airway. Had the patient been placed supine, his airway would probably have obstructed from the obvious bleeding, mobile midface, and facial swelling.

them to sit up. If the patient is combative despite adequate oxygenation, correction of hypovolaemia, and adequate pain relief, then early intubation and ventilation may be necessary to secure the airway and prevent loading. This reinforces the concept of the mechanism of injury in planning appropriate management for patients.

Beware the patient who keeps trying to sit up—they may be trying to clear their airway.

Clearing the cervical spine

This should take place as soon as possible due to the problems associated with prolonged spinal immobilization. Until then, the cervical spine needs to be protected (manual stabilization or collar, blocks, and tape). See ➔ Chapter 4.

Assessment of the front of the neck following trauma

This is often a forgotten site and requires careful examination. It should be regarded as a watershed between 'Airway' and 'Breathing' during the primary survey, as life-threatening problems in both can manifest clinical signs here. Assessment of the airway involves more than just looking into the mouth and nose. Poiseuille's law dictates that even a small change in the diameter of a tube can result in a significant change in flow through it. Although strictly applicable to fluid dynamics, this equation highlights the potential for problems to arise when there is swelling within the larynx and trachea. Although unusual, fractures of the larynx and hyoid do occur and may lead to substantial glottic swelling. Motorcycle helmet wearers, strangulation, and contact sports injuries are important clues from the history. A hoarse voice, haemoptysis, and crepitus in the neck are highly suggestive of these injuries and should be actively sought after. Carefully palpate the hyoid and larynx for signs of injury and look for external swelling which may reflect swelling internally. Useful clinical signs to look for include:

- Tracheal deviation or separation
- Laryngeal tenderness or crepitus
- Hyoid tenderness
- Surgical emphysema
- Distended neck veins
- Open wounds
- Significant swelling.

These may indicate the presence of significant and potentially life-threatening injuries.

Airway problems seen in facial trauma

Obstruction

This may be caused by dentures/loose teeth or severe fractures of the mandible or midface. The commonest causes are bleeding and/or saliva, notably when the patient is intoxicated or supine. Swelling is often an aggravating factor. Saliva and blood should initially be cleared by suction. If the bleeding is coming from an identifiable controllable source it should be stopped. However, it is usually generalized and from multiple sites. Nasal packs may be necessary (remember the possibility of skull base fractures). If bleeding continues, the airway should be protected with a definitive airway.

Displaced tissues

Midface fractures may collapse in on themselves, impinging on the posterior pharyngeal wall and resulting in obstruction. Much of the obstruction is due to the associated swelling in addition to loss of soft palate support, which progresses over several hours. Bilateral anterior ('bucket handle') or comminuted mandibular fractures can similarly displace resulting in loss of tongue support. The base of the tongue can then fall backwards into the pharynx. Swelling is again often associated. *All these effects are much more likely when patients are supine and there is alteration in their conscious level.* A definitive airway will therefore probably be required. Seek senior help quickly.

Soft tissue swelling

This inevitably occurs, especially with major injuries, often necessitating prolonged intubation or an elective tracheostomy. However, major swelling can also occur in the absence of any fracture, as occasionally seen in patients taking anticoagulants, or those with clotting abnormalities. Patients with cervical spine fractures may develop posterior pharyngeal swelling contributing to an obstructed airway. Penetrating and blunt (e.g. strangulation/hanging) neck trauma may also be associated with pharyngeal oedema and bleeding. *It is important to appreciate that swelling from whatever cause can take several hours to develop. Be wary and regularly re-examine the patient.* Of particular concern are those patients who have suffered facial burns. These are frequently associated with inhalation injuries, which can lead to rapid swelling that is not apparent on initial examination. Stridor is a particularly worrying sign and often necessitates early intubation.

Direct trauma to the airway will probably require placement of a definitive airway.

Initial management of the airway

Control of the airway can be lost easily and may be very difficult to secure following facial trauma and burns. Often early assistance from an experienced anaesthetist is required and should be anticipated well in advance of signs of impending obstruction. Occasionally an immediate surgical airway is required, notably when there is gross swelling in extensive facial injuries. Members of the trauma team should be competent in performing this.

All seriously injured patients should receive oxygen. The patient should be given high-flow oxygen (15 L/min) through a non-rebreathing mask, and the oral cavity/oropharynx carefully cleared with suction while further assessment takes place. The following steps may help. They will probably require the hard collar to be loosened—ask someone to support the head.

Simple techniques to maintain an airway

Chin lift and jaw thrust
These are commonly used techniques to maintain the airway but may be difficult to carry out in the presence of comminuted mandibular fractures. Both of these techniques have been shown to produce movement of the cervical spine and should therefore be performed with counter support from an assistant to the head to prevent this.

Reduction of displaced facial fractures
This may involve gentle manipulation of the midface and its temporary stabilization using bite blocks between the posterior teeth. Bridle wires may be passed to temporarily stabilize mandibular fractures.

High-volume suction
A wide-bore soft plastic sucker should be readily available to clear the mouth, nose, and pharynx of blood and secretions, taking care not to induce vomiting. Loss of the protective gag reflex should prompt consideration of an oropharyngeal airway or intubation.

Adjuncts to simple airway techniques

Oropharyngeal airway
This is often poorly tolerated and can precipitate vomiting and laryngospasm. If not placed correctly it can push the tongue posteriorly, causing airway obstruction.

Nasopharyngeal airway
This is better tolerated than an oropharyngeal airway but is associated with epistaxis. Concerns exist about the potential for intracranial positioning in patients with midface/anterior skull base fractures. In reality the risks are very low, and in experienced hands nasopharyngeal tubes can be safely passed in these patients.

Advanced airway techniques

A definitive airway may be defined as a cuffed tube in the trachea. It may be required if there is any doubt about the patient's ability to protect their own airway immediately or in the near future. In the emergency situation, it is important that the technique used is one with which the clinician is most confident; the trauma setting is not the time to attempt unfamiliar procedures.

Laryngeal mask airway

A laryngeal mask airway (LMA) can facilitate rescue ventilation when mask ventilation and tracheal intubation are unexpectedly difficult. However the airway is not formally protected and aspiration from vomiting can still occur. It is therefore not the first choice of advanced airway.

A guide to initial airway management for the non-airway specialist (i.e. most of us)
- Give high-flow oxygen (15 L/min) via a non-rebreathing mask.
- Get senior help.
- Consider jaw thrust with counter support of the head.
- Consider an oropharyngeal airway if the patient is unconscious and obstructing (GCS score <8). Do not use a nasopharyngeal tube.
- If the airway is patent but there is no spontaneous ventilation then manually ventilate with a self-inflating bag and mask. Call for urgent anaesthetic assistance.
- If the patient is unconscious, you are on your own, and you cannot ventilate with a face mask then insert a LMA. If the mask leaks, add more air into the cuff, up to a maximum of 30 mL.
- If experienced, consider orotracheal intubation. Be careful, however, not to extend the head.
- If you are unable to intubate and cannot ventilate the patient, then suction the mouth with a large-bore Yankauer sucker and perform a surgical cricothyroidotomy.

Tracheal intubation

Orotracheal intubation with in-line cervical immobilization is usually the technique of choice in the majority of cases. A cuffed tube in the trachea provides a definitive, protected airway. However, placement can be challenging in patients with facial trauma. Difficulties can result in aspiration, hypoxaemia, hypercarbia, and hypertension, all of which may significantly worsen any coexisting cerebral injury. In the absence of midface or craniofacial fractures, alternative techniques include fibreoptic-assisted oro- and nasotracheal intubation. These specialized techniques have been shown to be associated with less manipulation of the injured cervical spine. However, they require extensive training. The use of fibreoptic assistance is usually limited as the view is often obscured by blood.

Surgical airway

This is required when it is not possible to secure the airway by any other means within a safe period of time.

Needle cricothyroidotomy

This is rarely required as it is better to place a surgical cricothyroidotomy directly. However, in some circumstances it allows you to 'buy time' (approximately 30 minutes) while preparing for a surgical cricothyroidotomy. ATLS® recommendations are that oxygen is delivered at a rate of 15 L/min via a Y-connector. Carbon dioxide removal is inadequate with this technique

Surgical cricothyroidotomy

This is widely recognized as the preferred choice of emergency airway control when endotracheal intubation is not possible. The main advantage of this technique over a needle cricothyroidotomy is that a larger, cuffed airway can be placed, facilitating positive pressure ventilation and reliable expiration with removal of carbon dioxide. The key factor in performing a needle or surgical cricothyroidotomy is identification of the cricothyroid membrane. This should be possible, provided the anterior neck is not too oedematous.

Tracheostomy

This is considered inappropriate in the emergency setting as it is time-consuming, technically more difficult to perform, and requires a previously secured airway during the procedure. Only those surgeons with extensive experience of performing tracheostomy (under local anaesthesia) should undertake this. For the rest of us, perform a surgical cricothyroidotomy.

Percutaneous tracheostomy

This should only be performed by experienced practitioners familiar with the technique. It cannot be undertaken if the neck has not been cleared (the neck needs to be extended).

Primary survey: breathing

All patients must be given 100% oxygen.

Look for signs that the patient is having problems in breathing (i.e. using accessory muscles of respiration, tachypnoea, stridor, or wheeze). This rapid assessment of breathing in the trauma patient should include the following:

- Stand at the top or foot of the bed and look at the chest. You are more likely to see asymmetrical movement of the chest than standing beside the patient.
- Talk to the patient.
- Assess respiratory rate (should be less than 20 breaths/min).

- Pulse oximetry—this is a non-invasive method of continuously measuring the oxygen saturation of arterial blood. An oxygen saturation of 95% or greater by pulse oximetry is good evidence of adequate peripheral arterial oxygenation. Changes in oxygenation can occur rapidly and cannot be detected clinically. For this reason the patient should have continuous pulse oximetry.
- Check the position of trachea. Is the trachea deviated? If so, consider a possible tension pneumothorax.
- Auscultation of chest—is there equal and good air entry bilaterally throughout both lung fields? If not, look for one of the underlying common causes following trauma listed in the following 'Conditions affecting ventilation' section and manage accordingly.
- Comatose patients (head injury/drugs/alcohol) may be hypoventilating. Attach a pulse oximeter and get some blood gases.

Conditions affecting ventilation

If you are a member of the 'ATLS® Fan Club' you will remember life-threatening problems in the chest (mostly 'B' problems):
- Airway: foreign bodies in the chest—emergency bronchoscopy/aspiration/inhalation injury.
- Tension pneumothorax: needle decompression and formal chest drain.
- Large (massive) haemothorax: volume replacement and chest drain.
- Sucking chest wound (open pneumothorax): three-sided dressing initially then chest drain.
- Flail chest: analgesia, monitoring, and ventilatory support.
- Cardiac tamponade: drainage, analgesia, monitoring, and ventilatory support.

In the context of maxillofacial injuries, breathing problems may occur following aspiration of teeth, vomit, dentures, and other foreign bodies. *If teeth or dentures have been lost and the whereabouts unknown, a CXR and soft tissue view of the neck should be taken to exclude their presence in the pharynx or lower airway (Figure 2.3).*

Unfortunately, acrylic, from which 'plastic' dentures are made, is not very obvious on a radiograph and a careful search is necessary. All foreign bodies need to be removed.

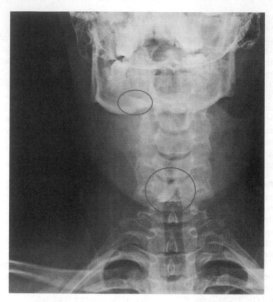

Figure 2.3 Contrary to popular belief, a CXR alone does not exclude loose or foreign bodies in the airway. A soft tissue view of the neck is often required (or look closely at the C-spine views).

Reproduced from *Atlas of Operative Maxillofacial Trauma Surgery: Primary Repair of Facial Injuries*, 'Initial Considerations: High- vs. Low-Energy Injuries and the Implications of Coexisting Multiple Injuries', 2014, Figure 1.27b, eds M. Perry and S. Holmes, Copyright © 2014, Springer-Verlag London. With permission of Springer.

Initial management of breathing problems

Breathing problems can occur following aspiration of vomit, teeth, dentures, and other foreign materials. If teeth or dentures have not been accounted for then a CXR *and a soft tissue view of the neck* is mandatory to exclude their presence in the pharynx or lungs. Unfortunately, fractured acrylic dentures may not be readily identifiable on plain radiography. CT may be required.

Summary of breathing management

- High-flow oxygen (15 L/min) through a non-rebreathing mask should be given to all patients initially.
- Rapid clinical examination and consider the six common differentials that can have an adverse effect on breathing. Treat accordingly.

- Call for anaesthetic help early. Tachypnoea and using accessory muscles of respiration can lead to patient exhaustion very quickly. If spontaneous ventilation is inadequate it will need to be supported as soon as possible. Intubation and ventilation is indicated in the following situations:
  - Apnoea
  - Inability to maintain an airway by other means
  - Protection of the lower airway from aspiration/vomit
  - Risk of losing the airway from swelling
  - Inability to maintain adequate ventilation by other means.

Primary survey: circulation

Hypovolaemic shock secondary to haemorrhage is responsible for up to 40% of the mortality following trauma. Following high-velocity or penetrating trauma, patients can quickly lose significant amounts of blood into several anatomical sites. Life-threatening blood loss from the face can also occur, but is uncommon.

The commonest cause of preventable death following trauma is hypovolaemia. Therefore any patient that is cold to touch and has a rapid pulse is in hypovolaemic shock until proven otherwise.

The important initial observations are:
- Pulse
- Skin colour
- Level of consciousness.

These are a good guide to the presence of shock. The earliest sign of blood loss is tachycardia. Caution should be taken particularly with the elderly, children, and athletes. These patients do not respond to blood loss in the same manner as other patients. A normal pulse rate is no guarantee that the patient is not actively bleeding.

Hypotension is a relatively late sign in hypovolaemic shock. If a tension pneumothorax has been excluded, all hypotensive trauma patients should be considered to be in severe hypovolaemic shock unless proven otherwise (ATLS®).

Key points in the management of blood loss
- Identify source of bleeding (internally or externally):
  - Identification may involve log rolling the patient early.
  - The main areas of bleeding are external wounds, chest, abdomen, retroperitoneum, pelvis, and long-bone fractures.
- Rapid assessment is the key to success. CT is increasingly being used in the overall evaluation of stable patients. Additionally:
  - CXR—identify pneumo/haemothoraces, mediastinal widening.
  - Echocardiography—rapidly diagnose a pericardial effusion.
  - FAST scan—useful to identify free fluid in abdomen and visualize solid organs (spleen, liver, and kidneys).
  - Pelvic X-ray—fractured pelvis.

- While the above-listed investigations are being performed, the following resuscitation measures need to be in place:
  - Two wide-bore cannulae, ideally in antecubital fossa.
  - Blood sent for group/save and crossmatch.
  - Begin resuscitation with 250 mL boluses of warmed crystalloid if shock is evident (or follow local protocol).
  - Surgical intervention or embolization may be required very early to control bleeding—involve the surgeons/radiologists early. They need time to set up.

Assessing patients in 'shock'
- Pulse
- Capillary refill
- Presence of cool, clammy peripheries
- Mental status
- Respiratory rate
- BP
- Urinary output.

ABGs are particularly useful in the evaluation of haemorrhagic shock. If the base excess reading is very negative and lactate is raised (lactic acidosis), this is an indication of tissue hypoperfusion.

All trauma patients should have good IV access and blood taken for crossmatch. Initially warmed crystalloid (this varies in different units) may be infused and the patient's response reassessed. *However, which fluid to use and how much to give are critical and may depend on where you work—find out what your local protocol is, fluid administration might be different (smaller boluses).* Be careful not to over-infuse. Aggressive fluid administration in the presence of 'uncontrolled' haemorrhage may result in further bleeding. Blood loss can result in acidosis, hypothermia, and dilution of clotting factors, sometimes referred to as the 'first biologic hit'. The site of blood loss must therefore be rapidly identified and controlled.

Sources of major blood loss
- External wounds
- Chest
- Abdomen
- Retroperitoneum
- Pelvis
- Limbs
- Face.

Major haemorrhage from head and neck injuries is uncommon. The chest, pelvis, and limbs can be quickly assessed clinically and then radiographically. The abdomen cannot however, especially in the unconscious patient and will require further investigations (ultrasound or CT). Immobilization of limb/pelvic fractures and a laparotomy to control bleeding should be regarded as part of 'C' and not be delayed. If a patient fails to respond to a fluid challenge, think of other causes (especially in injuries above the diaphragm)—cardiogenic, tension pneumothorax, cardiac tamponade, spinal, or septic.

Children, the elderly, athletes, and patients with pacemakers or on beta blockers may respond differently to blood loss. Blood loss in children is more significant.

Blood loss in facial trauma

Bleeding following maxillofacial injury is common but is not usually life-threatening. If the patient is in shock, look for another cause. Look carefully for occult bleeding elsewhere (consider chest, abdomen, pelvis, retroperitoneum, limbs, and open wounds). Nevertheless, life-threatening facial haemorrhage has been reported to occur in up to 10% of serious facial injuries. *Always consider facial bleeding in the awake supine patient—they may be swallowing blood which could go unnoticed.*

If bleeding is significant and obvious, it should be controlled in the primary survey. Bleeding from lacerations can usually be controlled by pressure applied either with a swab (take care with scalps if there is a risk of a skull fracture) or by placement of sutures to close lacerations. These are used to apply pressure and are not intended as definitive closure. Blood loss from the scalp, face, and neck can sometimes be profuse. With scalp lacerations, full-thickness bites are taken to close the aponeurosis using a continuous technique.

Midface bleeding

This can be troublesome. Bleeding arises from multiple sites within comminuted bones and torn mucosa. Concealed bleeding may occur in the supine patient, and may contribute to persisting shock. It may not be recognized until the patient vomits. Pressure can be applied to the nose with anterior and posterior nasal packs. Displaced/mobile midface fractures should be reduced. This requires an assistant to hold the head and protect the neck. Release the hard collar, but do not remove it (a well-fitting collar restricts mouth opening). Manually reduce the midface fractures to reduce the bleeding. Apply gentle suction to the nose and pharynx to look for active bleeding. If the bleeding is controlled, place mouth props to support the fracture, and reapply the hard collar. Surprisingly, this is not as painful as one might think. In selected cases, use of external fixators applied to the skull and maxilla may be necessary but this requires transfer to an operating theatre and considerably more time. This is rare.

Epistaxis (bleeding into the nasopharynx)

This may be controlled by passing an inflatable custom device (such as a Rapid Rhino™), and gently inflating the balloon. If not available, a practical alternative is to pass Foley catheters through each nostril until the ends are visible in the oropharynx. Inflate the catheters with 10 mL of sterile water and gently withdraw them into the nasopharynx. Apply a padded umbilical clamp across the catheter to prevent nasal alar necrosis and to keep the balloon from dislodging. Pack the anterior nasal cavity with a BIPP (bismuth iodoform paraffin paste).

Fractured mandible

Active bleeding from a displaced fractured mandible can be stopped by manually reducing the fracture and providing temporary fixation with bridle wires (0.4 mm orthodontic wire). These are passed around the teeth on either side of the fracture site. It is preferable not to use the teeth immediately adjacent to the fracture as they may be dislodged into the fracture when the wire is tightened.

Oral bleeding

This may be controlled with dental gauze packs and manual reduction of obviously displaced jaw fractures. The amount of blood loss is often overestimated as the patient often salivates profusely.

Bleeding from a 'hole' (e.g. following a gunshot or stabbing injury)

This can sometimes be stemmed by placing a urinary catheter in the hole and inflating it. Obviously be careful and think what may be in the depths of the hole!

If local pressure is not sufficient to stop haemorrhage from either soft or hard tissue injury, consider possible coagulation disorders. If these are normal, consider also the need for angiography and embolization or surgical ligation. This is rare.

Significant facial haemorrhage often requires urgent intubation. This facilitates control of the bleeding with packs etc. These injuries are also likely to swell considerably.

Surgical intervention

Surgical ligation of the external carotid (via the neck) and ethmoidal arteries (via the orbits) is more of historical interest and now very rarely undertaken. To do so requires a general anaesthetic and because of the extensive collateral supply will be necessary on both sides. The neck cannot be turned either, making this technically difficult. It is therefore generally time-consuming and not very effective. Alternatively, endoscopic techniques such as transantral and intranasal approaches may be used. These are of limited use in widespread facial fractures, where multiple bleeding points may be present both in bone and soft tissues. These techniques are best used in localized nasal injuries resulting in uncontrollable epistaxis.

Supra selective embolization

The use of supra selective embolization in trauma has now been reported to be very successful. It is increasingly used in extremity trauma, some solid organs, and bleeding secondary to pelvic fractures. Catheter-guided angiography is used to first identify and then occlude the bleeding point or points. This involves the use of balloons, stents, coils or polyvinyl alcohol (PVA).

Primary survey: disability

Head injury is a common cause of morbidity and mortality after trauma because of the resulting injury to the brain. The injury may be primary, occurring at the time of the traumatic episode. Other than preventive measures there is little that can be done about this. Secondary injury occurs later and can be due to reduced perfusion, inadequate oxygenation, and raised intracranial pressure (ICP)—all of which we can do something about.

Assessment begins with the Glasgow Coma Scale (GCS) (or AVPU) and pupillary responses. The GCS is a quick and simple method to determine the level of consciousness that is predictive of patient outcome. However, the GCS score cannot be accurately interpreted until A, B, and C are optimized. Changes in the GCS score with time are more significant than an individual reading. A decrease by 2 points (and the development of a dilated pupil) indicates a critical head injury. Remember, hypoglycaemia, alcohol, and drugs can also alter level of consciousness. However, a reduced conscious level following trauma should always be considered secondary to injury unless proven otherwise.

CT scanning is often required to assess head-injured patients. Patients must therefore be stable prior to transfer to CT. Remember, all facial injuries are technically head injuries. The head injury takes priority over the face in assessment.

Commonly associated problems include:
• Cervical spine injury
• Reduced airway protection
• Profuse bleeding
• Blindness.

Cerebrospinal fluid leaks

Facial fractures which extend into the base of the skull, (e.g. Le Fort II, Le Fort III, NOE, and occasionally fractures involving the mandibular condyle) can tear the dural lining and allow cerebrospinal fluid (CSF) to leak from the nose (rhinorrhoea) or from the ear (otorrhoea). Clear CSF tends to mix with blood and presents as a heavily blood-stained, watery discharge. This trickles down the side of the face. Peripherally the blood tends to clot while the non-clotted blood in the centre is washed away by CSF. This creates two parallel lines referred to as 'tramlining'. One quick test for CSF is the 'ring test' (allow drops to fall on blotting paper: blood clots centrally, the CSF diffuses outwards to form a target sign). Other laboratory tests include examining for eosinophils and sugar. This distinguishes CSF from mucous. More sensitive indicators include beta-2 transferrin and tau protein, although there is some delay in getting results back. Practically it is easier to simply assume that a leak is present. Tell the patient not to blow their nose for 3 weeks and refer to neurosurgeons.

Primary survey: exposure

Patients are exposed—'E'—to look for other injuries which may be hidden beneath their clothing. This is relevant only for major trauma patients or injuries that do not respond to initial treatments. Be mindful that some injuries may not be immediately apparent (a patient may have been stabbed during an alleged assault in addition to being beaten). If blood is visible on clothing, check underneath it.

Following major trauma, the patient is completely undressed during 'E' and examined from head to toe and from front to back. Remember to maintain spinal precautions during log rolling.

'E' also stands for environment—a naked patient can quickly become hypothermic, especially if they have lost blood. Cover all patients with warm blankets to prevent this.

When assessing facial injuries 'E' can also be a timely reminder for 'eyes'—once the life has been saved, the next priorities are sight- and limb-saving measures.

Reassessment of the multiply injured patient

This should be an ongoing part of the initial management. All interventions that have been undertaken should be reviewed—the condition of the patient should improve. If at any point during resuscitation the patient deteriorates, then reassess starting with the airway.

At the end of the primary survey, review the patient along with any results of investigations to ensure they are stable and life-threatening problems have been dealt with. Only then can a complete secondary survey examination be undertaken and attention to the face be drawn.

At some point the patient will need to be 'log rolled' onto their front allow inspection of the back. Timing depends on the likelihood of certain injuries, e.g. it may be necessary during 'B' if a penetrating lung injury is suspected (open pneumothorax).

Further detailed assessment (the 'secondary survey')

The secondary survey does not start until the primary survey has been completed and the patient is stable. This is a complete head-to-toe assessment of the patient. *It is at this point that most head, neck, and dental problems can be attended to.*

Antibiotics, steroids, and tetanus prophylaxis

Protocols may vary between different units. Antibiotics are usually given for fractures, which are compound (open) into the mouth or through the skin (e.g. mandible). Giving prophylactic antibiotics for CSF leakage is controversial and the opinion of a neurosurgeon should be sought. Tetanus prophylaxis should be considered especially in mucky wounds, which should be thoroughly cleaned as soon as possible. Steroids are sometimes given to reduce facial swelling, although their effectiveness is not proven if swelling has already occurred.

Vision-threatening injuries in facial trauma

In craniofacial trauma, the possibility of vision-threatening injuries should only be considered once A, B, C, and D have been managed. However, when examining the eyes during 'D', this can be a good time to make a mental note of any obvious ocular findings. A number of vision-threatening injuries require early diagnosis and treatment if sight is to be preserved. It takes only 1.5–2 hours of optic ischaemia for visual loss to be permanent. Ideally, visual acuity and testing for a relative afferent pupillary defect should be performed in all injured eyes if the condition of the patient allows this. These simple tests are useful because of their prognostic significance. Any patient requiring a brain CT with suspected periorbital/ocular injuries should also undergo imaging of the orbits at the same time. This will avoid unnecessary transfers later for further scans.

Vision can be threatened anywhere along the visual pathway from globe to cortex. The main (potentially treatable) causes to consider are:
- Direct globe injury
- Retrobulbar haemorrhage/orbital compartment syndrome
- Optic nerve compression/traumatic optic neuropathy
- Loss of eyelids/incompetent eyelids.

These are discussed in detail in ➔ Chapter 9 and ➔ Chapter 10.

Direct injury to the globe
This requires urgent ophthalmic referral.

Retrobulbar haemorrhage/orbital compartment syndrome
These are surgical emergencies which can result eventually in irreversible ischaemia of the retina and optic nerve. Treatment requires immediate relief of pressure.

Optic nerve compression/traumatic optic neuropathy
These occur when there is disruption around the optic canal resulting in compression or shearing forces to the optic nerve. Treatment is controversial and may be medical or surgical.

Loss of eyelids/incompetent eyelids
Inability to close the eyelids can result in drying out of the cornea and scarring. Immediate repair is not essential, but protection of the globe is.

The walking wounded

Minor injuries to the maxillofacial region are very common in the UK, around 80% occur in children. Major facial injuries are less frequently seen in the UK. MVCs now account for about 5% of facial trauma. This is partly due to seat belt and drink driving legislation.

In most emergency departments, patients attend as 'walking wounded', that is, with isolated, or multiple (but not life-threatening), injuries. Common causes include assaults, falls, and sporting injuries. Such patients should still undergo a primary survey, although this will not take long if the patient is well. Once this has been carried out, attention can then be focused on the maxillofacial region.

Assessment of the stable maxillofacial injured patient

Evaluation of the head and neck should be performed in a sequential fashion (soft tissues, facial skeleton, teeth). The scalp and face should be inspected for abrasions, lacerations, ecchymosis, and palpated for tenderness and step deformities. Intraoral inspection should assess the occlusion (bite) and look for loose/missing teeth and mucosal lacerations/ecchymoses. Assessment must include a thorough examination of the cranial nerves. More details of the examination of each anatomical region can be found in the relevant chapters in this book.

Many of these patients are the result of an alleged assault. A police report may be required at a later date. Therefore clear and accurate documentation of the initial clinical findings in the notes is very important.

'Soft tissue' injuries

The term 'soft tissue' refers to all non-bony structures including skin, fat, muscle, nerves, and vessels. Surgeons often refer to the 'soft tissue envelope' when talking about fractures. This is an important functional layer. *The success of fracture management is highly dependent on maintaining a good blood supply. This can only come from the soft tissues.* Crush and blast injuries can therefore have a major impact on prognosis, even if the soft tissues appear to be relatively undamaged.

Any wound that breaches the dermis will result in a permanent scar. The severity of the scarring depends on a number of factors (such as the trauma itself, the patient's age/health, and the management of the wound itself, including aftercare). The final cosmetic outcome is therefore partly outside our control. However, outcomes can be still be greatly influenced by careful surgical technique and gentle handling of the soft tissues. Optimal management of soft tissue injuries is therefore essential. Thorough wound toilet, judicious debridement, and meticulous tissue handling are all required to achieve the best possible aesthetic and functional outcomes. Even if the skin is intact following an impact, subsequent neglect or mismanagement of the injured site can still result in significant deformity or disability.

The very rich blood supply of the head and neck helps to defend this site against infection and promote healing. Despite high intraoral bacterial counts, infected wounds within the mouth are surprisingly uncommon. Saliva and exudates from around the gingiva contain antibodies and various growth factors, which facilitate rapid wound healing and prevent infection. Skin, however, does not have these protective mechanisms and infection may arise not only from external sources, but also from naturally occurring commensal organisms. This can be promoted whenever there is devitalized tissue within the wound, in which bacteria can proliferate. Penetrating injuries also need particular attention. Bacteria can be driven deep into the tissues and are then difficult to eradicate.

Initial assessment and management of soft tissue injuries

It is important to take sufficient time to make a careful assessment of any soft tissue injury. Before exploring any wounds, consider the possibility that this may produce further bleeding. If necessary, have the appropriate equipment to hand to control any bleeding. Be especially careful with scalp and neck wounds, and in children.

A good working knowledge of anatomy is essential to help assess for tissue loss or underlying injuries (e.g. parotid duct/nerve injuries).

When necessary, involve appropriate specialists (often maxillofacial/plastics/ENT/ophthalmology) according to local referral policy and at an early stage. Consider this with anything more complex than a superficial wound (abrasions).

Assessment

The following checklist may be helpful in the assessment of soft tissue injuries to the face:

- Control haemorrhage: apply pressure with a clean pad of gauze.
- Consider the mechanism of injury (incised vs crushed tissues).
- If sufficiently experienced, assess for any injuries to underlying structures, (dentition/bones/globe/lacrimal gland/eyelid levators/canthus/parotid duct/facial nerve/sensory nerves).
- Consider the possibility of underlying fractures. The mechanism of injury will give a good indication.
- Is there tissue loss, or is it just displaced? Rarely, is there true loss of tissue (usually seen following bites, blasts, or projectile injuries). More commonly, the tissues are present but are gaping, creating an appearance of tissue loss. *Where tissue is twisted, realign and support it as soon as possible.* Failure to do so may make the difference between an ischaemic, but recoverable area of tissue and an infarcted one. Tissue that is attached by even a small pedicle can do surprisingly well if realigned early. This is due to the excellent blood supply to the head and neck.
- Is any imaging required? Identification of foreign bodies often requires imaging. Plain films are often required, although CT may be needed to identify deeper foreign bodies and to help locate them precisely. In the presence of metallic foreign bodies, magnetic resonance imaging (MRI) is contraindicated. MRI is more useful in identifying

non-metallic foreign bodies such as plastic, but some materials may still be very difficult to see (notably vegetation such as twigs, etc.). Do not forget to ascertain if any teeth have been lost—a CXR and neck X-ray may be necessary.

- What is the anticipated extent of scarring? Risk factors for a poor cosmetic result include delayed presentation, contamination, tissue loss, crush injury, underlying fractures, and patients with chronic medical conditions. Patients in these categories should be referred to the appropriate specialists at an early stage.
- Consider if the wound can be managed properly under local or general anaesthetic.
- Document carefully—ideally, photograph the wound.
- Consider tetanus prophylaxis and antibiotic treatment.
- If there will be a delay before definitive management, gently clean and loosely close, or dress the wound appropriately.
- Warn all patients about scarring and subsequent deformity.

Management of soft tissue injuries: principles

Clean wounds should ideally be closed as soon as possible (within 12 hours) with meticulous care, precise haemostasis, and accurate repositioning of the tissues. When suturing an irregular wound, look carefully for recognizable landmarks—matching these will greatly facilitate accurate apposition of the remainder of the wound.

Suturing of the wound should be performed in layers. The underlying tissues are precisely aligned to eliminate any 'dead space' beneath the surface. Closing the skin only and leaving a potential space or cavity can predispose to abscess formation, and compromise wound healing. When closing the skin, the aim is to produce a neatly opposed and everted wound edge. A small amount of eversion is reported to compensate for depression of the scar during wound contraction.

Alternatives to sutures include metal clips, adhesive paper tapes, and skin adhesives (e.g. cyanoacrylate glue). These can be applied quickly, but accurate alignment of skin edges can be difficult. Metal clips tend to be reserved for lacerations involving the scalp. Adhesive paper tapes and skin glues are especially useful in children and those who will not cooperate. Care is required in both patient and wound selection. Only superficial facial or hairless scalp wounds should be considered. The final cosmetic results are less predictable with these techniques compared to carefully placed sutures, as the unsupported deep tissues may gape. Although apparently simpler, gluing can still be quite tricky—take care not to allow glue to enter the patient's eyes, ears, or mouth and be careful not to glue your glove to the patient. Although it can be removed, this can be very embarrassing (you will not be the first to do it).

If the wound edges are ragged, trimming the edges may convert an 'untidy' wound margin to a neat edge that can then be closed, giving a superior aesthetic result. However, trimming should be reserved for dead or obviously damaged tissues, and should be kept to a minimum. Wide excision of tissue from the face may lead to difficulties in achieving a good closure of the defect, particularly near the eyes, nose, and mouth. There should be no tension across the wound. In cases where tension is a problem, undermining of the skin, local flap closure, or skin grafts may be used. If doubt exists about viability, tissue is often left in place and inspected later. These cases often need to be referred.

Management of devitalized tissue/foreign bodies

Tattooing can occur when grit and debris are not completely removed from a wound. This subsequently goes on to heal with visible particles under the skin surface. Foreign material must therefore be removed by meticulous wound cleaning and careful debridement. It is essential to remove all foreign material and this may require prolonged but gentle scrubbing of the wound (scrubbing in itself is additional trauma). Regional nerve blocks or general anaesthesia may be necessary. Take care not to scrub too aggressively. Overenthusiastic scrubbing can cause further trauma to the wound and extend any zones of ischaemia, resulting in devitalization of tissue. Small fibres from the scrubbing brush can also be left in the wound, resulting in further foci for infection. If scrubbing is required, use a small toothbrush and apply gentle pressure. Be patient—removal of all dirt may take some time. For small pieces of grit, the tip of a pointed scalpel may be used.

Copious but gentle irrigation is the best way to clean a wound. Although a number of antiseptics are available, some are reported to harm tissues and can delay healing. Sterile saline solution or water are not harmful to wounds and are recommended by many authorities. If antiseptics are used to irrigate wounds, remember to protect the patient's eyes.

If the wound edges are ragged, or if there is any obvious devitalized tissue, careful trimming back to healthy bleeding tissue may be required. If wound contamination is extensive, clean and debride as far as possible then dress the wound and arrange for another wound inspection after 24–48 hours, ideally with wound closure during the same procedure.

It is important to document any tissue loss, ascertain the patient's tetanus status, and take a wound swab for microbiological culture. Antibiotics should be prescribed according to local protocols.

Management of bites and scratches

Whether animal or human in origin, these injuries must be considered as potentially serious injuries and managed expeditiously. Both can rapidly become infected if they are not treated properly. Dog bites can range from simple puncture wounds, to irregular tears, to missing chunks of tissue. The canines (the longest teeth) can penetrate deeply, taking bacteria deep into the wound. Depending on the patient (and the dog), underlying fractures have also been reported.

Unlike other sites on the body, bites and scratches on the face can often be closed primarily. This is due to the excellent blood supply and relatively good healing potential of the face, compared to elsewhere. However, these injuries must be thoroughly cleaned and irrigated prior to suturing and should be monitored closely for signs of infection. Antibiotics should be prescribed according to local protocol. All crushed and devitalized tissue should be carefully removed. Abscesses can develop in the deeper tissues. More unusual bites (e.g. farmyard animals, snakes, and spiders) require specialist knowledge due to the risks of exotic infections or venoms.

Suturing

Over the past 20 years, simple treatments in closing superficial skin wounds, such as adhesive strips and tissue glues have gained widespread popularity. Excellent cosmetic results have been achieved in appropriately selected cases. However, wounds that are deep (i.e. below the dermis) or those that occur along lines of skin tension still require 'deep' sutures to achieve adequate repair. These deeper sutures maintain continued support once the skin sutures have been removed.

Deep lacerations are therefore closed in layers (i.e. muscle to muscle, skin to skin). Not only does this provide prolonged support during healing but also the deep closure eliminates any 'dead space' beneath the surface. Closing the skin only and leaving a potential space underneath can predispose to haematoma or seroma formation. This may weaken the wound and may also become infected.

There are a number of suturing techniques available to close a wound (simple interrupted, horizontal/vertical mattress, subcuticular). All of these have a particular advantage in specific situations. However, for the non-surgical specialist we would recommend using a simple interrupted suture technique. This suture technique is easy to learn and gives an excellent cosmetic result.

Choice of suture

Many different suture materials are currently available. The choice depends on a number of factors, such as the characteristics of the wound (including whether the patient will tolerate suture removal), the period of time over which suture support is desirable (including whether the suture is to be removed or left to resorb), ease of use, and the surgeon's preference.

Sutures can be classified according to the number of strands they are comprised of (monofilament/multifilament), and their degradation properties (absorbable/non-absorbable):

- Monofilament sutures (e.g. nylon) consist of a single strand of material. The suture exhibits low resistance when passed through tissue and there is less harbouring of micro-organisms than multifilament strands. These properties make monofilament sutures an ideal choice for skin closure on the face where cosmesis is extremely important. However, the knots may be less secure than with multifilament sutures.
- Multifilament sutures (e.g. silk) consist of several strands braided together. Multifilament sutures have a high tensile strength and are easy to use. However, the braided nature of the material acts as a focus for micro-organisms which may cause infection.
- Absorbable sutures (e.g. Vicryl®) tend to be used to close the deep layers, or in areas where the aesthetic result is not the primary consideration. They gradually lose tensile strength as they are degraded. The rate of absorption depends on the suture calibre and the wound conditions. Unfortunately, with some larger sutures the rate of degradation may be so prolonged that persistence of the suture causes cross-hatching if used to close the skin. However, in children a very fine absorbable suture (Vicryl® Rapide 6/0) may be used. Depending on the site, additional support may be possible

using steri-strips supplemented with a fine layer of cyanoacrylate. This provides prolonged support, protects the wound, and avoids the stress of subsequent suture removal. The very fine sutures disintegrate over a period of days, leaving no suture marks.

- Non-absorbable sutures (e.g. nylon) need to be removed. This must be carefully timed to balance the needs of sufficient wound support against the risks of developing cross-hatching. Cross-hatching is difficult to improve and may require revision, with further excision and primary closure. Sutures (6/0 nylon) placed in the face are usually removed around 5 days after surgery, or even earlier in delicate tissues such as the eyelids. With neck lacerations, sutures (4/0 nylon) are often retained for longer (7–10 days). Scalp sutures (4/0 nylon) are similarly left for 7–10 days or an absorbable suture used instead.

How to suture (simple interrupted suture)

- Following skin preparation with an appropriate surgical antiseptic (such as chlorhexidine or iodine based), local anaesthetic is infiltrated around the margins of the wound.
- Explore wounds carefully and thoroughly—they are often deeper than you think.
- Thoroughly clean the wound (irrigate copiously, but gently scrub the tissue). Use the tip of a pointed scalpel blade to remove grit.
- Remove only dead tissue. Carefully excise wound edges. Try to ensure there is sufficient tissue to allow tension-free closure.
- Ensure meticulous haemostasis.
- Remove the suture from the packet with the needle holder. Never use your fingers to hold the needle. Never hold the tip of the needle with the holder—this will damage it.
- Place the needle holder two-thirds along the circumference of the needle from the tip.
- Insert the needle at 90 degrees to the tissue using counter pressure from the forceps. Pull the suture through to the other side and tie a knot.
- Avoid pinching the skin with the forceps. This can crush the tissue leading to necrosis.
- As a rule, the distance from the edge of the wound should correspond to the thickness of the tissues being sutured. Each subsequent suture should be placed approximately twice this distance apart.
- Align key anatomical landmarks first (vermillion border, eyebrow, eyelids, etc.). A temporary suture to approximate these landmarks may be helpful.
- Close in layers (mucosa to mucosa, muscle to muscle, and skin to skin). Skin sutures should not be relied upon to hold the wound closed in the presence of tension.
- Once the wound is closed, ensure none of the knots on the skin lie over the suture line.
- According to local protocol a topical antibacterial ointment (e.g. chloramphenicol) or adhesive strips (steri-strips) may be applied to the skin wound until the sutures are removed.
- Ensure follow-up is arranged for skin suture removal 5–6 days post wound closure if non-absorbable sutures have been used.

Which facial soft tissue wounds should I refer?

Follow your local referral guidelines. These may include:

- Involvement of key landmark sites such as the vermillion border, eyelids, eyebrow, ala of the nose and ears.
- Deep facial wounds particularly with clinical evidence of damage to the bones, nerves (e.g. facial nerve), or other structures (e.g. parotid duct).
- Animal/human bites.
- Oral lacerations.
- Burns.
- Wounds with associated tissue loss.
- Any penetrating neck wounds.
- Lack of resources (time, equipment, skills) to do a good job.

Management of intraoral soft tissue wounds

These tend to occur following blunt trauma, during which the tissues are either avulsed from points of attachment (degloving injuries), or are lacerated by underlying fractures or nearby teeth. Intraoral wounds need to be assessed carefully as they can often contain debris and can quickly become infected. Small wounds, including those of the tongue, can often be left and will heal uneventfully. Larger ones need repair.

Be careful with penetrating soft palate injuries in children. The typical history is a fall while running with a pencil or pen in the mouth. Although the palatal wound itself is usually small, carotid injury and delayed onset of stroke have been reported.

'Hard tissue' injuries (fractures)

Overview of the facial skeleton and clinical examination

The arrangement of the facial bones may be considered as comprising three areas:

- Upper third (frontal bone).
- Middle third—between the supraorbital ridges and the upper teeth. (2 maxillae, 2 zygomas, 2 lacrimal bones, 2 nasal bones, 1 vomer, 1 ethmoid).
- Lower third (mandible).

Some of these bones (ethmoid and orbital roof) are extremely delicate and so thin that on a real skull light can easily pass through. The remainder vary in thickness but often remain quite delicate (nasal, zygoma). The mandible is the strongest of the facial bones. It is a 'U'-shaped bone comprised of an outer dense cortical layer and delicate trabecular bone inside. The face is not solid but contains several 'cavities' such as the sinuses, orbits, oral, and nasal cavities. Around these the bones form a series of vertical struts known as 'buttresses'. As a result, these bones are very good at resisting vertically directed forces (e.g. during chewing) but are weak when resisting horizontal forces (i.e. during most injuries).

Upper-third injuries

This area comprises the cranial vault, skull base, and frontal sinus. Initial clinical assessment involves an evaluation of the GCS along with a thorough inspection of the skull for evidence of any hard/soft tissue trauma.

The gold standard imaging of upper third fractures is CT to include the cranial vault, skull base, orbits, sinuses, and temporal bone. Early discussion with a neurosurgical team is essential to guide management.

Cranial vault

The cranial vault is formed by the frontal, parietal, occipital, temporal, and greater wings of the sphenoid bone. Most fractures occur in either the frontal or parietal bone. Fractures can be open or closed, depressed or non-displaced. The main issue with these types of fractures is involvement of the brain and meninges. Patients can often be asymptomatic on initial evaluation. Involvement of the meninges can lead to CSF leaks (rhinorrhoea/otorrhoea). Depressed fragments of bone can lead to cerebral cortical lacerations or intra/extracerebral haematomas requiring emergency surgery.

Skull base

The bones forming the skull base are the frontal, sphenoid, temporal, and occipital bones. Skull base fractures are important in neurotrauma with approximately 50% of cases related to significant brain injury. They are generally the result of high-force impact, especially those of the middle cranial fossa and those that cross the midline. Clinical presentation can vary from asymptomatic to comatose.

As with all upper-third injuries, the initial assessment should involve an evaluation of the GCS. A complete neurological examination should then be performed.

Clinical features include:
- CSF rhinorrhoea/otorrhoea.
- Battles sign: ecchymosis in the mastoid region.
- Bilateral periorbital ecchymosis (panda eyes).

Frontal sinus

Most frontal sinus fractures are related to high-velocity impact such as road traffic accidents, assaults, and sport injuries. They often involve a combination of both the anterior and posterior walls of the sinus.

Clinical examination should include an assessment of any contour deformity over the frontal bone along with any lacerations or sensory deficit in this region.

Middle-third injuries

The middle third of the facial skeleton is a complex anatomical region which can be considered as being composed of several distinct areas. Injuries to each site will have their own structural, aesthetic, and functional characteristics, as well as their own surgical challenges. Although the term 'middle third' is commonly used to denote Le Fort fractures, injuries to this region are often much more widespread and complex. The term 'midface' is often used to refer collectively to those structures situated between the skull base and the occlusal plane. 'Middle-third fractures,' therefore overlap with fractures of the nose, naso-orbitoethmoid

(NOE) region, and zygoma. They may also extend upwards, into the anterior cranial fossa. The bones of the midface are important in maintaining the functions of the oral cavity, nasal cavity, and orbits. Not surprisingly, injuries here also have significant cosmetic implications. Fractures of the midface tend to result from high-energy impacts and can therefore be both life-threatening as well as disfiguring.

Clinical signs associated with middle-third fractures include:
- Facial swelling/deformity
- Subconjunctival bleeding
- Oronasal bleeding
- Palpable bony step deformity in the periorbital region
- Displacement or impaired movement of the globe, with diplopia
- Displacement of the medial canthal tendon (NOE fractures)
- Sensory impairment (infraorbital division of trigeminal nerve)
- A change in the occlusion (bite).

To assess a midface fracture radiologically, CT should be performed. For any patient that has suffered significant periorbital trauma, referral to an ophthalmologist at an early stage is important.

Clinical assessment of midface injuries

Clinical assessment of the injured midface should proceed in a sequential fashion following examination of the upper third of the facial skeleton. The neck should ideally have been 'cleared' first. This is discussed in ➡ Chapter 4, p. 106. It is important to be methodical as useful signs can be easily overlooked. Look for lengthening of the face or a 'dishface' deformity. Examination should also include the following:

Palpation of the bones
Palpate the midface skeleton at the following sites for tenderness, step deformities, or mobility:
- Infra/supraorbital rim
- Nose
- Zygomatic complex and zygomatic arch
- Maxilla.

Examination of the eye
- Visual acuity
- Visual fields
- Ocular movement
- Globe position/proptosis/enophthalmos
- Pupillary/relative afferent pupillary defect.

Examination of the ear
- Pinna particularly for a haematoma of the auricular cartilage.
- Tympanic canal for evidence of blood/CSF leaks.

Examination of the nose
Use a speculum to visualize the nasal airway. Look for septal haematoma and CSF.

Sensory and motor nerve examination
- Examine the sensory nerves of the face (supraorbital, infraorbital division).
- Examine the facial nerve.

Intraoral examination
- Posterior oropharyngeal collapse.
- Tenderness/step deformity along the maxillary buttress.
- Palatal haematoma/lacerations—these may indicate a split palate.
- Change in the occlusion (bite)—notably an anterior open bite.
- Apparent trismus—premature contacts in the molar region.
- Mobile dentoalveolar segments/missing teeth.
- Dentures—be careful. Loose fitting dentures can confuse even the experienced clinician. If broken, check all the pieces are present. If not, consider the possibility of aspiration.

Abnormal mobility of the midface
This can be detected by grasping the anterior maxillary alveolus and gently rocking the maxilla. At the same time the other hand palpates the sites of suspected fractures (nasal bridge, inferior orbital margins, or fronto-zygomatic sutures) (Figure 2.4).

Care is required if the neck has not been 'cleared'. If concerns exist about the neck this part of the examination is best deferred. Alternatively, the head must be fully supported. If the teeth and palate move but the nasal bones are stable, a Le Fort I fracture is present (or it is a denture). If the teeth, palate, and nasal bones move but the lateral orbital rims are stable, it is a Le Fort II fracture. If the whole midface feels unstable, it is probably a Le Fort III or some other complex fracture pattern. The level of a Le Fort fracture can be often determined by this examination. However, in practice, 'pure' fractures are uncommon, as other fractures of the facial skeleton are often present. The clinical picture can therefore be a little uncertain. This is not a major concern nowadays, since such high-energy injuries usually require a CT scan, which will ultimately define the fracture pattern.

Lower-third injuries
(See also ➲ Chapter 12.) Examination of the lower third of the facial skeleton is usually performed in conjunction with assessment of the midface.

Clinical assessment of mandibular injuries
Extraoral
- Assess for tenderness particularly around the chin and over the angles of the mandible on palpation.
- Look for swelling/bruising over the submandibular region.
- Examine the sensory division of the mental nerve (lower lip/chin).

Intraoral
- Assess the occlusion (bite).
- Look for bruising, particularly in the floor of the mouth and the buccal sulcus.
- Look for tenderness/mobility of the dentoalveolar segments. This is discussed further in the relevant chapter.

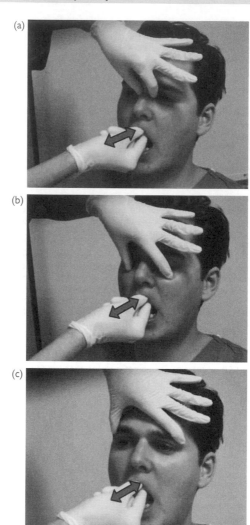

Figure 2.4 Clinical examination of the midface (take care with the cervical spine).

Some useful clinical signs and their significance

The usefulness of clinical signs can vary from those which only suggest an underlying pathology (*) to those which are almost pathognomonic (***). Their interpretation must be taken in conjunction with the history and likelihood of the condition being present.

General

- *Facial burns****
  - When associated with soot in the nose and mouth, singeing of the nasal vibrissae, *and* sooty sputum this represents a potential airway problem. There is also the risk of, and inhalation of, carbon monoxide and other toxins.
- *Facial nerve palsy***
  - Following head injury—fractured base of skull.
- *Horse voice/bovine cough****
  - Following a direct blow to the anterior neck may indicate disruption of the larynx. A bovine cough is where the vocal cords do not meet in the midline prior to the explosive expulsion of air. As a result the cough is relatively weak and ineffectual.
- *Wry neck (torticollis)**
  - Following trauma is due to muscle spasm. May occasionally be associated with dislocation of the posterior facet joints.

The face

- *Intercanthal distance***
  - Separation of the inner corners of the eyes. If greater than 30–32 mm (female) or 32–34 mm (male) the patient may have detached canthi secondary to an underlying NOE fracture. As well as an increased intercanthal distance, the medial canthus loses its pointed shape, becoming rounded. This can occur uni- or bilaterally. If unilateral, the distance from midline to canthus will be greater on one side. The interpupillary distance should be within normal limits. There may also be depression at the root of the nose.
- *Anterior open bite and elongated face***
  - If not pre-existing, is suggestive of posterior and inferior displacement of the maxilla following a Le Fort fracture. This results in posterior gagging of the molar teeth—an anterior open bite (AOB).
- *Septal haematoma****
  - Seen as a blue/reddened swelling on the septum on direct examination. Needs drainage as failure to do so can result in septal perforation, abscesses, and intracranial infection.
- *Numbness of the cheek**
  - Suggests a cheek or blowout fracture.
- *Numbness of the lower lip**
  - Suggests a mandibular fracture.

- *Anosmia**
  - Loss of smell due to tearing of olfactory nerves secondary to an underlying anterior cranial fossa floor fracture. Not reliably detectable in acute phase of injury.
- *'Bow-string' test***
  - Assesses for medial canthal detachment in NOE injuries—the lateral canthus is pulled laterally and the medial canthus observed. If this is detached it will also move laterally.

Within the mouth

- *Dysphagia**
  - Many causes. When related to submandibular, pharyngeal, or other posterior oral swellings it is a significant finding often requiring admission. Is often painful (odynophagia).
- *Inability to protrude the tongue***
  - When related to submandibular, sublingual, or other oral swellings it is a significant finding often requiring admission.
- *Trismus***
  - Limitation of mouth opening due to muscle spasm (usually masseter or medial pterygoid). May be seen following a direct blow. When related to submandibular, pharyngeal, or other posterior oral swellings it is a significant finding often requiring admission.
- *Guerin's sign****
  - Palatal bruising of the hard palate—underlying fracture involving palatine foramen.
- *Upper buccal sulcus bruising***
  - Fractured zygoma or unilateral Le Fort I or II.
- *Sublingual haematoma****
  - Bruising/bleeding under the tongue—fractured mandible (body/symphysis/parasymphysis).
- *Bleeding gums***
  - May indicate an associated fracture of the tooth or bone.
- *Change in the patient's bite****
  - If the occlusion has changed, it is likely that there is an underlying fracture of maxilla, mandible, or alveolar bone. Displacement of the zygoma may also flex the maxilla. This can sometimes result in diagnostic confusion. Subluxation of teeth may also produce a malocclusion although usually much more minor. If none of these are present, a malocclusion may be a result of a temporomandibular joint (TMJ) effusion/haemarthrosis.
- *'Cracked cup note'**
  - When percussing the maxillary teeth suggests a fracture.

The eyes

(See also ➲ Chapter 10.)
- *Visual acuity****
  - This is the single most sensitive indicator of visual impairment. It must be recorded in all patients with midface trauma. In patients who wear spectacles to correct short sight the recording must be

done with the spectacles on or through a pinhole. If the patient is unconscious, pupillary responses to light must be checked.
- All patients must have a documented visual acuity. Any decrease in visual acuity requires an ophthalmic opinion.

- **Pupillary responses****
  - Check direct response to light and consensual response. Responses should be equal on both sides and to direct and consensual stimulation. A pupil that reacts poorly to direct stimulation but briskly to consensual has an afferent pupillary defect.
- **Swinging flashlight test*****
  - Detects subtle defects to the optic nerve. Light is shone in one eye then swung to the other and back and forth. If the right eye has a problem, on shining the light in the right eye both pupils will constrict as the light moves to the left they will constrict further. As the light is brought back to the right the pupils will not respond or dilate a little.
- **Periorbital haematoma******
  - If the margins of this are well defined, this represents a fracture involving the orbit. Usually this means a fractured zygoma but can also include a blowout fracture, fractured base of skull (anterior cranial fossa), unilateral NOE or nasal bones.
- **Racoon (panda) eyes*****
  - Bilateral well-defined 'black eyes'—fractured base of skull (anterior cranial fossa), Le Fort III, or NOE fracture.
- **Lateral subconjunctival haemorrhage****
  - This indicates a fracture involving the orbit, usually the cheek or NOE region. There is no posterior limit to the haemorrhage.
- **Chemosis***
  - Swelling of conjunctiva is often seen in significant trauma. It looks a bit like frog's spawn. If no tear of conjunctiva is present, it will resolve. If a tear is present, it is important to rule out globe injury.
- **Hyphema****
  - Blood in anterior chamber seen as fluid level when patient is standing. Needs ophthalmic assessment and probably require admission and observation.
- **Iridodialysis***
  - The iris is detached from its root leading to a distorted pupil shape.
- **Dilated pupil (traumatic mydriasis)***
  - Spasm of the dilator pupillae. Can be seen following a direct blow to the eye. Not to be confused with a third nerve palsy.
- **Diplopia***
  - Double vision may be neurogenic, myogenic, or bony in origin. It may be temporary or permanent and should be reviewed. Depending on possible cause refer to ophthalmics or maxillofacial.
- **Unilateral restricted upward gaze****
  - Often a sign of a 'blowout' fracture, occasionally due to injury to ocular muscle or its nerve. Painful diplopia from a blowout may require urgent release.

- *Retraction sign****
  - When looking from the side of the patient, as they look upward the globe is seen to move posteriorly. This is a good sign for a blowout fracture. Entrapment of the fat and restriction of the inferior rectus muscle results in a shift of the axis of rotation of the globe from its centre to the point of entrapment. Thus the pull of the superior rectus results in a backward rotation of the globe.
- *Hypoglobus**
  - Inferior displacement of the globe seen in cheek complex fractures, where the bone and Lockwood's ligament drop down. May also be seen in large blowout fractures.
- *Enophthalmos**
  - Posterior displacement of the globe due to increased orbital volume. Seen in blowout fractures of the orbit and cheek fractures. Globe appears 'sunken in' with a deep supra tarsal groove.
- *Third nerve palsy****
  - Dilated pupil, the eye looks down and out, and ptosis. In severe head injuries this represents third nerve compression from an expanding intracranial lesion. The patient has a reduced GCS score.
- *Aqueous leakage****
  - A penetrating injury of the cornea.
- *Superior orbital fissure (SOF) syndrome***
  - (Lazy French Tarts Sit Naked In Anticipation!) Ophthalmoplegia, fixed dilated pupil, and ipsilateral forehead numbness—fracture extending into the SOF, or possible carotid aneurysm. This is usually part of a significant injury.
- *Orbital apex syndrome***
  - As in the SOF but here the patient has reduced visual acuity.
- *Periorbital oedema**
  - When infective in origin represents significant spread of infection. If the eye is closing the patient may probably need admission.

The ears
- *Haemotympanum***
  - Blood visualized behind the ear drum. Indicative of a fracture of the middle cranial fossa.
- *Battles sign****
  - Bruising around the mastoid region—fractured base of skull (middle cranial fossa).
- *CSF rhinorrhoea/otorrhoea****
  - 'Tramlining'—fractured base of skull. Blood mixes with CSF and leaks out. Along the edges the blood clots while centrally the CSF leak washes it away to form two parallel lines (like tramlines).
- *Bleeding from the ear***
  - May indicate a fractured base of skull or mandibular condyle. If the tympanic membrane is intact, the bleeding is local to the meatus, usually the anterior wall. This is often secondary to an associated condylar fracture. If the tympanic membrane is perforated the blood may be from a middle cranial fossa fracture.

Further reading

American College of Surgeons Committee on Trauma. *ATLS Advanced Trauma Life Support for Doctors.* 8th ed. Chicago, IL: American College of Surgeons; 2008. https://www.facs.org/quality-programs/trauma/atls

American Society of Anesthesiologists. Practice guidelines for the management of the difficult airway: a report by the American Society of Anesthesiologists Task Force on Management of the Difficult Airway. *Anesthesiology.* 1993;78:597–602.

National Audit Office. *Major Trauma Care in England.* 2010. http://www.nao.org.uk/wp-content/uploads/2010/02/0910213.pdf

Nottingham University Hospitals NHS Trust. *Major Trauma Clinical Guidelines.* 2011. https://www.nuh.nhs.uk/media/12076/MTguidelinesOct2011.pdf

Perry M. Advanced Trauma Life Support (ATLS) and facial trauma: can one size fit all? Part 1. Dilemmas in the management of the multiply injured patient with coexisting facial injuries. *Int J Oral Maxillofac Surg.* 2008;37:209–14.

Perry M, Morris C. Advanced trauma life support (ATLS) and facial trauma: can one size fit all? Part 2: ATLS, maxillofacial injuries and airway management dilemmas. *Int J Oral Maxillofac Surg.* 2008;37:309–20.

Perry M, Moutray T. Advanced Trauma Life Support (ATLS) and facial trauma: can one size fit all? Part 4: 'can the patient see?' Timely diagnosis, dilemmas and pitfalls in the multiply injured, poorly responsive/unresponsive patient. *Int J Oral Maxillofac Surg.* 2008;37:505–14.

Perry M, O'Hare J, Porter G. Advanced Trauma Life Support (ATLS) and facial trauma: can one size fit all? Part 3: Hypovolaemia and facial injuries in the multiply injured patient. *Int J Oral Maxillofac Surg.* 2008;37:405–14.

Chapter 3

The head

Common presentations

- Blackouts/fits (seizures)/faints
- Headaches (bilateral/generalized)
- Headaches (unilateral/focal)
- Trauma
- Loss of smell (see ➲ Chapter 7)
- Vertigo/loss of balance (see also ➲ Chapter 6)
- Visual disturbance.

Common problems and their causes

Blackouts/fits (seizures)/faints

Common
- Vasovagal
- Epilepsy/non-epileptic attacks
- Medical conditions (hypoglycaemia, cardiac disease, stroke, hypotension, etc.)

Uncommon
- Carotid disease
- Cervical spine disease in elderly.

Headaches (bilateral/generalized)

Common
- Tension headache
- Sinusitis
- Migraine
- Cervicogenic headache
- Analgesic misuse.

Uncommon
- Intracranial haemorrhage (ICH/SAH)
- Hydrocephalus
- Raised ICP (tumours/trauma)
- Intracranial infections (meningitis, encephalitis)
- Dural venous thrombosis (cavernous sinus/sagittal sinus).

Headaches (unilateral)

Common
- Trauma/post-concussion headache
- Infections (sinusitis/otitis media)
- Glaucoma
- Temporal (giant cell) arteritis
- Migraine
- Cluster headaches
- Tension headache/TMJ symptoms.

Uncommon
- Post-traumatic haematomas (extradural, subdural)
- Intracranial infections (meningitis can be localized, brain abscess, subdural empyema)
- Mastoiditis
- Brain tumours
- Referred dental pain
- Trigeminal autonomic cephalalgias
- ICH (may initially be localized).

Injuries

Common
- Blunt trauma
- Scalp lacerations.

Uncommon
- Impalement injuries
- Penetrating injuries
- Blast injuries.

Loss of smell
(See ⯈ Chapter 7.)

Common
- Upper respiratory tract infection/rhinitis/sinusitis
- Nasal polyps/hayfever/allergies
- Head/nasal/naso-orbito-ethmoidal (NOE) trauma (anterior cranial fossa).

Uncommon
- Tumours of the frontal lobe/esthesioneuroblastoma
- Multiple sclerosis
- Cushing's syndrome/diabetes
- Epilepsy
- Cranial radiotherapy
- Liver or kidney disease
- Parkinson's disease
- Alzheimer's disease
- Primary ciliary dyskinesia
- Meningioma
- Paget's disease of bone
- Primary amoebic meningoencephalitis
- Long-term alcoholism
- Kallmann syndrome—a genetic condition
- Sarcoidosis.

Vertigo/loss of balance
(See also ⯈ Chapter 6.)

Common
- Middle/inner ear conditions (see ⯈ Chapter 6).

Uncommon
- Meningitis
- Subarachnoid haemorrhage.

Useful questions and what to look for

Blackouts/fits (seizures)/faints

Ask about
- Onset
- Duration and frequency
- Exacerbating factors
- Nausea and vomiting
- Preceding or associated symptoms (aura/change in vision/jaw claudication)
- Detailed PMH (consider non-neurological causes).

Look for
- Reduced level of consciousness
- Visual disturbance
- Photophobia/papilloedema
- Heart murmurs/cardiac signs
- Autonomic symptoms
- Neck stiffness/dizziness on moving
- Focal neurological deficit/signs of injury
- Systemic symptoms (including BP and rash)
- Tongue biting
- Incontinence.

Headaches (all types)

Ask about
- Location/character
- Timing
- Onset
- Duration and frequency
- Exacerbating/relieving factors
- Nausea and vomiting
- Visual disturbance
- Preceding or associated symptoms (aura/jaw claudication/seizures)
- PMH (hypertension/diabetes)
- Diet (especially caffeine) and medication/drug intake.

Look for
- Reduced level of consciousness
- Photophobia/papilloedema
- Autonomic symptoms
- Neck stiffness
- Focal neurological deficit (especially abnormal/asymmetric pupils or CN III palsy)

- Systemic signs (including BP)
- Tenderness (frontal sinus/temporal artery/globe)
- Rash (meningitis/herpes zoster).

Injuries

Ask about
- When it occurred
- Mechanism of injury (blunt/penetrating)
- Loss of consciousness
- Other injuries (especially the neck)
- Progression of symptoms since injury
- Alcohol or drug use
- Medications (especially anticoagulants)
- Seizures
- Preceding headache.

Look for
- ATLS (as required)
- GCS
- Pupil responses
- Other injuries (notably neck/scalp/facial/ocular).

Loss of smell
(See ➜ Chapter 7.)

Ask about
- History of head/nasal injury
- Constant or intermittent
- Obstructed breathing through the nose
- Nasal discharge
- Headaches/visual problems
- PMH (many medical causes).

Look for
- Examine nose
- Cranial nerve examination
- Frontal sinus tenderness to percussion
- Vision and ocular movements.

Vertigo/loss of balance
(See also ➜ Chapter 6.)

Ask about
- Describe symptoms
- Duration: seconds, minutes, hours, days
- Associated symptoms (neurological or aural)
- PMH.

Look for
- General exam
- Otoscopy
- Neurological exam/eye movements.

Examination of the head

This is tailored according to the suspected pathology (injuries, infections, neurological). Various elements make up a comprehensive examination. *Neurological examination cannot be considered in total isolation from the rest of the body.* The following should all be considered.

Conscious level: the Glasgow Coma Scale

The GCS has three components (Table 3.1). A fully alert and orientated person has a GCS score of 15. A dead body has a GCS score of 3 (not zero).

Paediatric variation of the Glasgow Coma Scale
- Motor and eye opening same as adult.
- Verbal depends on age/ability—5-point scale:
  - Babbles/coos/words as per usual (5)
  - Less than usual ability or spontaneous irritable cry (4)
  - Inappropriate crying (3)
  - Occasionally whimpers/moans (2)
  - No response (1).

Cranial nerve examination

This should be undertaken routinely. With practice, a 'quick cranial nerve survey' can be undertaken in just a few minutes (see Table 3.2).

Table 3.1 Components of the Glasgow Coma Scale (corresponding score in brackets)

Eye opening (EO)	
EO spontaneously	(4)
EO to speech	(3)
EO to pain*	(2)
EO none	(1)

* Do not test with supraorbital pressure as patient will instinctively close their eyes.

Verbal response	
Orientated	(5)
Confused	(4)
Inappropriate words	(3)
Incomprehensible sounds	(2)
None	(1)

Best motor response	
Obeys commands	(6)
Localizes pain	(5)
Flexion to pain	(4)
Abnormal (spastic) flexion*	(3)
Extension to pain	(2)
None	(1)

Adapted from *The Lancet*, Volume 304, Issue 7872, Graham Teasdale and Bryan Jennett, Assessment of coma and impaired consciousness: a practical scale, pp. 81–84, Copyright (1974), with permission from Elsevier.

Table 3.2 Cranial nerve functions and their examination

Number	Nerve	Function	Test	Palsy
I	Olfactory	Smell	Various smell bottles, e.g. coffee, lemon (test each nostril separately)	Loss of small (anosmia)
II	Optic	Vision	Visual acuity, visual fields, pupillary responses, fundoscopy, colour vision	Blind eye, visual field defect or loss of acuity
III	Oculomotor	Eye movements	Eye movement in all directions, pupillary responses	Ptosis, eye deviated down and outwards, unreactive dilated pupil
IV	Trochlear	Eye movements	Eye movement down when looking medially	Inability to look down when looking medially
V	Trigeminal	Facial sensation Muscles of mastication	Sensation in 3 trigeminal divisions, corneal reflex, jaw movement	Loss of facial sensation, loss of corneal reflex Jaw weak & deviates to side of lesion on opening, wasting of mastication muscles (chronic)
VI	Abducens	Eye movements	Eye movement laterally	Inability to look laterally
VII	Facial	Facial movements Taste to anterior tongue	Facial movements Sweet, bitter, salt taste substances	Loss of facial movement UMN: forehead spared LMN: forehead affected Loss of taste
VIII	Vestibulo-cochlear	Hearing Equilibrium	Hearing, Weber's & Rinne's tests, balance & equilibrium	Deafness Nystagmus, loss of equilibrium
IX	Glosso-pharyngeal	Pharyngeal & posterior tongue sensation & taste Motor to upper pharynx	Pharyngeal sensation, gag reflex	Loss of gag reflex & pharyngeal sensation Deviation of the uvula.
X	Vagus	Visceral parasympathetic supply (extensive) Larynx & pharynx motor function	Pharyngeal movement, gag reflex Laryngoscopy	Loss of gag reflex & pharyngeal movement Hoarse voice, vocal cord paralysis
XI	Accessory	Trapezius & sternomastoid motor function	Trapezius & sternomastoid power	Weakness of trapezius & sternomastoid
XII	Hypoglossal	Tongue movements	Tongue movements	Tongue deviates to side of lesion

Peripheral neurological examination

This should also be undertaken routinely as part of the evaluation of the central nervous system (CNS). Deficits in the limb may also occur with spinal cord and peripheral nerve injuries (see also ➜ Chapter 4).

- Limb function:
  - Appearance (deformity, wasting, abnormal movement, fasciculations)
  - Muscle tone
  - Power in each muscle group
  - Limb reflexes
  - Sensation in each dermatome (touch, pain, vibration, temperature, proprioception).
- Coordination:
  - Romberg's test for equilibrium
  - Gait
  - Finger-nose/heel shin test
  - Cerebellar signs (dysdiadochokinesia).

Higher functions

- Language ability: expressive, receptive, and nominal dysphasia
- Reading ability: dyslexia
- Writing ability: dysgraphia
- Calculation ability: dyscalculia
- Object recognition: agnosia
- Ability to perform specific tasks: dressing, geographical (follow route), and constructional (copy drawing) apraxia.
- Memory test: immediate, short-term, long-term, verbal and visual memory (cannot be tested if confused or dysphasic).
- Reasoning and problem-solving ability.
- Mental state: degree of anxiety, mood, emotional behaviour, inhibition, speed of thought and response.

External examination of the head

Be methodical. Your examination will be guided by the suspected problem (trauma, sinusitis, headache, subarachnoid haemorrhage (SAH)):

- Inspection. Standing at a distance from the patient, take a general look at the head and neck. Note any asymmetry, lumps, trauma, scars, discolouration, and obvious neurological deficit.
- Function. Check eye movements, vision, and the cranial nerves.
- Palpation of the head. Depending on the presenting complaint, a thorough palpation of any visual findings is performed:
  - Scalp
  - Forehead. Percussion over the frontal sinus may elicit tenderness if there is sinusitis
  - Supraorbital ridges
  - Nasal bridge
  - Occiput
  - Neck.

Feel for tenderness, fluctuation, steps in bony continuity, and enlarged lymph nodes or swellings in the neck. *If there is an obvious exposed skull fracture do not manipulate it. Cover with a sterile dressing*

- Auscultation. Can be considered for vascularized lumps (e.g. haemangioma, arteriovenous malformation (AVM)) or following trauma (surgical emphysema/carotid bruit). A carotid cavernous fistula can cause an orbital bruit along with proptosis, chemosis, ophthalmoplegia and loss of vision
- *Don't forget to check for papilloedema.*

Some useful signs

Facial nerve palsy
Following a head injury this can indicate a fractured base of skull. Often with associated hearing loss.

Intercanthal distance
If greater than 30–32 mm (female) or 32–34 mm (male) the patient may have detached canthi secondary to an underlying NOE fracture. Check for CSF leakage

Anosmia
Loss of smell can occur due to tearing or infiltration of the olfactory nerves (anterior cranial fossa fracture or tumour). It is common after head injury as the olfactory nerves are vulnerable to injury as they run across the skull base anteriorly.

Racoon (panda) eyes
Bilateral, well-defined 'black eyes'—fractured base of skull (anterior cranial fossa), Le Fort II/III, or NOE fracture.

Third nerve palsy
Dilated pupil, the eye looks down and out, and there is ptosis. In severe head injuries this represents third nerve compression from an expanding intracranial lesion. The patient may have a reduced GCS.

Superior orbital fissure (SOF) syndrome
Ophthalmoplegia, fixed dilated pupil and ipsilateral forehead numbness—fracture extending into the SOF, or possible carotid aneurysm. This is usually part of a significant injury.

Orbital apex syndrome
As in the SOF syndrome but here the patient also has reduced visual acuity.

Haemotympanum
Blood visualized behind the ear drum. Indicative of a fracture of the middle cranial fossa.

Battle's sign
Bruising around the mastoid region—fractured base of skull (Figure 3.1).

CSF rhinorrhoea/otorrhoea
'Tramlining'—fractured base of skull (Figures 3.2 and 3.3).

Bleeding from the ear
May indicate a fractured base of skull or mandibular condyle.

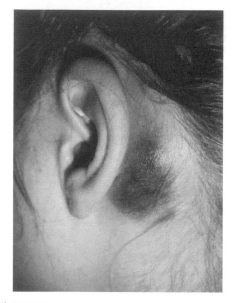

Figure 3.1 Battle's sign.

Reproduced with permission from Johnson, C., Anderson S. R., Dallimore J., et al., *Oxford Handbook of Expedition and Wilderness Medicine*, Second Edition, Plate 22, Copyright © 2015 with permission from Oxford University Press.

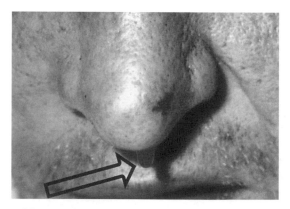

Figure 3.2 CSF rhinorrhoea.

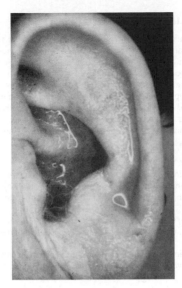

Figure 3.3 CSF otorrhoea.

Useful investigations

Laboratory tests

- A white cell count (WCC) should be taken in all suspected infections and patients presenting with severe headaches (for underlying infections).
- C-reactive protein (CRP) or erythrocyte sedimentation rate (ESR) are usually very high in temporal arteritis and should prompt administration of steroids and urgent referral.
- Lumbar puncture (LP) may be required for CSF analysis.
- Blood cultures in suspected meningitis/encephalitis.

CT/MRI scanning

These are now the investigation of choice in the assessment of most head-related problems, especially trauma and suspected space-occupying lesions. CT scanning is the mainstay of imaging in head trauma. Often the cervical spine is imaged simultaneously as there is a 5% risk of cervical spine fracture with a serious head injury.

Fresh blood can be seen on CT and therefore it is often a preliminary investigation in the assessment of suspected SAH.

CT angiography may be considered in carotid dissection or penetrating injury and CT venography for suspected cerebral venous thrombosis.

Head trauma: introduction

Head injuries are a common reason for attendance at the emergency department, particularly at night and weekends. A wide spectrum of severity is seen and it is important not to overlook the patient with a potentially serious intracranial injury. However, there are also other causes of an altered conscious level, in addition to head injuries. *Alcohol excess, drugs, hypoxia, hypotension, hypoglycaemia, and other metabolic disturbances should always be considered.* A systematic approach to trauma patients should be followed with airway, breathing, and circulation remaining the priority, even in patients with an apparently isolated head injury.

Terminology

'Primary' brain injury occurs at the time of the trauma. As clinicians there is nothing we can do about this. Prevention is the only way to reduce this. 'Secondary' brain injury occurs after the initial event and is due to complications such as hypoxia, hypercarbia, hypotension, raised ICP (haematomas or cerebral oedema), cerebral herniation, or infection. One way or another, these all result in either hypoxia or inadequate cerebral perfusion.

The aim of head injury management is to prevent secondary brain injury by regular observation and rapid correction if any deterioration occurs. This helps promote a physiological milieu that encourages natural recovery from the primary injury.

Primary brain injury

Primary brain injury can take the form of:

Cortical lacerations (burst lobe)

This also usually results in an acute subdural haematoma together with a cerebral haematoma and surrounding contusions. The affected brain usually swells markedly. A craniotomy is often necessary for evacuation of the subdural haematoma and debridement of the damaged brain. Prognosis is usually poor due to the extent of the primary brain damage.

Cerebral contusions

This is discussed under 'Intracranial haematomas' in 'Classification and common types of head (brain) injuries' topic later in this chapter, and occurs when the brain strikes the inner table of the skull.

Diffuse axonal injury

This consists of widespread disruption and shearing of axon sheaths following a high-energy impact. It is particularly associated with a rotational or deceleration element to the force. Concussion is a transient impairment of consciousness following a minor or moderate head injury is probably a mild form of diffuse axonal injury. The CT scan in diffuse axonal injuries can be normal, but more often shows a tight, swollen brain, with or without petechial haemorrhages. The degree of brain swelling usually increases over the first 48 hours post injury. The prognosis for diffuse axonal injury is poor and surgical options are limited.

Head injuries: pathophysiology

The brain is the most sensitive organ in the body to hypoxia and ischaemia. Therefore it is essential to maintain an adequate supply of well-oxygenated blood to the injured brain.

Autoregulation

This maintains a constant supply of blood to the brain between a mean arterial pressure of 50 and 160 mmHg. However, this mechanism can be impaired following head injury. The cerebral perfusion pressure (CPP) is the force driving blood through the brain and is normally over 70 mmHg. It is related to the mean arterial pressure (MAP) and intracranial pressure (ICP) by:

$$CPP = MAP - ICP$$

The effects of intracranial swelling and bleeding

Any developing intracranial mass lesion will initially be compensated for by displacement of venous blood and CSF, so the ICP will not rise. When this compensatory mechanism has been exhausted, the ICP will rise and the CPP will fall. The Cushing reflex then comes into play, increasing the systemic BP to maintain cerebral blood flow. The pulse rate falls due to a vagal reflex. When this compensatory reflex fails, progressive cerebral ischaemia will occur leading to cerebral infarction and brain death. A vicious circle becomes established with hypoxia, hypotension, and cell breakdown products, which worsen the cerebral oedema, contributing to further deterioration (Figure 3.4).

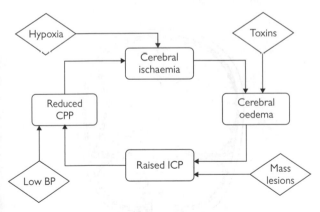

Figure 3.4 Pathophysiology of raised ICP.

Brain herniation

Three main types of herniation are commonly seen when a mass lesion develops intracranially (Figure 3.5).

Subfalcine herniation

One hemisphere is displaced beneath the falx, which is seen as midline shift on a CT scan. This can obstruct the foramen of Monro anteriorly, causing unilateral ventricular dilatation. It can also compress the posterior cerebral artery against the falx posteriorly, causing a posterior cerebral infarction.

Transtentorial herniation

The uncus of the medial temporal lobe herniates through the tentorial notch. This compresses the oculomotor nerve (dilated pupil), and the midbrain.

Tonsillar herniation

The cerebellar tonsils herniate through the foremen magnum causing brainstem compression (coning).

Criteria for admission (may vary with different units—check local policy)
- Skull fracture (proven or suspected)
- GCS score <15
- Focal neurological deficit
- Infants/elderly
- Suspected non-accidental injury
- Alcohol intoxication
- High-risk mechanism of injury
- Social (e.g. lives alone)
- Risk factors (e.g. warfarin/anticoagulants).

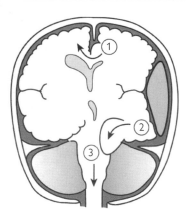

Figure 3.5 Brain herniation. (1) Subfalcine 'midline' herniation. (2) Tentorial herniation. (3) Tonsillar herniation.

Reproduced with permission from Smith J., Greaves I. and Porter K., *Oxford Desk Reference: Major Trauma*, Figure 8.11, p. 132, Copyright © 2010 with permission from Oxford University Press.

Assessment of head injuries

History
The following are important and should be determined in all cases:
- When it occurred.
- Mechanism of injury—suddenly stopping (a deceleration injury) will transfer more energy to the brain than a stationary person struck by a moving object (an acceleration injury).
- Loss of consciousness or seizure—any delayed loss of consciousness implies complications are developing. With children, was a cry heard immediately? This reduces the likelihood that there was loss of consciousness.
- Progression of symptoms since injury.
- Alcohol or drug use.
- PMH.
- Medications, especially anticoagulants.
- Preceding headache or other symptoms such as collapse leading to a fall.
- Period of retrograde or antegrade post-traumatic amnesia.
- Other injuries.

Examination
- Airway, breathing, and circulation status.
- *Always consider cervical spine injury with airway assessment.*
- Glasgow Coma Scale.
- Pupil responses: *unequal but reactive pupils occur in 20% of normal individuals.* A dilated unreactive pupil is usually on the side of a mass lesion (a true localizing sign). The usual sequence is initial pupillary constriction as CN III is irritated followed by dilatation as a palsy occurs.
- Focal neurology: cranial nerve and limbs. A hemiparesis can be caused by a mass lesion pressing on the opposite motor cortex, or a mass on the same side compressing the opposite cerebral peduncle against the edge of the tentorium (Kernohan's notch). Thus, a hemiparesis does not help in determining the side of a mass lesion and is considered a false localizing sign.
- Local signs of injury:
  - CSF rhinorrhoea or otorrhoea, bleeding from the ear: an open (compound) skull base fracture.
  - Battle's sign (bruising over the mastoid): a fractured petrous bone.
  - Panda eyes or periorbital haematoma (well-circumscribed periorbital bruising): an anterior fossa skull base fracture.
  - Scalp lacerations, abrasions, swelling.
- Examination for other injuries: this should be repeated when the patient has been stabilized (notably neck/scalp/facial/ocular).

Investigations
CT scanning is the mainstay of imaging in head trauma. Often the cervical spine is imaged simultaneously as there is a 5% risk of cervical spine fracture with a serious head injury. Today, skull X-rays have little role in current investigation of head injuries.

Classification and common types of head (brain) injuries

Head injuries are usually classified for management, epidemiological, and research purposes into minor, moderate, and severe, based upon the GCS score.

① Concussion

This is a temporary disturbance in brain function following relatively minor head injuries. Macroscopically, the brain structure remains undamaged. Typically the patient is 'knocked out' for several minutes. Prolonged episodes of unconsciousness are rare. In any event, the patient rapidly wakes up and makes a full recovery. So long as there are no other complicating medical or social factors such patients can go home providing they can be carefully observed. They should avoid a second concussion/head injury (if due to sports). Documented advice should be provided, including risks of complications and when they might need to return. 'Return to play' protocols are now widely used in contact sports.

Intracranial haematomas

The risk of harbouring an intracranial haematoma is related to the patient's level of consciousness and the presence of a skull fracture. One of several different types of haematoma might develop.

Cerebral contusions and haematomas

In cerebral contusions, blood is interspersed between the neurons and glia, whereas with cerebral haematomas, the bleeding forms a cavity within the brain. However, cerebral contusions can enlarge and result in a haematoma (Figure 3.6).

Contusions often occur at the poles of the brain due to a contrecoup injury, i.e. the contusion is in an area of the brain opposite the site of impact. These can be associated with marked oedema and a greatly raised ICP. Contusions are usually treated conservatively, but a lobectomy (or evacuation of an intracerebral haematoma) can be performed if the ICP cannot be controlled.

Extradural haematomas

Extradural haematomas are usually associated with a skull fracture or suture diastasis. The commonest site is temporal, due to a tear of the middle meningeal artery, but they can also occur in the frontal and occipital regions. They are rare in young children, as the skull fractures are not sharp enough to damage the artery, and in the elderly, as the dura is usually adherent to the skull. They classically present with delayed deterioration due to the dura being only slowly stripped from the skull. However, only a minority of patients are completely asymptomatic during this 'lucid interval'.

Extradural haematomas are biconvex (lens) shaped on CT scans and are mostly high density (Figure 3.7). Low-density areas within them are due to active bleeding.

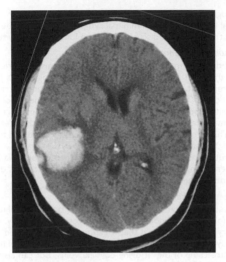

Figure 3.6 Intracerebral haematoma.

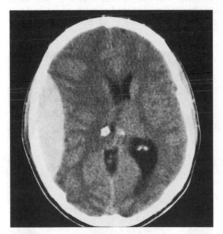

Figure 3.7 Extradural haematoma.

The prognosis is very good if they are treated early enough. Very small extradural haematomas with minimal symptoms can often be left alone (although they should be discussed with the local neurosurgical unit).

☺ Acute subdural haematomas

Acute subdural haematomas may occur due to tearing of bridging veins between the brain and skull. In such cases the prognosis is good with prompt treatment. Alternatively a laceration of the brain surface (burst lobe) may occur. This has a worse prognosis. There need not be a skull fracture with subdural haematomas. They are more common than extradural haematomas and can extend over a wide area of the lateral cortical surface. They are crescent shaped on CT scans as the blood follows the surface of the brain (Figure 3.8).

Thin acute subdural haematomas can be treated conservatively with close observation, but significant ones need a craniotomy as the clotted blood is too viscous to drain via burr holes.

① Chronic subdural haematomas

Chronic subdural haematomas are thought to be due to minor venous bleeding following a minor head injury several weeks previously. The head injury is often so trivial that it cannot be remembered in 50% of cases. They usually occur in the elderly who have a degree of brain atrophy and stretching of the bridging cortical veins, but can also occur in babies due to non-accidental injuries. They are often associated with coagulopathies and alcohol excess.

Chronic subdural haematomas can cause a wide variety of symptoms, including headaches, reduced consciousness, and focal neurology. *Therefore, consider this diagnosis in all elderly patients with intermittent*

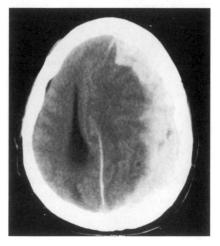

Figure 3.8 Acute subdural haematoma.

confusion or transient ischaemic attack (TIA)-like symptoms after trauma. Chronic subdural haematomas can be treated by burr hole drainage as the blood is liquid. They have a good prognosis but might recur, especially with a persistent coagulopathy.

☺ Penetrating head injury

A penetrating head injury is an open injury in which the dura mater has been breached. These are often caused by high-velocity projectiles but can also occur from objects such as knives, or bone fragments from an overlying skull fracture. Penetrating injuries are similar to closed head injuries (such as contusion or ICH) but have an increased incidence of infection. Haemorrhage may be harder to control. Initial management is the same as closed injuries although antibiotics should also be given.

Take care if exploring penetrating or open head wounds overlying a skull fracture, especially those in the midline. This can result in massive blood loss if a venous sinus has been torn.

Head injuries: initial management

① Scalp lacerations

Scalp lacerations should be thoroughly cleansed and closed urgently, in two layers if possible. The use of tissue glue may be acceptable for small lacerations. The possibility of foreign bodies or an underlying fracture should be considered and imaging may be necessary to confirm this. Also remember anti-tetanus prophylaxis. Scalp sutures can usually be removed after 7 days. Haemorrhage can be significant from these and can result in haemodynamic instability if neglected.

Potentially significant head injuries

Observations should be performed hourly initially, and half-hourly in higher-risk patients. Make sure the nursing staff know when to call for a medical review. Most patients can be discharged the following day if asymptomatic. Stable patients who need longer admission can have their observation frequency reduced to 2-hourly. Patients not admitted should receive written guidelines of when to return to hospital and should only be discharged with a responsible adult who can call for assistance if required.

Transferring patients

- Fully resuscitate in all patients before transfer—this may include a laparotomy/pelvic fixation etc. to stop bleeding as per ATLS® protocol.
- Intubate and ventilate comatose patients.
- If patients are being transferred for observation only, avoid intubation and sedation if safe to do so (discuss with neurosurgeons). This allows their conscious level to be assessed.
- Rapidly reverse anticoagulant medication to prevent further bleeding.
- IV mannitol can be given to buy time by reducing ICP. Maximum dose is 1 g/kg—in a 70 kg adult, this is 350 mL of 20% mannitol.
- Hypertonic saline is also increasingly used to reduce ICP, but always seek advice from ICU/neurosurgery before prescribing.
- Transfer promptly with an experienced anaesthetist.

☼ Head injuries in children

These can be difficult to assess. Many of the clinical features which would lead to concern in adults are often present, even following minor injuries (vomiting, drowsy, headaches, etc.). An infant can become haemo-dynamically unstable due to bleeding into a scalp haematoma. Consider the mechanism of injury, other injuries present, and whether the parents are capable of taking the child home for close observations. Interpretation of skull X-rays can be difficult as large fractures may be confused with wide sutures or vascular markings. If in doubt, refer or admit. *Non-accidental injury is the second most common cause of ICH in a child.* This should be considered if the history is inconsistent with the mechanism of injury, or if the child has had multiple attendances with injuries at different hospitals. Retinal haemorrhages, multiple old fractures, and cigarette burns are other signs.

Other issues

Post-concussion headache

This may have features of a tension-type headache but is often associated with dizziness and loss of concentration.

Driving

A significant head injury will often result in a restriction from driving for at least 6 months.

CSF leaks

CSF can leak from the nose (rhinorrhoea) or from the ear (otorrhoea). Clear CSF tends to mix with blood and presents as a heavily blood-stained, watery discharge. This trickles down the side of the face, where peripherally the blood tends to clot while the non-clotted blood in the centre is washed away by CSF. This creates two parallel lines referred to as 'tramlining'. One bedside test for CSF is the 'ring test' (allow drops to fall on blotting paper: blood clots centrally, and the CSF diffuses outwards to form a target sign). *Tell the patient not to blow their nose for 3 weeks.* If they do, the increased pressure can force air intracranially through the tear, which then cannot escape. This is the neurosurgical equivalent of a tension pneumothorax and results in tension pneumo-cephalus. CSF should test positive for glucose. Beta-2 transferrin is a more specific test for CSF.

Post-traumatic seizures

Risk factors include intracerebral haematoma, open depressed fractures with dural laceration, and focal neurological signs.

① Headache

Headache is a symptom, not a diagnosis. It can arise from a number of different conditions involving the head, neck, and beyond. These include the periosteum of the skull, muscles, nerves, arteries and veins, subcu-taneous tissues, eyes, ears, sinuses, and mucous membranes. There are a number of different classification systems for headaches. A useful one is from the International Headache Society. Treatment of a headache depends on the underlying cause. *Take headaches seriously.* Although most cases are benign and self-limiting, a few are due to serious pathology. The key is awareness of important causes and eliminating them from the differential diagnosis clinically and by investigation.

Some useful facts in diagnosing headaches

- Headache may not necessarily be a symptom of head pathology. Consider also the eyes (glaucoma), TMJs (TMJ dysfunction syndrome), sinuses (infection/tumours), neck (degenerative conditions), and systemic conditions such as hypertension and giant cell arteritis.
- Pain in the cheek, orbit, or forehead can occur with migraine.
- Unilateral headache is characteristic of classic migraine or cluster headache. The latter is usually frontotemporal, around the eye, or cheek.
- Bilateral pain over the forehead or temples which can affect the vertex, occiput, or eyes would be seen in tension headache.

Worrying features with a headache

- Associated fever
- Sudden onset
- Late onset (new headache in over 50s)
- Nausea or vomiting
- Stiff neck/photophobia
- Changes in personality or mental function/neurological deficit
- Change in usual pattern of headache/present on waking
- Pain that increases with coughing or movement
- Headaches becoming steadily worse
- Associated painful red eye/pain and tenderness near the temples
- Headaches in patients with cancer or impaired immune systems.

Headaches persisting for longer than 6 weeks with abnormal physical signs should be thoroughly investigated, including:
- FBC with ESR (to exclude temporal arteritis).
- CXR for bronchial carcinoma.
- CT or MRI brain to exclude space-occupying lesion.

Classification of headaches

The International Classification of Headache Disorders (ICHD) is a useful guide to the causes of headache and is accepted by the World Health Organization. It contains diagnostic criteria. Several groups are listed.

Primary headaches

These are the most common types and include tension-type headache and migraine. They have typical features. Rarer types include cluster headache (severe pains that occur in bouts), and hemicrania continua (a continuous headache on one side of the head).

Secondary headaches

These are classified based on their aetiology and not symptoms. There are more than 200 types. Causes include:

- Head or neck trauma
- ICH:
  - SAH
- Post craniotomy
- Ischaemic stroke or TIA
- Vascular malformations
- Arteritis:
  - Temporal arteritis
- Cerebral venous thrombosis:
  - Cavernous sinus or sagittal sinus thrombosis
- Low or high pressures of the CSF pressure:
  - Hydrocephalus
  - Benign/idiopathic intracranial hypertension
  - Post-LP headache
- Non-infectious inflammatory disease
- Intracranial neoplasm
- Substance ingestion or its withdrawal
- Intracranial infections: meningitis, brain abscess, subdural empyema
- Systemic infections
- Dialysis
- High BP
- Fasting
- Injury to facial structures including teeth, jaws, or TMJ.

This list is not complete but illustrates the diverse nature and potential seriousness of any patient you may encounter who has a headache. In the absence of identifiable pathology, management of headache is the treatment of its symptoms. Analgesia is often the initial treatment.

Assessing a patient with a headache

Ask about the following:

Character

- Severe, pulsatile headache is typical of common migraine.
- Throbbing, sharp, headache is described in classic migraine.
- Stabbing or burning pain is described in cluster headache.
- Pressure, or a 'band-like' tightness that varies in intensity, frequency, and duration is consistent with tension headache.

Timing

Headaches that are worst on wakening are typical of raised ICP. It can also occur with caffeine withdrawal.

Duration

Headaches at night for 1–3 weeks are features of cluster headaches.

Exacerbating or precipitating factors

- Straining, coughing, or sneezing can worsen headaches associated with raised ICP. Cough impulse headache is common in Chiari malformation.
- Stress, diet (chocolate, cheese, red wine), hormonal state (pre-menstrual, oral contraceptive pill), emotions, and barometric changes are associated with migraine. Caffeine withdrawal can cause severe symptoms, which are quickly relieved by ingestion of caffeine.

Onset

Sudden-onset headache is often termed thunderclap headache. The most concerning cause of this is a SAH.

Preceding symptoms

- Flu-like illness can precede temporal arteritis.
- Impending sense of ill health is a feature of classic migraine.
- Visual aura can precede migraine.

Other associated factors

Family history

Often seen in migraine.

Age

Temporal arteritis is seen in patients over 60. Migraine is more often seen in puberty.

Gender

Females are more likely to have SAH, migraine, venous sinus thrombosis, and tension headache; men tend to get cluster headaches.

Associated medical problems

Depression and anxiety often relate to tension headache; smoking and hypertension are risk factors for SAH and stroke. Pregnancy predisposes to thrombosis or pre-eclampsia.

Headaches: associated symptoms

Reduced level of consciousness

This is concerning when it is associated with a headache. It may reflect raised ICP. Urgent investigation and treatment are required. SAH, ICH, tumour, or intracranial infection are all possible diagnoses.

Visual disturbance

- Sudden irreversible loss of sight may occur within weeks of the onset of temporal arteritis. Often the presenting feature is of a visual field disturbance, which becomes progressively worse. Blindness is thought to occur as a result of ischaemic optic neuritis caused by arteritis of the ophthalmic arteries. Cavernous sinus thrombosis can also cause loss of vision as can pituitary apoplexy.
- Visual aura, such as flashing lights, are a feature of classic migraine.
- Loss of visual acuity or field constriction can be a feature of raised ICP and benign/idiopathic intracranial hypertension.
- Ophthalmoplegia can occur in pituitary apoplexy, cavernous sinus thrombosis, or in a cavernous carotid fistula.

Nausea and vomiting
These are often present in migraine but are seen with raised ICP.

Autonomic symptoms
Such as rhinorrhoea, unilateral nasal obstruction, a red eye (conjunctival injection), and lacrimation. These are often seen in trigeminal autonomic cephalalgias.

Photophobia
This is often seen in classic migraine but if seen with thunderclap headache, SAH must be considered. It also occurs in meningitis.

Neck stiffness
This can be due to meningism in meningitis and SAH.

Focal neurological deficit
Such as dysphasia, hemiparesis, or sensory disturbance, in association with a headache is a concerning finding. A brain tumour, SAH, or a stroke could be the cause. However, some migraines can cause temporary hemiparesis or hemisensory loss.

Jaw claudication
Pain on chewing due to temporal arteritis of the facial artery (rare).

Seizures
May be seen in brain tumours, SAH, or intracranial infection.

Systemic symptoms
Weight loss, arthralgia, and fever can occur in temporal arteritis.

Intracranial infections

Meningitis
Patients with meningitis can deteriorate extremely rapidly, so immediate attention is necessary. *Consider this in any irritable child with a non-blanching petechial rash.* Meningitis is inflammation of the linings of the brain and spinal cord (the meninges) with infection of the CSF. Most frequently, the pathogen is viral and may vary with age and social environment. Bacterial pathogens need urgent treatment.

Bacterial pathogens in meningitis
Neonatal
- *Streptococcus* (group B)
- *Escherichia coli*
- *Listeria monocytogenes*.

Children (<14 years of age)
- *Neisseria meningitidis*
- *Streptococcus pneumoniae*
- *Haemophilus influenzae*.

Adults
- *Neisseria meningitidis*
- *Streptococcus pneumoniae.*

Clinical features
- Pyrexia
- Tachycardia/tachypnoea/shock
- Headache
- Photophobia
- Irritability
- Seizures
- Vomiting
- Neck stiffness
- Positive Kernig's sign (a strong sign of meningeal irritation)—pain occurs with attempts at passive knee extension with the hips fully flexed
- Maculopapular rash (meningococcal meningitis)
- Deteriorating conscious level in late cases.

Management
- Resuscitation, IV fluids.
- Antibiotics should be given as soon as the diagnosis is suspected and continued until the CSF WCC is normal. Discuss choice with microbiologist/neurologist.
- Take throat swabs and blood for polymerase chain reaction (PCR).
- Blood cultures.
- CT scan to determine safety of LP and rule out other pathology.
- LP for CSF analysis.
- Contact tracing (local public health department)—for single cases treat close contacts only ('kissing contacts'). Usual regimens: rifampicin 600 mg twice daily for 2 days, ciprofloxacin 500 mg single dose.

☼ Subdural empyema

Most cases of subdural empyema are secondary to sinusitis or middle ear infection. Patients initially present with an illness similar to meningitis, but can develop a hemiparesis due to cortical venous thrombosis. Seizures are common.

Investigations and management
This should follow the same pathway as for meningitis, but a *LP should be avoided due to the risk of coning.* A CT scan will usually show a thin subdural collection, and pus can accumulate along the falx. The size of the collections is much less than with symptomatic chronic subdural haematomas.

Patients should be resuscitated and referred for prompt neurosurgical drainage of the pus, usually via a craniotomy. Efforts should be made to look for a source of infection and to treat it accordingly. Investigations such as an echocardiogram may be required.

⚙ Brain abscess

Sinusitis and middle ear infections are common causes of brain abscesses, following direct spread intracranially. Haematogenous spread of infection can also occur. Well-recognized causes include infective endocarditis and dental caries. However, in some cases the cause is never determined.

Clinical features
- Headache
- Vomiting
- Focal neurology
- Epileptic fits
- Deteriorating conscious level in late cases
- Pyrexia is often absent.

Investigations
- The WCC and CRP are often normal.
- CT scans show a ring-enhancing lesion with surrounding oedema. In contrast to gliomas, abscesses are usually perfectly circular with a wall of uniform thickness. Abscesses may be multiple.
- MRI—diffusion-weighted sequence can help differentiate from other pathology, such as tumour.
- *LP should not be performed due to the risk of coning.*

The diagnosis is usually suspected on the basis of an enhancing circular lesion on a CT scan of a patient with an infection elsewhere.

Management
Patients should be referred for prompt neurosurgical drainage. If their consciousness is deteriorating, patients should be fully resuscitated and consider administering steroids and mannitol prior to transfer.

⚙ Encephalitis

This is an acute inflammation of the brain and has both infective and non-infective causes. Encephalitis which is associated with meningitis is referred to as meningoencephalitis. Herpes simplex virus, poliovirus, and measles virus are common pathogens. Others rare types of encephalitis include Japanese encephalitis and equine encephalitis. Bacterial encephalitis may occur following spread of meningitis. Parasitic or protozoal infestations, such as toxoplasmosis, malaria, or amoebic infection, can also cause encephalitis. *Cryptococcus neoformans* causes fungal encephalitis in immunocompromised patients.

Clinical features
Whatever the cause, common symptoms include:
- Headache
- Fever
- Confusion
- Drowsiness, and fatigue
- Seizures, tremors, hallucinations, and memory problems may indicate advanced disease.

Children or infants may present with non-specific symptoms such as irritability, drowsiness, and fever.

Always check for a stiff neck—this indicates meningitis or meningoencephalitis.

Investigations
- CT scan is initially undertaken to exclude brain swelling. If there is no swelling a LP can be undertaken.
- CSF analysis usually shows increased amounts of protein and white blood cells with normal glucose. Specific diagnosis is made with detection of antibodies on PCR.
- Serological tests may show high antibody titres.

Management
- Patients should be resuscitated and referred urgently. Supportive treatment (IV fluids/sedation/mechanical ventilation) may be required.
- Antiviral agents (e.g. aciclovir for herpes simplex virus).
- Corticosteroids may be used to reduce brain swelling but this is controversial in the presence of infection.

:✪: Intracranial bleeding (non-traumatic)

:✪: Subarachnoid haemorrhage

Aetiology of spontaneous SAH
- 80% are from intracranial saccular (Berry) aneurysm. These often remain asymptomatic and are found in 2–3% of routine post-mortems.
- 15% have no identifiable cause
- 5% from other causes (e.g. AVM).

Up to 50% of aneurysmal SAH patients die within a month of the initial bleed. Untreated, the re-bleed rate over the first month approaches 50% and 80% of these patients die or become dependent. It is therefore vital not to delay the diagnosis, as patients are at risk of re-bleeding and death.

The risk of re-bleeding in AVMs is much less at around 6% in the first year and 3% for each subsequent year, so treatment can often be delayed.

Clinical features
- 'Thunderclap' headache—a sudden, severe occipital headache radiating over the head and down the neck
- Impaired conscious level
- Neck stiffness
- Photophobia
- Nausea or vomiting
- Seizure.

Unfortunately 'thunderclap' is a non-specific symptom and less than 25% of patients presenting with this symptom will actually have a SAH. The differential diagnosis is wide. *All patients with a sudden-onset headache should therefore be investigated for SAH, even if the headache has eased within a few hours.*

Investigation

A CT scan should be performed as soon as possible after the bleed. Delay in performing the scan reduces its diagnostic rate as the blood lyses. A normal CT scan does not rule out a SAH. LP and CSF spectrophotometry for bilirubin is required in all suspected cases if the CT scan is normal, but if performed too soon, the CSF can be normal, as bilirubin has not yet been produced from the blood breakdown products. The LP should not therefore be performed within 12 hours from the onset of headache.

Once SAH has been diagnosed, CT angiography or cerebral catheter angiography is performed to determine the cause (Figure 3.9).

Often CT angiography is performed as the first-line test.

Management

- Resuscitation, IV fluids, routine bloods including clotting studies.
- Analgesics, antiemetics.
- Oral nimodipine. This improves outcome by reducing the risk of ischaemic complications. It limits the normal surrounding vasoconstrictor response that occurs following a bleed.
- Aneurysms are secured by either surgical clipping or endovascular embolization. In many centres, practice has moved towards endovascular coiling as the mainstay of aneurysm treatment.
- AVMs can be excised, embolized, or treated with extremely high-dose, finely localized radiation (stereotactic radiosurgery), which leads to gradual obliteration over a 2-year period.
- If no structural cause is found on detailed angiography, the patient can be reassured that they are not at increased risk of further bleeds.

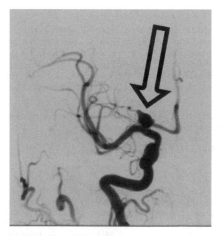

Figure 3.9 Angiogram showing berry aneurysm.

The prognosis for recovery from a SAH is closely associated with the GCS. A lower GCS will likely result in a worse outcome.

Complications of SAH

- Vasospasm—this results in stroke/death in 15% of patients with SAH. At day 7, up to 70% will have angiographic vasospasm, although this is only clinically manifest in 20–30%. The pathophysiology is poorly understood but the risk is increased with a heavy blood load. In patients who develop vasospasm, hypertensive therapy is often instituted when the aneurysm is secured. This involves transfer to level 3 care and an inotrope infusion. Direct angioplasty by intra-arterial nimodipine can also be tried.
- Hydrocephalus occurs in 25% of patients. This is often communicating and can usually be managed with LPs or an external ventricular drain. A shunt may be required.
- Seizures have been reported in 5–10% of SAH patients.
- Electrolyte problems—this is usually low sodium and often due to 'cerebral salt wasting'. It is treated with adding sodium orally or intravenously using 1.8% saline. Fluid restriction is dangerous as it may precipitate vasospasm.
- ECG/cardiac rhythm changes occur in >50% of SAH patients.
- Pulmonary oedema and pneumonia are common.

Spontaneous intracerebral haemorrhage

ICH, a form of stroke, is most commonly due to hypertension. Bleeding disorders, AVMs, aneurysms, tumours, and venous hypertension secondary to central venous thrombosis can also be responsible.

Clinical features

These include the following, but not all need to be present:

- Headache
- Loss of consciousness
- Focal neurological deficit.

Investigation/management

- Resuscitation, IV fluids, clotting studies.
- CT scan. This should be performed as soon as possible after the onset of symptoms, especially if the patient is unconscious or an aneurysmal SAH is a possibility.
- An LP is unnecessary and potentially dangerous.
- An angiogram should be considered, especially if the clot is close to the circle of Willis or Sylvian fissure (possible aneurysmal cause) in younger non-hypertensive patients (possible AVM), or if surgical evacuation is being considered.
- Neurosurgeons may consider ICH evacuation if the patient is deteriorating due to raised ICP and the clot is superficial.
- Stroke rehabilitation. This will be necessary in the majority of patients.

⊕ Hydrocephalus and raised intracranial pressure

⊕ Hydrocephalus

- Communicating: there is free flow of CSF from the ventricular system to the subarachnoid space.
- Non-communicating (or obstructive): there is an obstruction within the ventricular system so that the CSF cannot reach the subarachnoid space. *It is not safe to perform a LP in this group.*

Clinical features
- Headache
- Vomiting
- Visual disturbance/loss of upgaze
- Deterioration in consciousness.

Investigations

A CT scan will typically show ventricular dilatation. The fourth ventricle is usually dilated in communicating hydrocephalus, but may be small in non-communicating hydrocephalus. A MRI scan might be necessary, particularly if a third ventriculostomy is being considered, to visualize the basal cisterns.

Management
- Shunts: divert CSF into the peritoneum, or less commonly the right atrium or pleura.
- Third ventriculostomy: creates an internal bypass by forming a stoma between the floor of the third ventricle and the basal cisterns.
- External ventricular drainage: the CSF drains via a manometer to an external collecting system. This is usually performed if there is infection or bloodstained CSF preventing shunt insertion, or in an emergency when there is insufficient time to insert a shunt.

⊕ Raised intracranial pressure (intracranial hypertension)

Causes include:
- Masses (tumour, infarction with oedema, contusions, haematoma, or abscesses)
- Generalized swelling (ischaemia, acute liver failure, hypertensive encephalopathy, hypercarbia, and Reye's syndrome)
- Increase in venous pressure (venous sinus thrombosis, heart failure, or mediastinal obstruction)
- Obstructed CSF (aqueduct stenosis, Chiari malformation, meningeal disease)
- Increased CSF production (choroid plexus tumour)
- Craniosynostosis
- Idiopathic
- Management is directed at the cause. CSF diversion may be required.

Shunts and shunt complications

These are devices used in the management of hydrocephalus. They divert CSF into the peritoneum (or less commonly the right atrium or pleura) and maintain the ICP at the correct level. If a shunt fails to function correctly the ICP is affected. Total obstruction can result in rapid onset of symptoms and deterioration in consciousness. Shunts consist of:

- A ventricular catheter.
- A subcutaneous reservoir—for sampling CSF.
- A valve—this may have an incorporated reservoir, depending upon the type.
- A distal catheter—most commonly to the peritoneum (ventriculoperitoneal (VP) shunt), but occasionally to the right atrium via the internal jugular vein (ventriculoatrial (VA) shunt) or pleura.

Shunt assessment

- CT scan: to look at the ventricular size. It is most useful to compare the scan with a previous scan taken when the shunt was known to be functioning.
- However, in patients who have had multiple-shunt revisions, the ventricular wall can become stiff and the ventricles may not dilate.
- Shunt series: plain X-rays of the whole of the shunt to look for breakages, disconnections, or migration of the shunt from its usual location.
- Shunt tap: a needle is inserted into the subcutaneous reservoir under aseptic technique. This can exclude infection, reduce ICP by removing CSF, and also assess ventricular catheter patency.

Shunt obstruction

The commonest site of a blocked shunt is the ventricular catheter (due to choroid plexus), followed by the valve (due to CSF debris) and the distal catheter (due to omentum in VP shunts and clot in VA shunts). A blocked shunt usually presents with similar symptoms to the patient's initial presentation, but the symptoms often progress more rapidly.

CT scan usually confirms the diagnosis but if there is doubt, symptomatic patients should be admitted for observation until their symptoms have settled. If symptoms persist, the obstructed component, or the whole shunt, will need to be replaced. Attempts to clear the obstruction usually fail.

Shunt infection

Shunt infections usually develop within a few weeks of the last shunt operation and are due to contamination from skin bacteria. Patients can present with symptoms of a blocked shunt accompanied by a fever. They usually do not have meningism. An infected VA shunt will usually not block and so the infection may continue undetected for a long period.

The symptoms of an infected VA shunt usually consist of vague ill health and a low-grade temperature. Diagnosis is by a shunt tap, with CSF microscopy and culture. The CSF WCC might be normal, as CSF flow flushes the bacteria away from the ventricles. Antibiotics alone are usually insufficient to clear a shunt infection. Removal of the shunt and external ventricular drainage are often necessary, with a new shunt being inserted when the CSF is sterile.

Prophylactic antibiotics have not been shown to prevent shunt infections. New antibiotic impregnated or silver-lined shunt catheters are available.

☼ Shunt overdrainage

Occasionally a shunt will drain excessive CSF, so that the patient develops low-pressure headaches, which are worse when upright and are eased by lying down. If the ventricles are very large, the low pressure can cause them to collapse, tearing cortical bridging veins and causing subdural haematomas. These patients can have symptoms of raised ICP with a hemiparesis.

Low-pressure headaches are treated with reassurance and advising a high fluid intake. Caffeine can also be helpful. The shunt can be revised if the symptoms persist.

☼ Intracranial thrombosis

☼ Venous sinus thrombosis

Venous sinus thrombosis can affect any age and either sex, but most commonly affects young and middle-aged females. It can be caused by trauma with depressed fractures overlying the sinus, tumours invading the sinus, and post neurosurgery.

Clinical features
- Headaches, especially in the morning
- Visual disturbance
- Papilloedema.

Investigations
CT or MRI scans might show brain swelling. The 'delta' sign is a triangular filling defect in the sinus on a contrast CT scan. An occluded sinus is usually visible on MRI scans. Infarction or haemorrhage due to venous hypertension might also be visible.

Management
- Anticoagulation.
- Thrombolytic therapy may be given if the patient is deteriorating.
- CSF diversion: may be necessary later if intracranial hypertension results.

☼ Cavernous sinus thrombosis

Often fatal in the pre-antibiotic era, cavernous sinus thrombosis is essentially a septic thrombosis within the cavernous sinus. *It usually arises from an infection in the face (hence the advice not to squeeze spots!)*, most commonly the periorbital region, but it can also arise from paranasal sinus infection.

Propagation of an infected thrombus to the cavernous sinus occurs against venous flow, because of the absence of valves in the facial, angular, ophthalmic, and pterygoid plexus of veins. Thrombosis might spread to other venous sinuses and the infection may spread to cause subdural empyema or meningitis. Infective endocarditis and thrombosis of the internal carotid artery can also occur.

Clinical features
- Systemic upset: swinging pyrexia/tachycardia/rigors/sweats.
- Facial or periorbital pain.
- Venous obstruction: eyelid oedema/dilated facial veins.
- 'Pulsating exophthalmos': a transmitted carotid pulse with periorbital oedema.
- Blindness with papilloedema and retinal haemorrhages.
- Ophthalmoplegia: classically CN VI first followed by CNs III and IV.
- Obvious site of infection: usually unilateral initially; most commonly a periorbital cellulitis.
- Central signs: developing evidence of meningeal irritation.
- Bilateral signs develop with contralateral extension of thrombus.

Investigations
- CT or MRI scans: usually show brain swelling and possible local infection. An occluded sinus might be visible on MRI scans.
- Bloods including inflammatory markers and coagulation studies.
- Cerebral angiogram, with venous phase (if diagnosis uncertain).
- Investigations into the cause of the infection.

Management
- Antibiotics and drainage of any collection of pus.
- Anticoagulation.
- Thrombolytic therapy might be considered if the patient is deteriorating.

⊙ Cerebral tumours

There are a large number of different brain tumours and cysts, both benign and malignant. Commonly they present with one of three syndromes (or a combination of them):
- Raised ICP
- Progressive neurological deficit
- Epileptic fits.

Investigations

MRI scan is now the investigation of choice and will invariably be required before surgery, but a CT scan, without and with contrast, is usually the first-line investigation. Malignant tumours are seen as irregular enhancing lesions that might be cystic or solid, with mass effect and surrounding oedema. The three commonest tumours are:
- Metastases, which can be small, round 'cannon ball' lesions, usually multiple, at the grey–white mater junction and most commonly in the middle cerebral artery territory; if suspicious, a CT chest/abdomen/pelvis can be performed to search for a primary source.

- Gliomas, which are usually large irregular lesions with indistinct margins.
- Meningiomas, which have a dural attachment and homogeneous contrast enhancement.

Management
- Steroids to reduce vasogenic oedema—typically dexamethasone 4 mg four times daily. This is usually given with a proton pump inhibitor for gastric protection.
- Anticonvulsants should be given if the patient has had fits. Some neurosurgeons use prophylactic anticonvulsants.
- Neurosurgical referral. Excision of the tumour is the preferred treatment, but might not be possible due to the site of the tumour, the extent or nature of the lesion, or the frailty of the patient, in which case a biopsy or debulking may be performed or a palliative course of management without surgery.

In high-grade malignant tumours, patients will proceed to adjuvant therapy with radiotherapy with or without chemotherapy. There are advances in this field based on molecular profiling of tumours.

Emergency treatment
Rarely, if the patient is deteriorating rapidly, IV mannitol and a massive dose of dexamethasone should be given pending neurosurgical transfer and emergency surgery.

⊕ Extracranial causes of headache

⊕ Temporal arteritis
Temporal arteritis (giant cell arteritis) is a vasculitic disease predominantly affecting patients over 60 years of age. It is an important diagnosis in the elderly patient who presents with severe headache because of the potential for blindness if left untreated.

Clinical features
Patients present with a headache that is either a generalized 'tension' type or severe and well localized over the temporal arteries, often with burning or tenderness of the scalp. Jaw claudication on chewing can be another feature, thought to be due to involvement of the facial artery. There may also be weight loss, arthralgia, and fever.

Of great importance is the risk of sudden irreversible loss of sight which may occur within weeks of the onset of symptoms. Often the presenting feature is of a visual field disturbance, which becomes progressively worse. Blindness is thought to occur as a result of ischaemic optic neuritis caused by arteritis of the ophthalmic arteries.

Temporal arteritis generally affects medium and large sized arteries. Branches of the carotid arteries are the commonest sites of involvement, but the vertebral, meningeal, and intracerebral vessels can be involved leading to hemiplegia or epilepsy.

Investigations
- ESR is usually markedly raised in excess of 90 mm/hour in these patients.
- Temporal artery biopsy will help to confirm the diagnosis. However, the disease generally shows 'skip lesions' and therefore a negative biopsy does not exclude a diagnosis.

Management
The aims of management are to reduce the pain and prevent complications, particularly blindness. High-dose steroids are given urgently. Dosage can be titrated against the ESR, and clinical response, but it may be necessary to continue treatment for 2–3 years with a gradually reducing dose.

ⓘ Polymyalgia rheumatica

Polymyalgia rheumatica (PMR) is a condition of middle-aged/elderly patients which is associated with temporal/giant cell arteritis. It is characterized by
- Systemic upset—weight loss, fever, fatigue.
- Severe arthralgia with stiffness—usually bilateral and symmetrical.
- Elevated ESR.
- A rapid response to small doses of corticosteroids.

Around 50% of patients with temporal arteritis have symptoms of PMR, whereas 15–50% of patients with PMR have giant cell arteritis.

Glaucoma

(See ➲ Chapter 10, pp. 303–5.) Patients may complain of pain in and around the eyes. It is important to consider ophthalmic conditions, especially glaucoma.

ⓘ Frontal sinusitis

This is potentially serious due to the risk of intracranial infection. The frontal sinuses make up one of the four paranasal sinuses. They are formed by extension of the ethmoidal air cells, into which they drain. These sinuses are absent at birth, but become reasonably well developed by the age of 7, reaching their full size after puberty. In up to 4% of the population they can be absent. The right and left sinuses form a cavity within the frontal bone, which is highly variable in size and shape and rarely symmetrical. A midline septum separates the two. The average sinus volume is approximately 6–8 mL.

Each sinus is lined with ciliated mucus-secreting epithelium. Mucus drains into the middle meatus of the nose via the frontonasal ducts (or frontal sinus drainage pathways (FSDP)). The ducts pass through the ethmoid sinuses taking a variable pathway. (This is an important point to remember when managing apparently isolated NOE fractures. It is around the drainage of the frontal sinus that classification, management, and complications of these injuries are based.)

If free drainage of mucus from the frontal sinus is impaired, infection can occur, resulting in frontal sinusitis. Patients complain of frontal headache, which is tender to percussion. Untreated, the infection can spread intracranially or spread into the orbit (orbital cellulitis).

ⓘ Ethmoid sinusitis

This usually occurs with other sinus infections. Patients complain of deep-seated throbbing pain, deep to the bridge of the nose. The medial orbital walls are paper thin, so orbital cellulitis can rapidly develop.

Clinical presentation of frontal/ethmoid sinusitis
- Headache/facial pain.
- Sensation of dull, constant pressure over the affected sinus.
- Symptoms are usually localized over the involved sinus and are often made worse on bending, straining, or lying down.
- Nasal discharge.
- Halitosis.
- Post-nasal drip.
- Pott's puffy tumour is a rare clinical entity characterized by subperiosteal abscess associated with osteomyelitis. It is usually seen as a complication of frontal sinusitis or trauma predominantly in the adolescent age group.

Management of sinusitis
Antibiotics and in some cases, sinus washout with opening of the middle meatus, using functional endoscopic sinus surgery. Ephedrine nasal drops and menthol inhalations may help reduce congestion and improve sinus drainage.

ⓘ Drug/medication-induced headache

Many drugs can cause headaches among their side effects. Caffeine can result in severe pain sometimes on waking. Migraine sufferers are particularly vulnerable to a vicious cycle of pain requiring increasing medication, which then triggers more pain. Medication should be slowly withdrawn. In some cases prednisone may help control pain during this period.

ⓘ Ice-cream headache

Some patients are prone to develop sudden, sharp head pain within a few seconds of eating or drinking anything cold, which stimulates the palate. The pain usually lasts less than a minute and resolves completely. It is believed to result from either rapid constriction and swelling of the anterior cerebral arteries, or as a result of referred pain from the roof of the mouth to the head. Treatment is preventative measures (eat slowly).

ⓘ Primary sexual headache (coital cephalalgia)

In this condition, the pattern of headaches can be variable. Some appear suddenly and stop abruptly; others occur on a regular basis for a long period of time. Attacks may be mild or severe. The differential diagnosis is SAH as this has been precipitated by coitus in patients. Management includes avoiding/reducing activities which precipitate symptoms. Propranolol, indometacin, and calcium-channel blockers (e.g. diltiazem) may help.

Remember that carbon monoxide poisoning can also present with a headache.

⑦ Primary headaches

These are not emergency conditions but are included as they are within the differential diagnosis of headache.

⑦ Migraine

Migraine is a severe headache that may present as a facial pain affecting the cheek, orbit, or forehead. However, classical migraine with preceding visual disturbances and an aura rarely affects the face.

- 'Common' migraine is ten times more frequent and is described as a severe pulsatile headache invariably associated with nausea. Migraine is episodic in nature and is thought to affect approximately 10% of the population. It is more common in females (3:1), usually begins around puberty and continues into middle age, and there may also be a family history.
- Classic migraine is described as starting with an impending sense of ill health and a visual aura (e.g. flashing lights). The throbbing, severe, sharp unilateral headache is associated with anorexia, nausea and vomiting, photophobia. and withdrawal—the patient often wants to just go into a darkened room and sleep.

Associations have been made with such trigger factors as stress, diet (chocolate, cheese, red wine), hormonal state (pre-menstrual, oral contraceptive pill), emotions (anger, excitement), and barometric changes.

Some migraines can cause temporary hemiparesis (hemiplegic migraine) or hemisensory loss. This can result in diagnostic confusion.

Management

Recognizing and removing precipitating causes, and simple analgesics in the first instance. Antiemetics may also be used to reduce nausea. If attacks are frequent and affect routine daily activities then prophylactic treatment can be considered with, e.g. oral pizotifen at night, or daily beta-blockers. In severe cases, patients may be prescribed sumatriptan to use in the prodrome state. Avoid narcotics.

⑦ Cluster headaches

Attacks generally occur in clusters, usually at night for 1–3 weeks, every 12–18 months. More common in men between 20 and 40 years it may be precipitated by alcohol. Typically the patient is woken at night by a severe unilateral stabbing or burning pain which may be frontal temporal, around the eye or over the cheek. Nausea is not a common feature but there is frequently rhinorrhoea, unilateral nasal obstruction, and the eye may be red (conjunctival injection) with lacrimation.

Cluster headaches often respond to ergotamine. Other prescribed drugs include verapamil, topiramate, and lithium.

⑦ Tension headaches

Tension headaches are described as a feeling of pressure, or a 'band-like' tightness that varies in intensity, frequency, and duration. It is often felt bilaterally over the forehead or temples but may affect the vertex, occiput, or eyes. Commonest in middle-aged women with associated stress or depression, it may be chronic or episodic and is only occasionally helped with simple analgesics (NSAIDs).

⑦ Hemicrania continua

This is a persistent unilateral headache that is usually unremitting. The pain is usually moderately severe, unilateral, and continuous, without pain-free periods. There may also be lacrimation, nasal congestion, or ptosis. The cause of hemicrania continua is unknown and there is no definitive diagnostic test for it. However, it generally responds only to indomethacin, which must be continued long term.

The back of the neck

Common presentations

- Injuries
- Lumps
- Pain/stiffness
- Vertebrobasilar insufficiency (dizziness/blackouts)
- Neurological symptoms.

Common problems and their causes

Injuries

Common
- Neck sprain ('whiplash').

Uncommon
- Fractures of cervical spine
- Dislocations of cervical spine
- Hanging.

Pain/stiffness

Common
- Non-specific neck pain
- Neck sprain ('whiplash')
- Torticollis
- Degeneration/cervical spondylosis
- Cervical radiculopathy.

Uncommon
- Rheumatoid arthritis
- Bone disorders
- Infections
- Tumours
- Carotid artery dissection
- Retropharyngeal abscess.

Miscellaneous conditions

Common
- Lumps (lymphadenopathy, lipoma, sebaceous cyst)
- Vertebrobasilar insufficiency.

Uncommon
- Cervical cord myelopathy/myelitis (non-traumatic).

Useful questions and what to look for

Injuries

Ask about
- When it occurred
- Mechanism of injury (what happened)
- Where they are sore
- Any loss of consciousness or signs of head injury
- Any peripheral neurological symptoms
- Progression of symptoms since time of injury
- Any other injuries (remember the entire spine).

Look for
- Other injuries following ATLS® principles
- Peripheral neurological deficit
- Bony tenderness (as necessary)
- Priapism (as necessary).

Pain/stiffness

Ask about
- Onset, duration, and progression
- Character/distribution (localized vs generalized)
- Possible causes (injury, posture, sleeping, sports)
- Peripheral neurological symptoms
- Symptoms in other joints.

Look for
- Range of motion
- Tenderness (midline vs muscles)
- Peripheral neurological deficit.
- Other joints
- Neck masses/swellings.

Lumps

Ask about
- Onset, duration, and progression
- Painful/painless
- Any other lumps
- Previous excision of skin or scalp lesions/malignancies
- Exposure to pets and other animals/recent travel abroad
- Systemic features (infection/lymphoma/malignancy).

Look for
- Assess character of lump (size, mobility, tenderness, etc.)
- Overlying skin (erythematous, blanching, fistula, induration, etc.)
- Head and neck exam for primary malignancies (nodes and scalp)
- Palpate other lymphatic sites (inguinal, axillary, supraclavicular)
- Examine liver and spleen.

Dizziness/blackouts (suspected vertebrobasilar insufficiency)

Ask about
- Any precipitating events (head turning, chest pain, etc.)
- Other neurological symptoms (especially cerebellar or visual)
- Headaches
- Neck pain/stiffness
- Any injuries following blackouts
- Past medical/drug history.

Look for
- Peripheral neurological deficit
- Symptoms reproduced by careful neck movements
- Consider ECG monitoring
- Other possible causes (cardiac, CNS, diabetes, etc.)

Neurological symptoms

Ask about
- Onset
- Preceding injury
- What the patient was doing when the symptoms began
- Determine whether pain/paraesthesia/paralysis
- Aggravating and relieving factors
- Any other neurological symptoms
- Weight loss
- Fevers
- PMH.

Look for
- Range of motion
- Tenderness (midline vs muscles)
- Peripheral neurological deficit
- Symptoms reproduced by careful neck movements.

Examination of the cervical spine following trauma

Examination depends on the presenting symptoms and what associated pathology/injuries are suspected. Patients may walk into the accident and emergency department with a relatively minor complaint, or they may arrive on a spine board, with total spinal immobilization.

Low-risk factors for cervical spine injury

- Simple rear-end MVC where the car wasn't forced into the car in front, hit at a high speed, or by a large vehicle.
- Ambulatory at any point after the injury.
- Sitting in the emergency department.
- Absence of midline spinal tenderness.
- Delayed onset of neck pain.

Examination of the *non-injured* neck, or the neck following *minor* injuries

Although the ATLS® protocol dictates complete immobilization of the spine, this is clearly not necessary (or practical) in every patient who complains of neck pain. The trick is to know which patients do and which ones do not need this. Knowing the mechanism of injury or any preceding symptoms, while maintaining a high index of suspicion, will allow most cases to be managed appropriately. *If in doubt, err on the side of caution and seek advice.* Useful clues include:

- Age: young patients are more commonly associated with trauma and congenital malformation, older ages with degenerative causes (be cautious with older patients as minor trauma can result in significant injuries).
- Position: are they standing, sitting, or lying down. Have they been fully mobile since the problem commenced?
- Posture: do they turn their head to see you or does their whole body turn? Have they developed neck stiffness and if so how severe is it?
- Clothing: Velcro®-style fastening vs tiny intricate buttons (may indicate pre-existing neurological problems).
- Does the patient use any walking aids, standing frame, soft collar etc.? These also give clues about pre-existing pathology.
- The hands: are these the hands of a rheumatoid patient?

Examination of the non-injured neck (or a neck following minor injuries) can be considered under three elements: look, feel, move.

Look

- Can they look up or is there a cervical spondylosis?
- Can you see an incision from a surgical approach to the cervical spine?
- How flexed is the cervical spine?
- Note any thoracic kyphosis, muscle bulk, and skin changes.
- Are they in pain?

Feel

Most palpation in the cervical examination can be performed from behind. It is often less tiring for the patient, and easier for you, if they are sitting down. Start at the occiput, working your way down over the erector spinae and spinous processes. The highest bone you will feel will be C2. Work down to T1, the most prominent bone in the neck. C7 may also be prominent. To work out if you are on T1 or C7, ask the patient to extend the neck slightly: C7 glides back, T1 does not. Palpate laterally, around and over trapezius into the supraclavicular fossae. Palpate along the sternomastoid muscle, feeling for swellings, spasm, and tenderness. If symptoms suggest, continue advancing until your fingers meet in the midline anteriorly and then examine the front of the neck (see ➲ Chapter 5).

Move (only possible if a spinal injury is not suspected)

Always start with active (patient-initiated) movement to avoid hurting the patient. If necessary, ask the patient to put a tongue depressor in their mouth to act as a guide to the range. Ask the patient to hold their head in a comfortable position. Note if it differs from the neutral position. Ask the patient to put their 'chin on chest' for forward flexion—this is usually about 75 degrees (but varies with age). Then 'Look up at the ceiling' for extension, usually about 50 degrees. Assess lateral flexion: 'Put your right ear on your right shoulder' and the opposite for the left. Look at the rise of the shoulder and compare sides. The range of motion is usually about 90 degrees. Assess rotation: 'Put your chin on your right shoulder'. This is just short of 90 degrees. Passive movement is very useful but should only be done by experienced clinicians. This can assess the static elements of the neck (ligaments, joint capsule) and mobility motion (cadence of motion).

Power

Once you have assessed the control of the neck, assess the power of the neck muscles in all the planes of movement: 'Push against my hand'.

Neurology

Comprehensive neurological examination of the upper and lower limbs is required. Remember tone, power, sensation, coordination, proprioception, and reflexes. Are the limbs held flaccid or is there a spastic posture? Coordination and proprioception expose central pathology, chronic alcohol abuse, infarct, metastasis, cord compression, etc.

Assessing a potential spinal injury patient and imaging

As with any injured patient start with assessing Airway, Breathing, and Circulation and addressing any issues encountered. Spinal assessment falls at the end of D for disability, provided the spine has been immobilized, which should be done alongside the assessment of the Airway. Unlike almost any other fracture (Look, Feel, Move, then X-ray), when there is suspected trauma to the cervical spine you may need to image first.

However not all cases need imaging. In some patients, clinical examination alone may be able to 'clear' the neck. Commonly used guidelines are the National Emergency X-Radiography Utilization Study (NEXUS) Low-Risk Criteria and the Canadian C-Spine Rules (or a combination of both). Applying these will help determine the need for imaging. If a patient does not fulfil any of the criteria for imaging in the guidelines and has only experienced low-risk factors then their collar can be removed and the neck carefully assessed. *Low-risk patients who can rotate their head >45 degrees bilaterally should be considered not to have any significant spinal injury. Imaging is not required. However, if the patient cannot reach 45 degrees or has severe pain >7/10 or neurological symptoms, imaging is required.*

If imaging is required, plain films or CT may be undertaken, depending on the overall condition of the patient. If the patient requires a head or thoracic spinal CT, the cervical spine is commonly included during this. Otherwise plain films may initially be taken. When plain films are used, the lateral view is particularly important and this should be obtained first as part of the initial radiographic survey, along with a pelvic and CXR (ATLS® protocol). Anteroposterior and odontoid peg views will also be required. *These are just guides. Always follow your hospital or local protocols.*

Indications for cervical spine imaging following blunt force trauma
- If GCS score is <15.
- Patient is intoxicated.
- If patient complains of focal neurological deficit, paralysis, or paraesthesia in their arms or legs.
- Patients with unexplained hypotension (systolic BP <90 mmHg) or hypo/hyperventilation (respiratory rate of <10 or >24 breaths/min).
- Urgent identification of C-spine injury is required (e.g. patient going for surgery).
- Severe neck pain >7/10.
- Patients with a high-risk mechanism of injury and either severe thoracic back pain >7/10 or visible injury above the clavicles.
- Patients with neck pain and any of the high-risk factors listed in the next box.

High-risk factors for cervical spine injury
- Age >65.
- Sustained axial load to the head (e.g. diving).
- Fall >1 m or >5 steps.
- MVC with combined speed of >65 mph.
- A rollover MVC or ejection from a vehicle.
- A MVC involving recreational motor vehicles.
- Accident as a cyclist.
- Injury sustained over 48 hours ago.
- Re-attendance with same injury.
- Known spinal disease.

How to 'clear' the cervical spine following trauma

'Clearing' a neck is more than just ruling out fractures. It also includes ruling out ligamentous injuries. This requires more than simply looking at a series of plain films. The following is a guide only. This applies to those patients in whom imaging is not indicated, based on the NEXUS Low-Risk Criteria or Canadian C-Spine Rules (or a combination of both), or in whom imaging has been taken but it has not identified any fractures or signs of soft tissue injury. However, always follow your local protocol if available.

- Assess the neurological state of the limbs:
  - Tone (lower motor neuron (LMN), damaged peripheral nerve = flaccid; upper motor neuron (UMN) lesion = increased).
  - Power.
  - Sensation (soft touch and pinprick).
  - Reflexes (look for reduction or absence, compare sides).
  - Proprioception (posterior columns) and coordination should ideally be included, but are probably seldom performed.
- Examine relevant imaging.
- Are there any other distracting injuries (especially head, neck, thoracic, and upper limb injuries)?
- Has analgesia (opiates) been given?
- Is there any spinal pain?
- Is the patient mentally alert (head injury, alcohol, drugs, etc.)?

If all the above are normal/excluded, take the front of the collar off. Instruct the patient not to move their head and ask an assistant to support the head. Instruct the patient to keep their head very still and not to nod or shake it.

- Assess for spinal tenderness. Ask the patient to answer yes or no to whether the area pressed is tender. Feel for any swelling, steps, or crepitus.
- Assess active movement (i.e. ask the patient to move their neck—do not move it yourself). Lateral flexion first, then rotation, then lift head off bed. Take your time—the neck will be a bit stiff at first if they have been immobilized for some time.

If the patient complains of any neurological symptoms or pain, the neck is not cleared—replace immobilization and refer. Consider also the mechanism of injury and the possible need to image the entire spine. If the patient can move their neck freely without pain or neurological symptoms then the neck has been cleared and the collar can be removed. Advise the patient to inform if symptoms develop.

Assessment of known spinal-injured patient

When a spinal cord injury is identified, the patient must be immobilized, and transferred carefully. A full neurological examination should be carried out. Assess and record each of the following:

- Tone: by passively moving the arms and legs. Tone can be increased in UMN lesions, or reduced in LMN lesions, i.e. damaged peripheral nerves. A spinal injury can produce a mixed picture.
- Power: each individual myotome should be tested. The patient's effort is graded on a scale of 0–5:
  - Grade 5: muscle contracts normally against full resistance.
  - Grade 4: muscle strength is reduced but muscle contraction can still move joint against resistance.
  - Grade 3: muscle strength is further reduced such that the joint can be moved only against gravity with the examiner's resistance completely removed. As an example, the elbow can be moved from full extension to full flexion starting with the arm hanging down at the side.
  - Grade 2: muscle can move only if the resistance of gravity is removed. As an example, the elbow can be fully flexed only if the arm is maintained in a horizontal plane.
  - Grade 1: only a trace or flicker of movement is seen or felt in the muscle or fasciculations are observed in the muscle.
  - Grade 0: no movement is observed.
    (Medical Research Council (MRC) scale for muscle strength, © Crown Copyright.)
- Reflexes: look for reduction or absence, by comparing both sides. Reflexes can be hyperreflexic in UMN lesion, or reduced in LMN lesions. An upgoing (extensor) Babinski reflex is a sign of a UMN lesion. There can be a mixed picture in spinal cord injuries depending on the nerves or tracts damaged.
- Sensation: pain (pinprick), temperature (spinothalamic tract), fine touch, and proprioception (dorsal column).

Neurological injuries

These can be considered as:
- Complete or
- Incomplete.

Or anatomically as:
- Anterior cord syndrome (motor function lost but sensation is preserved).
- Posterior cord syndrome (seldom seen).
- Central cord syndrome (upper limbs affected more than lower).
- Brown-Séquard syndrome (ipsilateral loss of motor and proprioception, with contralateral loss of pain and temperature sensation).

Useful investigations

Plain films
The indications for cervical spine imaging following blunt force trauma have been listed previously. This list combines the two main guidelines: the NEXUS Low-Risk Criteria and the Canadian C-Spine Rules.

CT scanning
Three-view plain X-rays are used in the majority of circumstances. However, CT should be used in the following circumstances:
- Patient with a GCS score <13
- Intubated patients
- Inadequate plain film series
- Abnormality or suspected abnormality on plain film
- Patient is being scanned for head injury or trauma series.

CT is also recommended in the following:
- Patients with dementia
- Patient with neurological signs likely to be of C-spine origin
- Patients with severe neck pain >7/10
- Patient with significantly reduced range of movement
- Patients with known vertebral disease.

CT may also be used in the evaluation of non-traumatic symptoms and signs, such as neck pain, stiffness, lumps, and neurological symptoms if MRI is not available.

MRI imaging
MRI should be used in patients with neurological signs likely to be cervical spine in origin and those patients with suspicion of vertebral artery injury. It is also useful as further imaging in those patients with severely restricted neck movement or neck pain with normal CT scans. However, in many centres MRI scans are not available out of hours and therefore plain films and CT scans are used as a stopgap. In those patients where MRI is indicated, it should be carried out at the first opportunity as its sensitivity may fall after 48 hours.

Cervical spine plain film interpretation in trauma

In trauma, the key image is the lateral cervical view and this should be obtained first as part of the initial assessment. However, before a cervical spine can be cleared radiologically, adequate anteroposterior and odontoid peg views are also required. Peg views usually require the patient to open their mouth. For that to be possible, the collar must be loose. For this reason these views may be initially deferred. Do not interfere with the immobilization until you have seen the lateral film, unless the situation demands that you need to. Assessment of plain films can be considered under the following headings.

Adequacy

First determine whether the film is adequate. Do not feel embarrassed in rejecting a film and asking for improved views. All radiographers involved in trauma know how difficult it is to obtain good films and there a number of different views they can use to help. An adequate lateral film shows all seven of the cervical vertebrae, skull base, and the superior aspect of T1.

Interpreting the lateral view

This is a difficult radiograph to interpret, and deserves time. Consider things in a logical order. A useful approach is Alignment, Bones, Cavities, and Disc (ABCD).

Alignment

The cervical spine has a natural curvature (cervical lordosis). This may be lost if there is muscle spasm. There are four curves to follow. Let your eyes follow your index finger as you trace each one out. This allows you to concentrate on specific areas in turn, rather than be flooded with information all at once. Each curve should be smooth and unbroken (Figures 4.1 and 4.2):

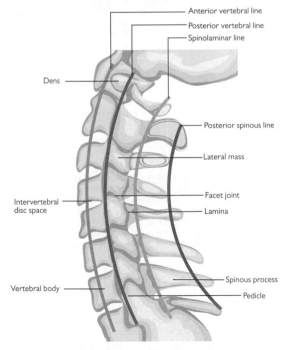

Figure 4.1 Lateral cervical spine.

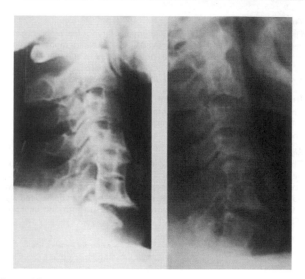

Figure 4.2 Note the angulation of C6 on C7 is greater than 11 degrees.

- Anterior line of the vertebral bodies
- Posterior line of the vertebral bodies
- Bases of the spinal processes (this may show a slight step of <2 mm at the level of C2)
- Tips of spinal processes.

Bones

Examine in turn:
- Vertebral body: below C2 these should have a fairly uniform rectangular shape. Examine for any cortical discontinuity, change in height, or wedging >3 mm between anterior and posterior height.
- Atlas and axis (C1 and C2): in adults the posterior aspect of the anterior part of C1 should be no more than 3 mm from the anterior aspect of the odontoid peg on the lateral film. The posterior aspect of the peg should make a continuous line with the posterior part of C1.
- Posterior elements: the facet joints, lamina, and spinal processes should all be examined for fractures.

Cavities

The pre-vertebral soft tissue shadow should be:
- <7 mm (or 30% of vertebral body) at levels C1–4 and
- <22 mm (or 1 vertebral body width) at C5–7.

An increase in this results from swelling and can be from an occult fracture or underlying ligamentous injury.

Discs
Intervertebral disc spaces should be of even height and shape.

Interpreting the anteroposterior view

The spinal processes should all be in line with an equal gap between them. No single space should be 50% greater than the one above or below it. Each vertebral body should have a spinal process and two facet joints; these can form a picture like an owl. Make sure each 'owl' has a beak and two eyes. Some people have a normal variation of a bifid spinal process—this can sometimes be mistaken for a fracture.

Interpreting the open mouth peg view

An adequate view includes the odontoid peg, lateral masses of C1, and their relationship to the lateral masses of C2 (Figure 4.3). The following should be true:

- There should be an equal distance between the peg and the lateral masses of C1. This can sometimes be affected by rotation but can also be associated with subluxation.
- The lateral masses of C1 should align with the lateral masses of C2 with no overhang (this can indicate a burst fracture).
- The peg should have a smooth cortex with no steps or disruptions.

There are three different Peg fractures
- Avulsion of the tip (stable)
- At base of peg (unstable)
- Extends in vertebral body (unstable).

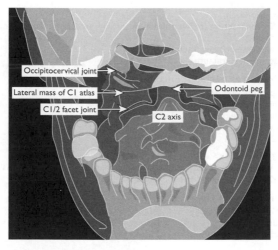

Figure 4.3 Open mouth 'peg' view.

Specific injuries to the neck

Serious injuries can be either bony or ligamentous in origin. The latter is especially important since the patient may have a normal looking X-ray. *So long as the spine is correctly immobilized, imaging can wait if necessary until more pressing injuries are dealt with. Full C-spine immobilization includes not just the neck, but immobilization of the entire spine.* Movement lower down the spine will result in a degree of movement in the neck. Injuries of the cervical spine may also be associated with spinal injuries elsewhere, which also need to be protected.

Following significant injuries, most patients arrive supine with:

- Spine board: solid inflexible plastic board with straps that hold the patient rigid across the chest, pelvis, and legs.
- Blocks: usually foam-filled rubber-coated blocks about the size of a shoe box, on both sides of their head, preventing the neck from rotating; they are radiolucent to allow radiographic examination of the spine.
- Tape: often simple Elastoplast®-type tape, but more commonly two purpose-made straps, one across the mandible, the other across the forehead, holding the head down on to the spinal board.
- Hard collar: stiff plastic collar that prevents flexion, extension, and lateral flexion of the neck. The patient cannot open their mouth.

Go to your emergency department, and ask to see these items. Become familiar with how they are applied and taken off.

☼ Fractures of the atlas (C1)
- Posterior arch
- Anterior arch
- Jefferson fracture (blowout fracture through anterior and posterior arches)
- Transverse process fracture
- Lateral mass fracture.

☼ Fractures of the odontoid peg (C2)
- Tip of the odontoid process
- Through the base of the odontoid
- Through the odontoid and extends into the body of the vertebra
- Fracture associated with unilateral or bilateral facet dislocation of C2 on C3.

Hangman's fracture
This is a fracture of the C2 posterior elements produced by extension and distraction (Levine classification).

☼ Fractures of the vertebral body
- Wedge compression
- Burst
- Tear-drop (Figure 4.4).

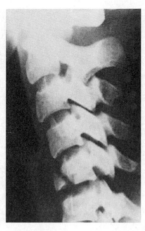

Figure 4.4 Tear-drop fracture of C6.

Facet joint injuries

- Occipito-cervical dislocation
- Atlanto-axial subluxation (odontoid distance is >3 mm)
- Unilateral facet dislocation (25% displacement of the upper vertebra on the lower, or malalignment of the spinous processes on the anterior-posterior film)
- Bilateral facet dislocation (50% displacement of the vertebra) (Figure 4.5).

SCIWORA (spinal cord injury without radiological abnormality)

Patients can occasionally sustain significant spinal cord injuries without any changes radiologically. This is more common in the paediatric population (due to increased elasticity of the ligaments), but can also occur in adults with underlying bone disease of the neck. If suspected an MRI should be carried out—this can reveal haematoma or oedema within the cord.

Neck sprain ('whiplash')

This is a very difficult diagnosis to prove (or disprove) or quantify, and is a potential minefield when it comes to litigation. It is a sprain of the surrounding neck muscles, notably trapezius and the deep extensors. 'Whiplash' is a controversial term. Anyone who has had a neck sprain will appreciate how painful it is. Muscle fibres are torn, resulting in intense painful spasm. The neck is held still by this spasm and the muscles feel hard. Sometimes the head is rotated to one side due to the pull of the sternomastoid. Radiographs can be difficult to interpret as spasm can distort the normal position of the neck, twisting it or straightening

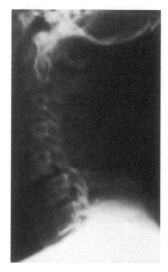

Figure 4.5 Bilateral facet dislocation of C5 on C6. Note 50% overlap.

its natural lordosis. *Loss of the normal curvature of the cervical spine on a lateral view suggests muscle spasm and therefore injury. This is a useful radiographic sign.* If a significant neck injury cannot be ruled out, CT is required. Management involves analgesia (NSAIDs) and physiotherapy. Pain may get worse before it gets better but should improve 3–4 days post injury.

☼ Hanging

Some patients may attempt (and fail) to commit suicide by hanging themselves. This can result in several injuries depending on the method/ equipment used:

- Upper airway injury and asphyxiation
- Cerebral hypoxia from carotid occlusion
- Cerebral oedema and ischaemia from jugular vein occlusion
- Carotid sinus reflex resulting in bradycardia and cardiac arrest
- Vertebral artery injury
- Cervical fracture with spinal cord injury.

If a rope is used, the location of the knot is a major factor in determining the mechanics of any injury. The face may be engorged and cyanotic with petechiae in the eyes. Forensic experts may be able to tell if hanging is attempted suicide or attempted homicide by the ligature mark. If the hyoid bone is broken, this may be a clue to manual choking. Take photographs and keep any ligature/rope for the police.

⚙ Spinal cord injury/lesions

Spinal cord injury can vary widely, with symptoms that include pain, paralysis, and incontinence. It can range from 'incomplete', with varying effects, to 'complete', with total loss of function below the level of the lesion. Spinal cord injuries have many causes, but are usually associated with major trauma from MVCs, falls, sports injuries, and violence. However, they can also be of a non-traumatic origin, secondary to malignancy, infection, intervertebral disc disease, and spinal cord vascular disease.

Classification

The International Standards for Neurological Classification of Spinal Cord Injury (ISNCSCI) is a useful classification. Traumatic spinal cord injury can be classified into five categories:

- A: 'complete' spinal cord injury where no motor or sensory function is preserved in the sacral segments S4–S5.
- B: 'incomplete' spinal cord injury where sensory but not motor function is preserved below the neurological level and includes the sacral segments S4–S5. This is usually a transient phase.
- C: 'incomplete' spinal cord injury where motor function is preserved below the neurological level and more than half of the muscles below the neurological level have a power grade of less than 3.
- D: 'incomplete' spinal cord injury where motor function is preserved below the neurological level and at least half of the key muscles below the neurological level have a muscle grade of 3 or more.
- E: 'normal' where motor and sensory scores are normal.

(Reproduced from 'International Standards for Neurological Classification of Spinal Cord Injury: Cases with classification challenges', S. C. Kirshblum, F. Biering-Sorensen, R. Betz, et al., *The Journal of Spinal Cord Medicine*, 37, 2, 2014, reprinted by permission of the publisher (Taylor & Francis Ltd, http://www.tandfonline.com).)

It is important to determining the exact 'level' of injury. This is described according to the vertebral level at which the injury occurs. While the prognosis of complete injuries is poor, the symptoms of incomplete injuries can vary, making it difficult to predict outcome.

⚙ Cervical injuries

These usually result in tetraplegia. However, depending on the location and severity of injury some function may be retained:

- Injuries at C3 vertebrae and above often result in loss of breathing, necessitating intubation and ventilation.
- Injuries at, or below, C4 variably affect the upper limb.

Additional features include:

- Reduced ability to regulate heart rate, BP, sweating, and body temperature.
- Autonomic responses to pain are impaired.

Initial management

Initial management of spinal cord injuries involves protecting the cord and minimizing secondary inflammation which may cause further damage. Traction should not be used (do not pull on the neck). The neck should be immobilized above and below the suspected level of injury.

In the early stages of injury, patients may develop neurogenic shock, respiratory failure, and pulmonary oedema. Careful assessment for these should be made. The mean arterial BPs must be carefully maintained (of at least 85–90 mmHg) using IV fluids, transfusion, and vasopressors under specialist advice. Later complications include pressure sores, pneumonia, pulmonary emboli, and deep venous thrombosis. Appropriate preventive measures should therefore be commenced. *The role of high-dose steroids is controversial so seek advice before giving these.* When trauma has not been involved, a careful search for the underlying pathology (notably tumours or disc protrusion) is made. Specific treatment varies depending on the cause as well as its location and severity of signs. Traumatic spinal cord injuries require considerable physiotherapy and rehabilitation. Experimental treatments include controlled hypothermia and stem cells technology, although these are still in the early stages of research.

Spinal cord syndromes

A number of spinal cord syndromes have been described. These occur as a result of injury to some of the ascending and descending tracts of the spinal cord, while others remain intact and functional. Knowledge of spinal cord anatomy helps interpret these findings.

Central cord syndrome (CCS)

CCS is a form of incomplete spinal cord injury characterized by weakness in the arms and hands while the legs are involved to a lesser extent. It is usually caused by injury to the cervical or upper thoracic regions of the spinal cord. It occurs as a result of ischaemia, haemorrhage, or necrosis in the central portions of the spinal cord. The more peripheral corticospinal fibres for the legs are therefore spared.

Underlying causes include atherosclerosis, trauma, emboli, and diseases of the aorta. CCS often occurs in older patients with cervical spondylosis following a hyperextension injury, so should be considered in any elderly patient presenting with facial injuries who has fallen 'flat on their face'. However, it also may occur in younger patients. CCS accounts for approximately 9% of traumatic spinal cord injuries and is generally associated with a more favourable prognosis compared to the other syndromes. In many cases neurological symptoms improve with conservative management (immobilization of the cervical spine with a neck collar for approximately 6 weeks). Surgical intervention (stabilization or decompression) may be required if there is instability of the cervical spine or if symptoms progress.

Anterior cord syndrome/anterior spinal artery syndrome/Beck's syndrome

This is often associated with flexion-type injuries to the cervical spine, causing damage to the anterior portion of the spinal cord. Other causes include atherosclerosis, aortic aneurysms, dissections, direct trauma to the aorta, and surgery to the mediastinum. These can damage or obstruct the branches of the aorta that supply the anterior spinal artery, which itself supplies the anterior portion of the cord. Acute disc hernia-tion, cervical spondylosis, kyphoscoliosis, and neoplasia can also result in occlusion of the anterior spinal artery. Rarer causes include vasculitis, polycythaemia, sickle cell disease, decompression sickness, cocaine use, and connective tissue disorders.

Below the level of injury, motor function (corticospinal tract), pain sensation, and temperature sensation (spinothalamic tract) are lost. However, touch, proprioception, and vibration sense remain intact (dor-sal columns). Areflexia, a flaccid anal sphincter, urinary retention, and intestinal obstruction may also occur. Treatment depends on the primary cause. Prognosis is generally poor. The mortality rate is approximately 20%, and 50% of individuals show very little or no change in symptoms.

Posterior cord syndrome/tabes dorsalis

This can also occur, but is very rare. It is caused by an injury or lesion affecting the posterior spinal artery in the posterior portion of the spi-nal cord. This results in loss of proprioception below the level of injury. Motor function, sense of pain, and sensitivity to light touch remain intact. Tabes dorsalis is demyelination secondary to an untreated syphilis infection.

Brown-Séquard syndrome

This usually occurs when the spinal cord is hemisectioned or injured on one side, usually from a penetrating wound (e.g. gunshot or knife injury). Rarer causes include tumour, multiple sclerosis, and tuberculosis (TB). On the ipsilateral side of the injury there is loss of motor function, pro-prioception, vibration, and light touch. Contralaterally, there is a loss of pain, temperature, and crude touch sensations. Treatment is directed at the cause.

① Syringomyelia

This refers to the formation of a cyst or cavity (syrinx) within the spinal cord. This expands over time, compressing the spinal cord (Figure 4.6).

Symptoms include pain, paralysis, weakness, and stiffness in the back, shoulders, and extremities. Syringomyelia may also cause loss of the abil-ity to feel extremes of hot or cold, especially in the hands. When syrinxes affect the brainstem, the condition is called syringobulbia.

Arnold–Chiari malformation

This is the most common cause of syringomyelia. A congenital abnormal-ity of the brain causes the lower part of the cerebellum to protrude into the cervical portion of the spinal canal. A syrinx may then develop in the cervical region of the spinal cord.

Acquired syringomyelia

Syringomyelia may also occur as a complication of trauma, meningitis, haemorrhage, a tumour, or arachnoiditis. Here, the syrinx develops in the part of the cord previously damaged by one of these conditions. It can then expand.

Investigations include MRI and myelography. Referral to a neurosur-geon is required. Treatment includes drainage of the cyst and placement of a shunt.

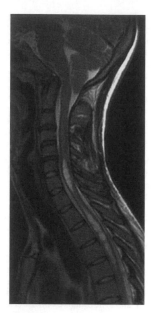

Figure 4.6 Spinal cord sagittal T$_2$-weighted (a) and T$_1$-weighted (b) magnetic resonance images from a patient with Arnold–Chiari type I malformation and syringomyelia.

Reproduced with permission from Filippi M., *Oxford Textbook of Neuroimaging*, Figure 26.4, p. 328, Copyright © 2015 with permission from Oxford University Press.

☼ Acute spinal cord compression

This is a neurosurgical/spinal emergency. Urgent referral and management are essential to minimize permanent loss of function.

Causes of spinal cord compression

- Trauma
- Tumours (benign or malignant): bone tumours, primary or metastatic tumours, lymphomas, multiple myeloma and neurofibromata
- Prolapsed intervertebral disc
- Extradural or subdural haematoma (following recent epidural, lumbar puncture, spinal surgery, or anticoagulant therapy)
- Inflammatory disease, especially rheumatoid arthritis
- Spinal infections (bacterial, TB, fungal, vertebral osteomyelitis, discitis or epidural abscess)
- Spinal manipulation.

Symptoms that suggest spinal compression include:
- Insidious progression
- Neurological symptoms: gait disturbance, clumsy or weak hands, or loss of sexual, bladder, or bowel function
- Neurological signs:
  - Lhermitte's sign—flexion of the neck causes an electric shock-type sensation that radiates down the spine into the limbs
  - UMN signs in the lower limbs
  - LMN signs in the upper limbs
  - Sensory changes are variable.

Cervical spine compression can result in quadriplegia if untreated. Compression above the level of C3, C4, C5 (level of the phrenic nerve) causes paralysis of the diaphragm and artificial ventilation is required. Sphincter disturbances are late features of cervical cord compression. There may also be loss of autonomic activity with lack of sweating below the level, loss of thermoregulation, and hypotension. *Always check and document bladder/bowel function, sphincter tone, and check for saddle anaesthesia (cauda equina).*

Management

Initial measures are supportive and the prevention of further injury. The neck should be immobilized and urgent imaging (CT or MRI) undertaken. Urgent referral to a spinal unit/neurosurgeon is required. Occasionally clinical oncology may be involved if surgery is not an option and the cause is a radiosensitive tumour. Steroids may help, depending on the underlying cause and should be discussed with the specialist. Depending on the extent of neurological deficit patients may require IV fluids and catheterization.

Spinal cord compression due to metastases

This can occur in around 5% of patients with cancer. Spinal pain is often present for several months before paraplegia. The thoracic spine is most commonly affected in metastatic cancers.

Differential diagnosis of neck pain

Neck pain is a common problem. Like a headache, in most cases the cause is not serious. However, the patient still needs careful assessment. The differential diagnoses include:
- Simple neck pain: acute neck strain, postural neck ache, or whiplash
- Headache
- Referred pain, e.g. from the shoulder
- Degenerative disc disease/cervical spondylosis
- Traumatic prolapsed intervertebral disc
- Malignancy: primary tumours, secondary deposits, or myeloma
- Infections: discitis, osteomyelitis, or TB
- Fibromyalgia
- Vascular insufficiency
- Psychogenic neck pain
- Inflammatory disease: rheumatoid arthritis
- Metabolic diseases: Paget's disease of bone, osteoporosis.

① Acute torticollis (wry neck)

This refers to a dystonic condition resulting in an abnormal positioning of the head. It has many causes, the most common being muscular irritation, often the sternocleidomastoid (SCM) and trapezius. These will usually settle spontaneously within a couple of days. Treatment includes simple analgesia and NSAIDs. Diazepam can also be used to improve symptoms by helping muscle relaxation. Physiotherapy can be very helpful.

Other rarer causes include infections involving ears or throat (e.g. otitis media and retropharyngeal abscess), tardive dystonia, secondary to medications such as antiemetics and antipsychotics, and posterior fossa tumours compressing the nerve supply to the neck.

① Vertebrobasilar insufficiency (beauty parlour syndrome)

This condition refers to the temporary onset of vertigo-like symptoms as a result of decreased blood flow in the posterior circulation of the brain. This supplies blood to the medulla, cerebellum, pons, midbrain, thalamus, and occipital cortex. Symptoms vary accordingly, but commonly include vertigo. Patients may suddenly become weak at the knee and crumple (a 'drop attack'). The differential diagnosis is large and includes labyrinthitis, vestibular neuronitis, and benign paroxysmal positional vertigo as well as cardiac causes and strokes/TIAs. Eagle syndrome is a rare condition which also presents with neurological symptoms occurring on head rotation (see ➜ Chapter 5, p. 173).

In vertebrobasilar insufficiency, osteophyte formation in the cervical spine occurs with increasing age and gradually compresses the vertebral vessels. This is made worse by any associated atherosclerosis, so this condition is commonly associated with diabetes, smoking, and hypertension. Occlusion of the vessels can result in positional-dependent vertigo or blackouts in which specific movement of the neck results in the symptoms. This is a useful clinical sign but be careful when eliciting it! Magnetic resonance angiography (MRA) may be used to identify vertebrobasilar stenoses or occlusions, but is not often required.

Management

Treatable coexisting problems should be managed (e.g. diabetes, hypertension). An appropriate exercise regimen can also be designed in order to avoid excessive pooling of blood in the legs. To prevent drop attacks, patients are advised to 'go to the ground' shortly after feeling dizzy or if they experience changes in vision. Patients may be started on an antiplatelet agent or anticoagulants once haemorrhage has been excluded with imaging.

⑦ Lump(s) in the back of the neck

Lumps are also discussed elsewhere (see ➲ Chapter 5). An isolated palpable lymph node in the back of the neck is usually non-neoplastic in nature.

An overview of the posterior triangle anatomy

Boundaries
- Front: posterior border of the SCM muscle
- Back: anterior border of the trapezius muscle
- Below: the lateral part of the clavicle.

The posterior triangle is a spiral that passes from its apex at the back of the skull down to its base in the front at the root of the neck. Its roof is formed by the investing layer of deep cervical fascia, and its floor by the prevertebral fascia.

Contents of importance

- Third part of the subclavian artery: runs very low in the posterior triangle at the level of the clavicle; just above the clavicle the suprascapular and transverse cervical vessels pass.
- External jugular vein: runs through the anterior/inferior part of the triangle to drain into the subclavian vein which lies more inferiorly and is not included in the posterior triangle.
- Occipital, transverse cervical, suprascapular, and subclavian arteries.
- Accessory nerve emerges from the posterior border of the SCM at the junction of its upper and middle thirds. It runs vertically down (over levator scapulae) to enter the anterior border of the trapezius usually 5–6 cm above the clavicle.
- Cervical plexus branches:
  - Muscular branches
  - A loop from C1 to hypoglossal
  - C2/3 branches to SCM and C3/4 to trapezius
  - Inferior root of ansa cervicalis
  - Phrenic nerve (C3, C4, C5)—runs from lateral to medial over scalenus anterior
  - Cutaneous branches
  - Lesser occipital nerve (C2)—posterior part of the neck to the superior nuchal line, and behind the auricle
  - Great auricular nerve (C2 & 3)—skin over the angle of the mandible and parotid gland, and the auricle
  - Transverse cervical (C2 & 3)—skin in the midline of the neck
  - Supraclavicular nerve (C3 & 4)—root of neck/upper chest.
- Brachial plexus trunks: the three trunks of the brachial plexus along with the cervical plexus are held down to the prevertebral muscles by the covering of prevertebral fascia that forms the floor of the posterior triangle. Strictly speaking they are not contents of this triangle, but are mentioned, however, because of their anatomical importance in penetrating injuries.

- Omohyoid muscle: posterior belly. From its origin at the hyoid bone it passes deep to the SCM, coming to lie over the carotid sheath. As it overlies the internal jugular vein the fibres form a flat tendon (the 'intermediate tendon') that is a useful marker during neck dissections to the vein's position. The muscle is held down to the clavicle at the intermediate tendon by a fascial sling.
- Cervical lymph nodes: level V.

Common lumps in the back of the neck

- Skin lumps (sebaceous cyst, skin tags, etc.)
- Lymph node (usually benign if solitary)
- Lipoma.

Diseases of the mastoid process and parotid tumours (in the parotid tail) may cause confusion in diagnosis. These are strictly not part of the posterior triangle, but if large enough may appear to be involving it.

The front of the neck

Common presentations

- Cough (chronic/severe)
- Difficulty breathing (stridor) (see also ➲ Chapter 8)
- Difficulty swallowing (dysphagia) (see also ➲ Chapter 8)
- Foreign body ingestion and aspiration
- Haemoptysis (coughing up blood)
- Hoarse voice/loss of voice
- Injuries
- Lumps and swellings
- Pain on swallowing (odynophagia) (see also ➲ Chapter 8).

Common problems and their causes

Cough (chronic/severe)

Common
- Infections (especially upper respiratory tract infections (URTIs))
- Gastroesophageal reflux
- Air pollution/reactive airway disease
- Foreign body
- Lung diseases (bronchiectasis, cystic fibrosis, interstitial lung diseases, and sarcoidosis)
- Lung tumours
- Diseases/stimulation of the external auditory canal (vagal stimulation)
- Cardiorespiratory diseases (heart failure, infection, infarction, asthma)
- Post-nasal drip.

Uncommon
- Angiotensin-converting enzyme (ACE) inhibitor
- Psychogenic/habit
- Occupational (factory workers).

Difficulty breathing (stridor)

Common
- Foreign body
- Spreading infection (e.g. tonsillitis, quinsy, epiglottitis, retropharyngeal abscess, croup)
- Airway oedema (e.g. trauma, anaphylaxis)
- Obstructive sleep apnoea (stertor due to upper airway collapse)
- Laryngitis
- Tumour/polyps
- Reinke's oedema
- Gastroesophageal reflux.

Uncommon
- Epiglottitis (children)
- Mediastinal mass
- Subglottic stenosis
- Thyroiditis
- Vocal cord palsy
- Tracheo/laryngomalacia
- Congenital anomalies in infants and children
- Vascular anomalies.

Difficulty swallowing (dysphagia)
(See also ➲ Chapter 8.)

Common
- Cerebrovascular accident
- Tumour
- Neurological diseases, e.g. Parkinson's disease, multiple sclerosis (MS), amyotrophic lateral sclerosis
- Globus.

Uncommon
- Oesophageal atresia
- Paterson–Kelly syndrome
- Benign strictures
- Oesophageal diverticula (pharyngeal pouch)
- Scleroderma
- Diffuse oesophageal spasm
- Webs and rings.

Foreign body ingestion and aspiration

Common
- Fish bones
- Peanuts
- Coins (most common object in children)
- Meat (food bolus commonest in adults).

Uncommon
- Dentures
- Many miscellaneous items.

Haemoptysis (coughing up blood)

Common
- Chest pathology (bronchitis, pneumonia, TB, bronchiectasis, pulmonary embolism, cystic fibrosis)
- Sinusitis
- Tumours (lung/upper aerodigestive tract)
- Cardiac (congestive cardiac failure and mitral stenosis)
- Trauma.

Uncommon
- Hereditary haemorrhagic telangiectasia
- Goodpasture's syndrome
- Wegener's granulomatosis
- Foreign body in the respiratory tract
- Sarcoidosis
- Bleeding diathesis (warfarin, antiplatelet drugs).

Hoarse voice/loss of voice

Common
- Prolonged excessive shouting/singing
- Laryngitis (viral, bacterial, fungal)
- Vocal fold paralysis
- Reinke's oedema (secondary to smoking)
- Hypothyroidism (laryngeal myxoedema)
- Gastroesophageal reflux disease (GORD)
- Injury.

Uncommon
- Psychological
- Laryngeal cancer
- Benign neoplasms (cysts, nodules, polyps, and ulcers, papillomatosis, haemangioma)
- Congenital disorders
- Adductor spasmodic dysphonia and muscle-tension disorders
- Vocal fold granulomas and caustic inhalation injuries
- Endocrine: adrenal, pituitary, and gonadic disorders
- Neuromuscular: MS, Parkinson's, stroke, Guillain–Barré syndrome, myasthenia gravis
- Connective tissue disorders (rheumatoid arthritis, systemic lupus erythematosus (SLE)).

Injuries

Common
- Blunt trauma—bruising and oedema
- Smoke inhalation
- Superficial lacerations.

Uncommon
- Fractured larynx
- Trachea avulsion
- Surgical emphysema
- Penetrating injuries
- Blast injuries.

Lumps and swellings (lateral side of neck)

Common
- Lymphadenopathy (inflammatory, infectious, reactive, tumour)
- Abscess (Ludwig's)/deep neck space infections
- Submandibular gland enlargement (tumour, infection, stone)
- Thyroid enlargement
- Parotid gland (tail).

Uncommon
- Plunging ranula
- Branchial cleft cyst
- Pharyngeal pouch
- Laryngocoele
- Teratoma and dermoid cyst
- Carotid body tumour
- Carotid artery aneurysm
- Cystic hygroma
- Cervical rib
- Torticollis.

Lumps and swellings (midline of neck)

Common
- Submental lymph node
- Thyroid enlargement
- Thyroglossal cyst (children and adolescents).

Uncommon
- Dermoid cyst (sublingual)
- Plunging ranula
- Laryngeal swellings (bursitis, chondroma, etc.)
- Thymic cysts
- Superficial swellings (sebaceous cyst, dermoid cyst, lipoma, abscess, etc.).

Pain on swallowing (odynophagia)
(See ➔ Chapter 8.)

Common
- Ingestion of very hot or cold food or drink
- URTIs/epiglottitis
- Drugs
- Ulcers.

Uncommon
- Immune disorders
- Neurological disorders
- Tumour.

Useful questions and what to look for

Cough (chronic/severe)

Ask about
- Post-nasal drip and nocturnal cough
- Full cardiac and respiratory history
- Recent URTI/sore throat
- Heartburn
- Change in voice
- Occupation
- Otalgia/discharge/irritation
- Diseases of the external auditory canal (e.g. wax)
- Medications (especially ACE inhibitors).

Look for
- Full cardiorespiratory exam
- Neck masses
- Examine fauces/cords for ulcers, infection, granuloma, etc.

Difficulty breathing (stridor)
(See also Chapter 8.)

Ask about
- Onset and duration
- Constant vs intermittent
- Dysphagia, drooling, hoarseness, airway, bleeding, weight loss, odynophagia, cough (barking cough), sleep pattern (snoring, daytime somnolence), choking (GORD, foreign body)
- Recent URTI, fever, cough, sore throat
- Allergy
- Recent trauma, caustic ingestion
- Previous airway surgery
- Medications (medicine allergies, ACE inhibitors)
- History of sarcoidosis, connective tissue disorders, granulomatous diseases, asthma, cardiac and pulmonary problems
- Complete perinatal history in infants and feeding difficulties (regurgitation, worse with feeding).

Look for
- Assess airway/respirations/cyanosis
- Oral cavity (macroglossia, tonsillar hypertrophy or infection)
- Cranial nerves
- Trachea midline, goitre, palpable laryngeal fractures
- Examine tracheal stoma (if relevant)
- Cutaneous lesions (haemangiomas)
- Nasoseptal deformities, nasal masses
- Chest (cardiorespiratory)
- Consider laryngoscopy/bronchoscopy depending on cause.

Difficulty swallowing (dysphagia)

(See also ⊃ Chapter 8.)

Ask about
- Onset and duration
- Progressive or static
- Difficulty initiating a swallow
- Coughing/choking, frequent chest infections
- Weight loss
- Gurgly or wet voice after swallowing
- Odynophagia.

Look for
- Complete neurological exam
- Examine fauces/cords/chest
- Neck masses.

Foreign body ingestion and aspiration

Ask about
- Description of object (if sharp may need retrieval)
- Dysphagia
- Pain (mouth, throat, chest, abdomen)
- Fever
- Choking, stridor
- Wheezing, hoarseness.

Look for
- Airway patency
- Assess chest and abdomen
- Examine neck/fauces/cords (but avoid manipulation).

Haemoptysis (coughing up blood)

Ask about
- Full cardiac and respiratory history
- Quality of blood (fresh/streaks/clots)
- Recent URTI/sore throat
- Change in voice
- Weight loss
- Occupation
- Smoking
- Medications.

Look for
- Full cardiorespiratory exam
- Neck masses
- Examine fauces/nose/postnasal space.

Hoarse voice/loss of voice

Ask about
- Onset and duration
- Time course, periodicity (morning hoarseness with GORD and evening hoarseness with voice abuse)
- Voice abuse
- Recent URTI, fever, sore throat, cough
- Smoking or alcohol abuse
- PMH of neuromuscular disorders, hypothyroidism
- Previous laryngeal trauma, surgery, or airway manipulation
- Odynophagia, dysphagia, aspiration, weight loss, hearing loss, heartburn.

Look for
- Assess perceptual quality of voice (pitch, loudness)
- Neck masses
- Thyroid masses
- Indirect or direct laryngoscopy (vocal fold motion, lesions, and competence)
- Complete neurological exam.

Injuries

Ask about
- When it occurred/mechanism of injury (blunt/penetrating)
- Other injuries
- Progression of symptoms since time of injury
- Hoarseness
- Pain
- Haemoptysis
- Difficulty swallowing
- Odynophagia
- Haematemesis.

Look for
- Airway obstruction
- Signs of blood loss/active bleeding
- Other injuries
- Site and estimate depth (root of neck can also involve the chest and arm)
- Lacerations, bubbling wounds
- Haematomas—?pulsatile
- Subcutaneous emphysema/laryngeal crepitus
- Diminished pulses
- Neurological impairment (Horner's syndrome, brachial plexus, spinal cord, CNs)
- Peripheral pulses (distal carotid, superficial temporal, brachial) and bruit.

Lumps and swellings

Ask about
- Onset, duration, and progression
- Painful/painless
- Recent URTI, toothache/carious teeth, sinus infection, otitis media, or other head and neck infection
- Exposure to pets and other animals
- Recent travel abroad
- Previous excision of skin or scalp lesions/malignancies
- Smoking and alcohol abuse
- Fever, postnasal drip, rhinorrhoea, otalgia, night sweats, weight loss, malaise, dysphagia, hoarseness.

Look for
- Assess character of lump
- Solitary versus multiple
- Overlying skin (e.g. erythematous, blanching, fistulas, induration, necrotic)
- Head and neck exam for primary malignancies (nasopharynx, oral cavity, base of tongue, tonsillar fossa, nasal cavity, external ear canal, scalp, thyroid, and salivary glands) or infections
- Other lymphatic sites (e.g. inguinal, axillary, supraclavicular)
- Examine chest, liver and spleen.

Pain on swallowing (odynophagia)
(See also Chapter 8.)

Ask about
- Onset and duration
- Precipitating factors
- Difficulty breathing
- Sore throat
- Haemoptysis/haematemesis.

Look for
- Examine chest
- Neck masses
- Examine fauces
- Complete neurological exam.

Examination of the front of the neck

In order to examine the neck thoroughly (usually a lump or lumps), the patient must be comfortable and the neck relaxed as much as possible. They must be sitting upright with their neck fully exposed, so that you can see the clavicles fully (Figure 5.1).

When examining the neck consider also the surrounding structures (especially the mouth, teeth, throat, and skin) for infections and tumours. These may need to be examined as well.

Look

Start by standing back and simply observing the patient from the front and then the lateral views.
- Is there an obvious lesion/lump (see later in topic)?
- Does the ear lobe stick out (parotid swelling)?
- Get the patient to drink some water (if not an emergency)—does the lump move on swallowing (attached to the tongue or upper airway)?
- Get the patient to stick out their tongue. If a lump moves up it will be attached to it somewhere (classically seen in thyroglossal cysts).
- Is the overlying skin affected (tethered or a discharging sinus)?
- Look at the scalp, face, and in the mouth—are there any lesions that could cause inflammatory or metastatic lymphadenopathy?
- Is there evidence of systemic disease (e.g. anaemic, cachexia, thyroid)?

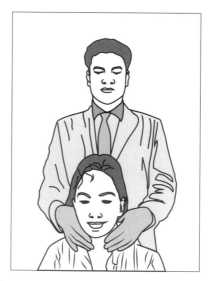

Figure 5.1 Examination of the neck is best done standing behind the patient.

Feel

Examine as many necks as possible until you are familiar with what is 'normal'. All necks have irregularities, palpable lumps, depressions, etc., which are normal findings (for instance, you can often feel prominent submandibular glands in the elderly). Only when you are familiar with the normal are you likely to pick up abnormal findings. There are different ways to examine the neck. Some clinicians feel both sides simultaneously for asymmetry, others feel each side in turn—that way you can laterally flex the neck and feel deep into the submandibular triangle. Try both and decide for yourself but don't throttle the patient! *Beware of putting pressure on bilateral prominent carotid bodies simultaneously. This can cause vagal stimulation and induce vasovagal syncope in elderly patients.*

Standing behind the patient, gently but firmly rest your fingertips under the lower border of the mandible under the chin. Palpate the submental area moving back to the submandibular areas, feeling for abnormal or painful masses. In some patients the submandibular gland hangs lower than normal. This is sometimes referred to as a 'ptotic' submandibular gland. It is commonly found in elderly patients and can often be confused with an enlarged lymph node. Feel along the side mandible as well as below, lymph nodes are commonly found in the lower face (the bucco-facial node), but should be considered as part of the neck. Palpate the depression behind the ramus, below the ear lobe—an important site for parotid swellings. Follow on by feeling down the anterior border of the SCM to the sternal notch, and then staying in the midline move back superiorly to the submental area where you started. Palpate the posterior triangle behind the SCM, the supraclavicular areas, and the occipital scalp. After laterally flexing the neck, gently grab the SCM and try to feel deep to it—this is an important and often missed area of examination. It is where many lymph nodes lay.

Assessing a lump

If there is a lump, note:
- Site
- Size
- Shape
- Surface
- Temperature
- Tethering
- Transillumination—cystic hygromas (congenital cavernous lymphangioma) transilluminate brilliantly
- Colour
- Consistency
- Pulsatile
- Auscultation—listen over the mass with a stethoscope. Is there a bruit?

What are you feeling for?
Lymph nodes are part of the immune system and are often enlarged when fighting infections. Infected lymph nodes tend to be:
• Firm
• Tender
• Enlarged
• Warm.

Inflammation can spread to the overlying skin, causing erythema. Untreated, the node can become necrotic, resulting in abscess formation. Following infection, lymph nodes can sometimes remain permanently enlarged, but are usually non-tender, small (<1 cm) and have a rubbery feel.

Malignant nodes are often:
• Firm
• Non-tender
• Adherent
• Fixed to the surrounding tissues.

The location of the lymph node may help to determine the site of malignancy. Diffuse, bilateral involvement suggests a systemic malignancy (e.g. leukaemia) or infection, while those localized on one side are more likely associated with a local problem.

Other important 'lumps' to consider include the thyroid and submandibular glands and the tail of the parotid (just below the ear lobe). In thin necks the hyoid bone can sometimes be palpable, as well as the carotid.

Useful investigations

Laboratory tests

A complete blood count with differential is usually required for any infective, inflammatory, systemic, or neoplastic pathologies.

Monospot, purified protein derivative (TB), HIV testing, cat-scratch, toxoplasmosis, mumps titres, and Epstein–Barr virus serology are commonly required in the assessment of lymphadenopathy.

Thyroid function tests should be taken for any thyroid lump or enlargement.

Plain films

These may be required to identify some foreign bodies. A CXR by itself may overlook small objects. Air trapping is a clue to the presence of radiolucent foreign bodies. Consider a CXR *and soft tissue neck* in both anteroposterior and lateral views, to locate the foreign body. The trachea is wider on the anteroposterior direction, whereas the oesophagus is wider on a lateral projection. Mediastinitis, haemothorax, and pneumothorax are worrying signs. These require further evaluation and urgent referral. *Beware: most fish bones and non-metallic objects are radiolucent and therefore may not be seen on X-ray.*

Orthopantomography (OPT)—this is required in the assessment of lymphadenopathy or swelling in the upper neck. Dental infections are a common cause.

A cervical spine X-ray may show a bony cervical rib or prominence of the anterior tubercle of the 7th cervical vertebra (with a fibrous band).

CT/MRI

CT is the diagnostic test of choice to evaluate laryngeal fractures (hyoid bone, thyroid, and cricoid cartilage).

CT/MRI of the neck provides greater differentiation of abscess, neoplasms, vascular lesions, haematomas, or congenital abnormalities. The chest may need to be included depending on the suspected pathology or injuries.

Angiography

This may be required urgently following trauma (penetrating injuries). If bleeding is active, selective embolization may be necessary.

Angiography is also occasionally undertaken in the assessment of vascular swellings (alternatively computed tomography angiography (CTA) or magnetic resonance angiography (MRA) may be performed).

Direct visualization techniques

- Fibreoptic nasopharyngoscopy (laryngoscopy). This can assess airway patency, visualize endolaryngeal lacerations, laryngeal oedema, and haematomas. It can also assess vocal fold mobility, supraglottic structure, and be used to examine a tracheal stoma.
- Rigid oesophagoscopy. This requires admission and general anaesthesia. It is usually indicated for foreign bodies that remain in the oesophagus for >2 days and large objects in the oesophagus. Batteries need immediate retrieval.
- Rigid bronchoscopy. This requires admission and general anaesthesia. Because this involves sharing the airway, anaesthesia is complicated. It may sometimes be needed in an emergent airway crisis.
- Flexible bronchoscopy can be undertaken in awake, cooperative patients. It enables visualization of the upper airway.

Ultrasound

This is useful in defining cystic or solid masses. When combined with Doppler it defines vascular lesions. It may also be used to look for calculi in the submandibular gland or duct.

Fine-needle aspiration

Fine-needle aspiration (FNA) can provide fluid for culture and sensitivity and is often used for discrete nodules or non-resolving masses suspicious for malignancy (>2 cm, non-tender, asymmetric neck masses). *Open (incisional) biopsy of suspicious lumps carries a risk of tumour seedling and should not be performed.*

Miscellaneous investigations (in outpatients)
- Videostroboscopy: used to examine vocal fold mucosa for anatomical defects, mechanical disturbances and vocal fold mucosal wave dynamics.
- Acoustic analysis: measures fundamental frequency, pitch period fluctuations or jitter, amplitude fluctuations or shimmer.
- Aerodynamic studies: these measure the mean transglottal airflow rate, glottal resistance, and subglottal pressure.
- Perceptual testing: assesses the qualitative rating of voice features.
- Laryngeal electromyography (EMG).
- Modified barium swallow and oesophagram: for oesophageal pathology, reflux, aspiration, and vascular abnormalities.
- Pulmonary function tests and flow–volume loops: identify level of obstruction and assess for intrinsic lung disease.
- Magnified airway (fluoroscopy): a dynamic evaluation of airway, assesses vocal fold motion.
- Sialography: this visualizes ductal anatomy (stones, trauma, fistulas, Sjögren's disease). It is contraindicated in acute infections.

:☠: Injuries to the front of the neck

Applied anatomy of the larynx

The larynx is a semi-rigid structure consisting of a horseshoe-shaped hyoid bone and collection of small cartilages connected by fibrous tissue.

It contains the vocal cords, 'supraglottic', and 'subglottic' spaces. The 'paraglottic' space lies between the lining mucosa and cartilages. This space is potentially very distensible from bleeding and oedema. The cricoid cartilage lies below the larynx and is the only complete ring in the respiratory tract. Airflow through a tube varies in a way similar to Poiseuille's law: flow = $p\pi r^4/8ln$, (where p is the pressure, r is the radius of the tube, l is its length, and n is the coefficient of viscosity). Small changes in the radius (e.g. from swelling/oedema) can therefore have profound effects on the flow of air through the larynx. This is important at the vocal cords, the narrowest part of the upper airway, where the mucosa can swell considerably. The hyoid bone is most commonly fractured following attempted strangulation. A fracture separating the cricoid from the trachea is referred to as laryngo-tracheal separation and is most commonly due to a clothesline-type injury.

Zones of the neck

The neck is divided into three zones:
- Zone I is located below the cricoid cartilage.
- Zone II is between the cricoid cartilage and the angle of mandible.
- Zone III is located above the angle of the mandible.

Injuries in zones I and III may require evaluation with CT or angiography as surgical exploration is difficult and risky. Zone II injuries may require CTA, MRA, oesophagoscopy, bronchoscopy, barium swallow, ultrasound, or angiography depending on the injuries suspected.

Symptoms of neck injury
- Laryngotracheal injury: hoarseness, stridor, airway obstruction, subcutaneous emphysema, pain, haemoptysis. The recurrent laryngeal nerve may also be injured.
- Oesophageal or hypopharyngeal injury: dysphagia, odynophagia, haematemesis, subcutaneous emphysema.
- Vascular injury: shock, haematoma, diminished pulses, stroke (hemiplegia).
- 5–15% of aerodigestive injuries are asymptomatic (may be missed).

Initial considerations

Neck trauma can be potentially life-threatening. Generally in penetrating injuries/lacerations, if the platysma muscle has not been breached, there is a low risk of serious injury. *Therefore, never explore a neck wound under local anaesthetic if you think it is deep to the platysma.* Many important underlying structures are at risk, especially when the injury is at the root of the neck. *Pharyngoesophageal injury is often missed and requires a high index of suspicion to diagnose.*

Blunt trauma to the front of the neck has a higher risk of laryngeal fractures than penetrating injuries. Paediatric laryngeal fractures are rare because of the elasticity of cartilage and higher position of the larynx in the neck. But significant swelling can still occur. Common causes of injury include:
- MVCs
- Sports (e.g. martial arts and racket sports)
- Assaults, knife wounds
- Attempted suicide
- Inhalation of smoke, hot air, or steam.

Types of injury that may occur following blunt trauma

- Oedema/haemorrhage. Oedema rapidly occurs particularly after thermal Inhalation. Early intubation is often necessary.
- Fractured larynx. In young patients, the larynx is elastic and tends to flex. In older patients the calcified cartilages tend to fracture.
- The hyoid bone is commonly fractured following attempted strangulation or hanging. Fractures may lacerate pharyngeal mucosa.
- The trachea can be avulsed from the cricoid cartilage (laryngo-tracheal separation) most commonly from a clothesline-type injury. Total separation is usually rapidly fatal—the trachea retracts substernally and the larynx migrates superiorly. However, with partial separation, the airway may remain patent, although it is still at high risk.
- Surgical emphysema of the neck and face may be seen after penetrating or blast injuries.
- Carotid injury is uncommon but can result in delayed dissection or rupture.
- Oesophageal injury is uncommon but rupture and mediastinitis may occur. It is an injury that is often not considered.
- Cervical spine injury should also always be considered.

Types of injury that may occur following penetrating trauma

These are highly varied depending on the method of injury (slash, stab, clothesline, projectile), direction, and depth of wound. Transverse wounds are especially worrying as many of these may be simultaneously involved. The following functional structures are all at varying degrees of risk:

- Airway
- Vascular
- Nerve(s) (hypoglossal, vagus, recurrent laryngeal, facial, brachial plexus, spinal cord)
- Thorax (lungs, pleura, mediastinum)
- Lymphatic (thoracic duct)
- Oesophageal/pharyngeal
- Cervical spine
- Muscles (SCM and prevertebral).

Assessing injuries to the front of the neck

Injuries to the front of the neck require careful assessment. Be methodical. Always start using ATLS® guidelines, paying particular attention to the airway. Consider the site and possible depth of injury (especially with penetrating injuries). Think of the various anatomical structures that may be injured and how these may be detected.

Remember that injuries to the root of neck can also involve the chest and arm.

Overview of symptoms

- Vascular structures: active bleeding, hypovolaemia, haematoma (expanding or pulsatile), peripheral pulses (compare with other side—distal carotid, superficial temporal, brachial, or radial), bruit
- Larynx/trachea, oesophagus: haemoptysis (ask patient to cough and spit on paper), air bubbling through wound/subcutaneous emphysema, hoarseness, pain on swallowing, haematemesis
- Cranial nerves: facial, glossopharyngeal (check midline position of soft palate), recurrent laryngeal (hoarseness, ineffective cough), accessory (shrug the shoulder), hypoglossal
- Spinal cord and brachial plexus, assess peripheral neurology
- Horner's syndrome (miosis, ptosis, anhidrosis, enophthalmos).

Assessing direct injuries to the larynx

The main concern is sudden loss of the airway. Consider the following:

- Mechanisms of injury: assaults, 'clothesline injury,' strangulation, penetrating injuries (gunshot wounds, knife).
- Development of oedema, and haematomas. This can occur even if there are no obvious fractures of the larynx.
- Obvious injuries to the larynx have a high risk of airway compromise—ask for immediate help.

- Hyoid and thyroid fractures may lacerate pharyngeal mucosa, which may be asymptomatic.
- Cricotracheal separation is highly unstable. Be careful during examination.
- Pharyngoesophageal tears are often missed.
- Recurrent laryngeal nerve injury.

Investigations

These are tailored to the injuries suspected. CT (with contrast) is usually a good starting point and can rapidly assess both the neck and thorax. Always follow local policy. Useful investigations include:

- Fibreoptic nasopharyngoscope: allows visualization of the endolarynx with minimal risk to airway, evaluates mobility, lacerations, airway patency, laryngeal oedema, and haematomas.
- CT of neck: diagnostic test of choice to evaluate laryngeal fractures (hyoid bone, thyroid, and cricoid cartilage).
- Oesophagram with water-soluble contrast (avoid barium as there is a risk of mediastinitis if there is a leak).
- Direct laryngoscopy and oesophagoscopy.

Management principles

- Protect the airway and stabilize the cervical spine (ABCs): endotracheal intubation may precipitate an airway crisis. In some cases a surgical airway under local anaesthesia may be safer. Get senior help.
- Laryngeal/tracheal injury: seek senior anaesthetic help early as swelling may result in delayed obstruction. These require urgent referral.
- Pharyngoesophageal injury: primary closure if <24 hours, otherwise consider drainage procedure, reconstruction, or oesophagectomy.
- Vertebral artery injury: embolization is preferred due to difficult exposure and control. If this fails, consider surgical repair.
- Carotid injury: associated with high mortality (10–20%); primary repair is the treatment of choice, otherwise consider patch grafting, by-pass grafting, or ligation (avoid ligation if suspected stroke).
- Spinal/brachial plexus injury: these require referral to a specialist unit. Protect the neck/arm, to avoid movement. Document deficits.
- Remember the chest, especially with penetrating injuries.

Non-surgical management

This may be possible with small soft tissue injuries (haematomas), and stable laryngeal fractures with an intact endolarynx. Patients are admitted for observation with a tracheostomy set at bedside. They should be kept NBM, with the head of the bed elevated, voice rest, and given humidified air. Prophylactic antibiotics, antireflux medications, and systemic corticosteroids may also be required.

Indications for surgical exploration include:

- Airway: compromise, hoarseness, progressive surgical emphysema
- Breathing: pneumothorax, pneumomediastinum
- Circulation: expanding haematoma, pulse deficit, active bleeding, haemoptysis, haematemesis

- Specific injuries: (bullet, knife, other); suspected foreign body
- Specific laryngeal findings: disrupted anterior commissure, exposed cartilage, progressive subcutaneous emphysema, fractured/dislocated laryngeal skeleton, dislocated arytenoids, vocal fold immobility.

Urgent tracheostomy under local anaesthesia may rarely be required to protect the airway. Ideally laryngeal injuries should be repaired within 2–3 days to avoid infection and necrosis. Endoscopic repair may be attempted for smaller mucosal disruptions and repositioning of arytenoids.

Beware of the patient who presents with surgical emphysema following blunt neck trauma. If untreated, this can result in tension pneumothorax or cardiac tamponade.

Difficulty breathing, noisy breathing, and upper airway obstruction

Not all noisy breathing is stridor. Moist sounds such as bubbling of secretions in the larynx or pharynx are common and not significant.

⬤ Stridor

Stridor is an abnormal, high-pitched, musical breathing sound caused by a narrowing of upper airway. Children are at high risk because they have narrower airways. *In young children, stridor should be regarded as an emergency and treated immediately.*

⬤ Stertor

Stertor is a low-pitched snoring or snuffly sound produced by vibrations of tissues in the nasopharynx, pharynx, or soft palate.

Stridor and stertor are both due to turbulence of the air flow within a partially obstructed respiratory tract (Table 5.1). Bernoulli's theorem—if air passes through a narrow tube, its velocity increases at the narrowing and its pressure falls. This results in collapse of the airway.

Table 5.1 Noisy breathing and the possible site of airway obstruction

Site of obstruction	Characteristics of stridor
Nasopharyngeal	Stertor with no gurgling
Oropharynx	Gurgly stertor with hot potato voice
Supraglottic	Inspiratory stridor with hot potato voice
Glottic	Inspiratory with hoarseness
Subglottic/trachea	Biphasic stridor with barking cough
Tracheobronchial	Expiratory stridor with wheezing

Assessment of stridor

This is tailored according to the suspected cause:
- Head and neck examination: oral cavity (macroglossia, tonsillar hypertrophy, or infection), complete neurological exam (cranial nerves), evaluate for external compression (trachea midline, goitre, palpable laryngeal fractures).
- Nasal exam/nasal endoscopy, for deformities/masses.
- Fibreoptic laryngoscopy: assess patency, vocal fold mobility, supraglottis, examine tracheal stoma (retroflex to access subglottis).
- Cardiac and pulmonary examination (wheezing, chest pain).
- Direct laryngoscopy: evaluation of the glottis and supraglottic.
- Bronchoscopy (rigid bronchoscopy for instrumentation).
- CXR and plain neck films: screening films for laryngotracheal structural defects, intrinsic lung and mediastinal disease.
- CT/MRI of the neck/chest.
- Arteriography: indicated if vascular abnormalities are suspected.

Upper airway obstruction

Upper airway obstruction (UAO) is a life-threatening emergency that requires prompt diagnosis and treatment. There are many causes, see Table 5.2. Severe UAO can be surprisingly asymptomatic at rest if it develops gradually. Sudden clinical deterioration is unpredictable.

Table 5.2 Causes of upper airway obstruction based on aetiology

Traumatic causes	Infections	Iatrogenic causes	Tumours	Angio-oedema
Laryngeal stenosis	Suppurative parotitis	Tracheal stenosis post-tracheostomy	Laryngeal tumours (benign or malignant)	Anaphylactic reactions
Airway burn	Retro-pharyngeal abscess	Tracheal stenosis post-intubation	Laryngeal papillomatosis	C1 inhibitor deficiency
Acute laryngeal injury	Tonsillar hypertrophy	Mucous ball from transtracheal catheter	Tracheal stenosis (caused by intrinsic or extrinsic tumours)	ACE inhibitors
Facial trauma (mandibular or maxillary fractures)	Ludwig's angina	Foreign bodies		
Haemorrhage	Epiglottitis	Vocal cord paralysis		
	Laryngitis			
	Laryngo-tracheo-bronchitis (croup)			
	Diphtheria			

Patients with possible UAO must never be sedated until the airway is secured. Sedation may precipitate acute respiratory failure. Some pharmacological interventions (adrenaline (epinephrine), steroids, and heliox) provide temporary support but cannot significantly improve mechanical causes of UAO.

☼ Croup (laryngotracheobronchitis)

This is an acute viral infection of the upper airway. There is swelling inside the throat, which produces the classical symptoms of a 'barking' cough (worse on crying), stridor, and hoarseness. It may produce mild, moderate, or severe symptoms, often worse at night. Diagnosis is often clinical but the causes previously listed must be carefully excluded. Management includes keeping the child as calm as possible, steroids, and adrenaline (epinephrine) in severe cases. Check oxygen saturation. Severe croup may require admission. Inhalation of hot steam or humidified air may soothe symptoms. Refer to paediatrics for advice.

☼ Epiglottitis (supraglottitis)

(See ➔ Chapter 8, pp. 246–7.) This is a potentially life-threatening disorder. It is typically caused by *Haemophilus influenzae* type B. Non-infectious causes of epiglottitis may include trauma, inhalation and chemical burns, or be associated with systemic disease.

(see http://www.rch.org.au/clinicalguide/guideline_index/Acute_Upper_Airway_Obstruction/; http://www.das.uk.com/guidelines/guidelineshome.html).

Initial management of stridor

These patients can rapidly deteriorate, so call for senior help urgently.

- Evaluate the airway: quickly determine severity of obstruction and stability of airway (acute vs chronic, progression of stridor, dyspnoea at rest vs with exercise).
- Establish the airway: complete anoxia can result in death in 4–5 minutes. Following injury, secure the airway without moving the cervical spine. Do not precipitate an airway crisis. *Any attempt at endotracheal intubation should also have a backup plan for an emergent surgical airway.* Initially suction blood clots and secretions from the oropharynx (remove foreign bodies and teeth). Overcome pharyngeal collapse with jaw thrust and chin lift. Masked ventilation may provide adequate oxygenation until able to secure.
- Administer oxygen. Masked ventilation may adequately improve oxygenation until help is available to secure airway. After establishing a secure airway, ease of ventilation and maintenance of oxygenation should be reassessed.
- In some cases heliox (80% helium, 20% oxygen) may be used to provide short-term oxygenation in stable airway obstructions. The O_2 concentration may be increased to 40%. Helium has a lower molecular weight (decreased density) allowing easier passage past narrow obstructions.

- Consider humidification, corticosteroids, nebulized adrenaline (epinephrine), and antibiotics.
- Once the airway is secure, further imaging may be required to identify the precise cause of obstruction (if not apparent).

☉ Subglottic stenosis

The subglottic area is circumferentially bound by the cricoid cartilage and is the narrowest part of the upper airway in infants (whereas the glottis is the narrowest in adults). It is a complete non-pliable ring, unlike the trachea, which has a posterior membranous section, and the larynx, which has a posterior muscular section. Narrowing of the subglottic area may be congenital or acquired. Acquired stenosis (subglottic stenosis (SGS)) is caused by either infection or trauma. Iatrogenic injuries play a major role.

Congenital

Stenosis can be either membranous or cartilaginous. Membranous stenosis is usually circumferential and may extend upward to include the true vocal folds. In cartilaginous stenosis, thickening of cricoid cartilage is seen. This is less common than membranous stenosis.

Acquired

Historically, acquired SGS has been related to infections such as TB and diphtheria which are very rare now. Stenosis today is more often caused by endotracheal intubation or high tracheotomy tube placement. Irritation causes inflammation which progress to ischaemia, ulceration, and granulation tissue, resulting in stenosis and occlusion of the airway. Additional factors include systemic illness, malnutrition, anaemia, and hypoxia. Often, SGS has an insidious onset, and early manifestations are mistaken for other disorders (asthma, COPD). Patients with mild stenosis are usually asymptomatic, and only diagnosed following difficult intubation during anaesthesia. Symptoms otherwise include dyspnoea, stridor, hoarseness, brassy cough, recurrent pneumonitis, and cyanosis. The Cotton–Myers grading classifies obstruction into grade I (0–50%), grade II (51–70%), grade III (71–99%), and grade IV (100% of the lumen, i.e. no detectable lumen) (data from *Annals of Otology, Rhinology & Laryngology*, 103, 4, Charles M. Myer, David M. O'Connor, Robin T. Cotton, 'Proposed Grading System for Subglottic Stenosis Based on Endotracheal Tube Sizes', pp. 319–323. Copyright (1994) Sage Publications).

Management

Medical therapy is almost always unsuccessful. For mild or granular stenosis, serial endoscopic dilation with or without steroid injections may be sufficient. Carbon dioxide laser and topical mitomycin C are showing promising results with endoscopic approaches. Reconstruction may be necessary for mature and circumferential stenosis which is severe (>70% luminal obstruction). The goals of open reconstruction are preservation of the voice by expanding the subglottic airway and stabilizing the expanded frame. Various procedures exist using grafts and stents.

✪ The acutely swollen neck

Ludwig's angina

This is a rapidly spreading, tense cellulitis of the submandibular, sublingual, and submental spaces bilaterally. When advanced it is an obvious diagnosis, with gross swelling both in the neck and the mouth. Earlier infections still need to be treated seriously and need urgent referral. *Ludwig's angina is a potential airway emergency which if not diagnosed and treated quickly has a mortality rate of around 75% within the first 12–24 hours.* With aggressive surgical intervention, good airway control, and antibiotics this rate has now dropped to 5%.

Usually the cause is a submandibular space infection secondary to an infected wisdom tooth. Other causes include tonsillitis, infected mandibular fractures, and submandibular sialadenitis. From the submandibular space, the infection spreads to the ipsilateral sublingual space around the deep lobe of the submandibular gland. It then passes to the contralateral sublingual space and thence to the adjacent submandibular space. The submental space is also affected by lymphatic spread. Infection can also originate in the sublingual space and spread laterally to both sides.

Left untreated, oedema and cellulitis spread backwards in the space between the hypoglossus and genioglossus to the epiglottis and larynx, resulting eventually in respiratory obstruction.

Clinical features
- Systemic upset.
- Massive firm swelling bilaterally in the neck.
- Swelling in the floor of the mouth, forcing of the tongue up onto the palate.
- A 'hot-potato' voice. This term is used to describe the characteristic pattern of speech, which has been likened to a person speaking with a hot potato in the mouth. It has several causes in addition to Ludwig's angina.
- Difficulty in swallowing and drooling.
- Inability to protrude the tongue.
- Eventually this leads to difficulty breathing.

Indicators of severe infection in the neck
- Difficulty breathing
- Shock
- Pyrexia
- Malaise
- Dysphagia/drooling
- Trismus
- Dysphonia
- Inability to protrude the tongue
- High WCC.

Management
The first consideration is the airway which can rapidly obstruct. *Difficulty in breathing, swallowing, or talking, and gross swelling are all indications to call for senior help (often anaesthetic) urgently.* Refer to maxillofacial or ENT team urgently. Further management includes IV fluids (patients often present after a few days, having not been able to drink), IV antibiotics (e.g. penicillin and metronidazole), together with surgical drainage of the submandibular and sublingual spaces and removal of the underlying cause. If there is respiratory difficulty, give oxygen. These cases are commonly associated with self-neglect (including alcohol and smoking) and immunosuppression (e.g. diabetes).

☼ Infections deep in the neck

These can be easily overlooked. They usually arise following penetrating injuries, untreated tonsillitis or wisdom tooth infections. *Once established, the infection can rapidly spread throughout the neck into the chest and become life-threatening.* When this occurs mortality is high. In the early stages diagnosis can be difficult.

Applied anatomy
The neck may be regarded as containing superficial and deep fascial planes. These divide it into several specific compartments. Terminology can be confusing.

Superficial cervical fascia
This does not play a major role in deep neck infections. It encircles the neck, blending with the fascia overlying the platysma muscle. Superiorly it blends with the muscles of the face comprising part of the 'SMAS' (superficial muscular aponeurotic system). This layer is important in certain types of 'face lift' procedures.

Deep cervical fascia
This is subdivided into three additional layers:
- The most superficial layer of the deep cervical fascia is also known as the investing cervical fascia. This encircles the neck like a stocking, attaching to and enclosing the SCM, trapezius, and omohyoid muscles and the parotid and submandibular glands. Posteriorly it attaches to the superior nuchal line. It can only distend a small amount.
- The middle layer of the deep cervical fascia is also known as the visceral layer. It encircles the strap muscles and the viscera of the neck (larynx, pharynx, trachea, and thyroid gland). Part of this layer covers the pharyngeal constrictors and the buccinator muscle—the buccopharyngeal fascia.
- The deep layer of the deep cervical fascia is also called the prevertebral fascia. It lies just anterior to the prevertebral muscles of the spine allowing the pharynx to glide over them during neck movements and swallowing.

These deep fascial planes divide the neck into several compartments, called 'fascial tissue spaces'. In the early stages of infection, the fascial layers limit the spread of infection to within the associated compartment. However, untreated infection will eventually perforate the fascia and spread more rapidly. Both the middle and deep layers pass into the chest (Figures 5.2 and 5.3). *One fascial space (the retropharyngeal) also passes into the mediastinum. Deep neck infections can therefore result in mediastinitis.*

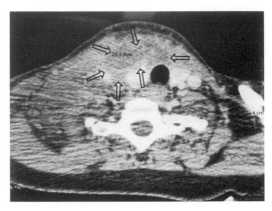

Figure 5.2 CT scan showing large abscess deep to the SCM muscle.

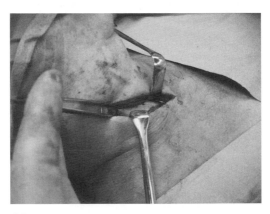

Figure 5.3 Operative finding showing a huge collection of pus.

Commonly infected fascial tissue spaces in the neck

The mylohyoid muscle has been described as the 'diaphragm' of the mouth, separating the oral cavity from the neck. It creates two large (and two of the most commonly involved) spaces. These are the sublingual space above the muscle and the submandibular and submental spaces below it.

Submandibular space

This is triangular in shape, bounded superiorly by the mylohyoid muscle medially and the mandible laterally, and the deep cervical fascia below. It contains lymph nodes, the superficial lobe of the submandibular glands, and blood vessels. It communicates with the sublingual space above, and the deep pterygoid space posteriorly.

Surgical access can be made 2–3 cm below the lower border of the mandible (to avoid injury to the mandibular branch of the facial nerve). Skin and subcutaneous tissues are incised. Blunt forceps penetrate the deep cervical fascia, aiming towards the mandibular border.

Submental space

This is contained by the two anterior bellies of the digastric muscles. Above is the mylohyoid muscle, and below the deep cervical fascia covered by platysma and skin. It contains submental lymph nodes and communicates posteriorly with the submandibular space.

Surgical access is obtained behind the chin prominence in the neck.

Signs and symptoms in deep neck infections

These can be deceptive. Fever, malaise, dehydration, and lethargy are common and patients rapidly become very ill. *A very high WCC (>20) is an ominous sign and often indicates tissue necrosis and a high risk of mortality. Pain on swallowing should be taken seriously.* It can be so severe that the patient sits drooling, and unable to swallow their own saliva. There may be cellulitis. Deep-seated abscesses do not fluctuate. Instead swelling presents with a 'dough-like' consistency. Initially the fascia may direct swelling medially, compromising the airway. Other important signs of symptoms include dysphagia and trismus. Untreated (if airway obstruction or sepsis does not kill the patient), erosion into the carotid vessels can result in septic emboli and stroke.

Management

Assess immediately for airway obstruction and when necessary consider urgent intubation or a surgical airway. *Get senior help.* Once the airway is secure, assess the patient's haemodynamic status and give fluids. Often they have sat at home for a few days unable to eat and drink so will probably be at least mildly dehydrated. These patients need to be admitted urgently. Start IV antibiotics. Consider immunosuppression (diabetes, alcoholics, long-term steroids, HIV etc.)

CT of the neck and chest is usually required to determine the extent of infection. Aggressive surgical drainage and removal of dead tissue is usually required, even if there is only cellulitis. By opening tissue planes not only is pus released but tissue perfusion is improved by reducing tension. The surgical approach depends on the location of the abscess. Some can be drained intraorally, eliminating a scar. However, drainage via a neck incision is more common, with placement of large drains.

There is some evidence that hyperbaric oxygen may be beneficial, but this is a controversial issue. Only in very mild cases can patients be managed conservatively, if so they must be watched very closely. In selected cases ultrasound guided aspiration may avoid aggressive surgery.

Choice of antibiotics
Since many infections originate as dental, pharyngeal, or tonsillar infections, coverage should include organisms known to affect these areas. Most infections will be mixed and will include Gram-positive cocci and anaerobes. If necessary, discuss with maxillofacial/ENT or microbiology.

Some specific types of neck infection

☼ Necrotizing fasciitis
This is a rare but potentially life-threatening mixed infection, characterized by necrosis of the fascia and subcutaneous tissues.

Untreated, the condition can spread rapidly with a mortality approaching 40%. Although it is more commonly seen in the groin, it can occur in the neck where it is nearly always due to an underlying dental infection. Patients often have an underlying predisposition such as diabetes, alcoholism. or chronic malnutrition.

Clinically the overlying skin is often pale and mottled or may appear dusky due to thrombosis of underlying vessels. Blisters and ulceration may develop. Complications include:
• Systemic toxicity
• Lung abscess
• Carotid artery erosion, with haemorrhage or septic emboli
• Jugular vein thrombosis and mediastinitis.

Treatment involves IV antibiotics, wide surgical debridement. and in some cases hyperbaric oxygen. Any underlying predisposition must be managed as well.

① Acute bacterial submandibular sialadenitis
The majority of these infections are secondary to a calculus (stone) in the duct. Other causes include surgical scarring or strictures secondary to radiation or other causes of chronic fibrosis. The whole gland swells up and there is malaise, pyrexia, and pain. Submandibular calculi are opaque in 80% of cases, so a radiograph may aid in the diagnosis. Antibiotics are required. If the stone is easily felt in the mouth it can be removed intraorally. If the infection leads to a collection, then incision and drainage of the submandibular space must be carried out, and the gland removed on an elective basis later. Mumps virus infection involving the submandibular gland is rare but has been reported.

⑦ Chronic submandibular sialadenitis (Kuttner's tumour)

This results from repeated episodes of acute sialadenitis. The structure, parenchyma, and function of the gland are gradually destroyed. The gland ends up feeling very hard to palpation. Treatment is by surgical excision.

⑦ Lump(s) in the neck

An important consideration

One of the most important considerations in an adult presenting with a lump in the neck is that it may be a metastatic lymph node. In such cases the primary cancer is often in the upper respiratory or alimentary tract. The risk is high in smokers and heavy drinkers. The primary tumour must then be found quickly (by imaging, examination under anaesthesia, and panendoscopy). Around half of malignancies can be found by careful clinical examination alone. Endoscopy of the upper aerodigestive tract will find it in another 10–20%. FNA cytology of a lump may be useful.

There are many different causes for a lump in the neck, but by far the commonest is an enlarged lymph node (benign or malignant).

Some key points
- In patients over 40, 75% of lateral neck masses are caused by malignant tumours.
- In the absence of obvious infection, a lateral neck mass is malignant until proven otherwise (metastatic squamous cell carcinoma or lymphoma).
- Open biopsy of a node should be avoided (risk of tumour seeding).

Applied anatomy

The neck is the link between head and trunk. It therefore contains vital neurovascular structures within a relatively confined space. The surrounding musculoskeletal system not only protects these structures, but also allows mobility of the head while helping in breathing, swallowing, and speech. The neck has an extensive lymphatic supply with around 300 lymph nodes distributed on both sides.

Triangles of the neck
The neck is divided into anterior and posterior triangles by the obliquely running SCM muscle (Figure 5.4). These are further subdivided into submental, submandibular, carotid, muscular, occipital, and subclavian triangles . . . but these subdivisions are often regarded as unnecessary from a clinical perspective.

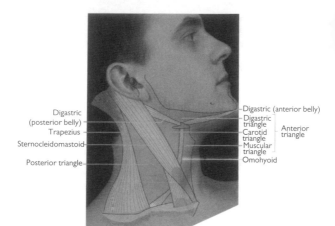

Digastric (posterior belly)

Trapezius

Sternocleidomastoid

Posterior triangle

Digastric (anterior belly)
Digastric triangle
Carotid triangle
Muscular triangle
Omohyoid

Anterior triangle

Figure 5.4 Triangles of the neck.

Reproduced from Ellis H. and Mahadevan V., *Clinical Anatomy*, Thirteenth Edition, Figure 187, copyright (2013) with permission from John Wiley and Sons.

Overview of the anterior triangle

The anterior triangle is bounded superiorly by the inferior border of the mandible; posteriorly by anterior border of the SCM muscle; and anteriorly by the midline. This may be further subdivided into submental, digastric, carotid, and muscular triangles by the digastric muscle and the hyoid bone. Clinically this subdivision is not necessary.

Contents of importance

- Suprahyoid muscles: digastric, stylohyoid, geniohyoid, mylohyoid (forming the diaphragm of the floor of the mouth).
- Infrahyoid muscles (the 'strap muscles'): sternohyoid, omohyoid, thyrohyoid, sternohyoid.
- Carotid sheath: runs from the level of the sternoclavicular joint to the bifurcation of the common carotid artery (at the level of the upper border of the thyroid cartilage at C3 vertebra).
- Common carotid artery dividing into internal carotid (no extra-cranial branches) and external carotid artery.
- Internal jugular vein (IJV): surface markings run from the ear lobe to the sternal end of the clavicle. The deep cervical lymph nodes are adjacent to the vein throughout its course. On the left-hand side the thoracic duct crosses behind the vein at the level of C7 vertebra.
- Anterior jugular veins: commencing beneath the chin, running inferiorly to the suprasternal region.
- Vagus nerve, runs in the groove between the common carotid artery and the IJV.

- Phrenic nerve 'C3, C4, and C5 keep the diaphragm alive'.
- Hypoglossal nerve: emerges between the internal carotid artery and the IJV in the upper part of the neck. It lays on the carotid sheath deep to the posterior digastric and passes forwards beneath the tendon of digastric to provide motor innervation to the tongue.
- Cervical lymph nodes: levels I to IV.
- Submandibular salivary gland: this comprises a large superficial part and smaller deep part that wraps around the posterior border of mylohyoid. Its duct runs forwards in the floor of the mouth, crossing the lingual nerve, to open in the anterior floor of mouth.
- Parotid: the lower pole, or tail, can pass into the neck, just below the earlobe. The lower branches of the facial nerve pass through and both can be injured by penetrating injuries in this region.
- Thyroid: a bi-lobed endocrine gland united in the midline by its isthmus, overlying the second to fourth tracheal rings. Pathological enlargement of the gland may displace other structures in the neck.
- Parathyroids: small glandular tissue lying on the posterior aspects of the lateral thyroid lobes—normally four (90% of population).
- Trachea: continues from larynx at the level of C6. A vital site for urgent and elective surgical airways.
- Oesophagus: behind the trachea, a continuity of the pharynx at the level of C6. The recurrent laryngeal nerves run on each side in the groove between the oesophagus and trachea.

Overview of the posterior triangle

The posterior triangle is a spiral that passes from its apex at the back of the skull to its base in the front at the root of the neck. It is bounded anteriorly by the posterior border of SCM, posteriorly by the anterior border of the trapezius muscle, and below by the lateral part of the clavicle. Its roof is formed by the investing layer of deep cervical fascia, and its floor by the prevertebral fascia.

Contents of importance

- Third part of the subclavian artery—runs very low in the posterior triangle at the level of the clavicle; just above the clavicle the suprascapular and transverse cervical vessels pass.
- External jugular vein—runs through the anterior/inferior part of the triangle to drain into the subclavian vein which lies more inferiorly and is not included in the posterior triangle.
- Occipital, transverse cervical, suprascapular, and subclavian arteries.
- Accessory nerve emerges from the posterior border of SCM at the junction of its upper and middle thirds. It runs vertically down (over the levator scapulae) to enter the anterior border of trapezius usually 5–6 cm above the clavicle.
- Cervical plexus branches:
  - Muscular branches
  - A loop from C1 to hypoglossal
  - C2/3 branches to SCM and C3/4 to trapezius
  - Inferior root of ansa cervicalis

- Phrenic nerve (C3, C4, and C5)—runs from lateral to medial over scalenus anterior.
- Cutaneous branches
- Lesser occipital nerve (C2)—posterior part of the neck to the superior nuchal line, and behind the auricle
- Great auricular nerve (C2 and C3)—skin over the angle of the mandible and parotid gland, and the auricle
- Transverse cervical (C2 and C3)—skin in the midline of the neck
- Supraclavicular nerve (C3 and C4)—root of neck/upper chest.
- Brachial plexus trunks: the three trunks of the brachial plexus along with the cervical plexus are held down to the prevertebral muscles by the covering of prevertebral fascia that forms the floor of the posterior triangle. Strictly speaking they are not contents of this triangle, but are mentioned, however, because of their anatomical importance in penetrating injuries.
- Omohyoid muscle: posterior belly. From its origin at the hyoid bone it passes deep to the SCM, coming to lie over the carotid sheath. As it overlies the IJV the fibres form a flat tendon (the 'intermediate tendon') that is a useful maker during neck dissections of the vein's position. The muscle is held down to the clavicle at the intermediate tendon by a fascial sling.
- Cervical lymph nodes: level V.

Miscellaneous anatomical structures and an overview of causes of lumps

Sternomastoid muscle

This muscle arises from the manubrium sterni and the medial clavicle. It passes superoposteriorly as a fleshy belly, which inserts into the mastoid process and the superior nuchal line of the occipital bone. The triangular gap between the two heads of origin of the SCM overlays the IJV—this site may be used for central venous access.

The strip of anatomy deep to the SCM should not be forgotten. Essentially the lower half covers the carotid sheath containing the common carotid artery, the IJV, and the vagus nerve, and the upper half lies over the emerging cervical plexus.

Omohyoid

The omohyoid muscle consists of two bellies, an inferior belly from the scapula, which ends in a middle tendon, and a superior belly, which continues from the tendon to the hyoid bone. The middle tendon, situated deep to the SCM, is attached by fascia to the manubrium, first costal cartilage, and clavicle.

Platysma

The platysma is a subcutaneous, quadrilateral muscular sheet which arises from the skin over the deltoid muscle and the pectoralis major and is inserted into the lower border of the mandible and the skin around the mouth. It is supplied by the cervical branch of the facial nerve. It raises the skin, thereby probably relieving pressure on the underlying veins.

Causes of lumps in the neck

Not all lumps in the neck are lymph nodes. Although lymphadenopathy is the commonest cause of a neck lump, it is important to be mindful of other causes:

- Developmental: branchial cyst, haemangioma, laryngocoele, teratoma, thyroglossal duct cyst, cervical rib
- Skin and subcutaneous tissues: sebaceous cyst, lipoma
- Infected lymph nodes:
  • Viral: Epstein–Barr virus, HIV
  • Bacterial: *Staphylococcus*, TB, cat scratch, *Brucella*
  • Protozoa: toxoplasma, leishmaniasis
  • fungal: histoplasmosis, blastomycosis, coccidioidomycosis
- Neoplastic lymph nodes: lymphoma, metastasis
- Granulomatous lymph nodes: sarcoid, foreign body reaction, etc.
- Paraganglioma, vascular tumours, etc.
- Carotid sheath: aneurysm, carotid body tumour, vagal or sympathetic neuroma
- Salivary gland (parotid or submandibular):
  • Infective: sialadenitis, sialolithiasis
  • Autoimmune: Sjögren's syndrome, neoplastic
- Miscellaneous: AIDS-related disease, Kawasaki disease, plunging ranula, thyroid, parathyroid, thymus, subclavian aneurysm.

Assessing a neck lump

History

Even with an obvious lump, take a full medical history. This will ensure that coexisting diseases and other possible causes of the lump are not overlooked. TB, for example, is still a common cause of cervical lymph adenopathy and can affect the administration of general anaesthesia. Smoking and alcohol are important in head and neck malignancy. Some animals (cats) can pass on infections (toxoplasmosis). Travel abroad may result in unusual infections.

Useful information when diagnosing neck lumps

Age

This may be a useful guide:

- <16 years: cervical lymphadenopathy secondary to infection is the commonest cause of neck lumps in this age group, followed by congenital and developmental lesions. Neoplastic disease can still occur (leukaemia/lymphoma) but is less common.
- 16–40 years: inflammatory lesions are still the most common followed by developmental lesions. Neoplasia is next most common with benign disease seen slightly more than malignant disease.
- >40 years: neoplasia is the most common cause of neck swellings with malignant disease predominating.

How long has the lump been present?
Was it acute in onset or a gradual increase over many months or years? Developmental lesions tend to gradually increase in size becoming increasingly troublesome. Inflammatory causes tend to develop rapidly and are often associated with pain.

Is it painful?
Cervical lymphadenopathy secondary to infection and inflammatory salivary gland disease often present with painful swellings. Metastatic lesions in the neck are rarely painful unless associated with secondary infection or malignant invasion of local nerves.

Does it vary in size?
Has the lump gradually increased in size, or does it increase and then decrease in size at different times of the day? Ask particularly about mealtimes as obstructive sialadenitis secondary to sialolithiasis (salivary stones) is quite common and often presents as submandibular swelling worse at mealtimes.

Does the patient have foul breath (halitosis) or a foul taste in their mouth?
Submandibular gland infection may discharge pus in the mouth, resulting in a foul tasting discharge. Similarly, a pharyngeal pouch can become secondarily infected as a result of food stagnation; the patient (usually elderly) will present with halitosis, dysphagia, and a painful neck swelling just anterior to SCM.

Ask about sore throat, unilateral hearing loss, earache, and hoarseness
These may indicate underlying malignancy.

Other symptoms of systemic upset
Are there other infective symptoms present: malaise, fever, and lethargy? Cervical lymphadenopathy may represent a generalized viral infection, e.g. glandular fever (late teens).

Has the patient travelled overseas recently?

Are there other features of malignant disease?
Weight loss/cachexia, lethargy, malaise. Generalized lymphadenopathy, sweating, skin itching associated with lymphoma.

Are there features of thyroid disease?
Thyrotoxic (tremor, tachycardia/atrial fibrillation, perspiration, lid lag, thyroid eye disease, bruit), hypothyroid (dry hair/skin, xanthelasma, puffy face, croaky voice).

Examination
Examine the entire head and neck including the throat, mouth, and teeth (infections and malignancy). This is discussed in detail in the relevant chapters. You may also need to examine other body sites and systems (lymphadenopathy, abdominal masses, liver, spleen, etc.). Fibreoptic nasendoscopy may also be required to assess the nasopharynx for occult primary tumours. This requires specialist training.

Neck node levels
Clinically, the deep cervical lymph nodes are divided into five levels. This classification is important in the management of some cancers of the head and neck.

Investigations
These are tailored according to the suspected cause.

Plain films
OPT and CXR are usually required to assess the dentition and look for lung pathology (tumours/infections).

CT scanning
CT scanning is exceptionally useful in assessing the extent of neck swellings particularly invasion into deeper tissues. However, artefact produced by metal in dental restorations often cause problems when investigating lesions in the floor of the mouth and upper neck.

MRI
MRI is useful in the head and neck as it produces images with excellent soft tissue definition. It is particularly useful in the assessment of salivary glands and other neck masses. Remember that its use is contraindicated in patients with metal implants such as aneurysm clips or cardiac pacemakers.

Fine-needle aspiration
A fine-bore needle ('green' gauge) attached to a 20 mL syringe is passed into the mass while it is immobilized between the fingers of the other hand. Negative pressure is applied by withdrawing the plunger of the syringe, thus collecting cells from the lesion into the needle/syringe. The sample is placed on a microscope slide and viewed by a histopathologist. Comment can then be made as to whether the cells show malignant features or not. This is quite an 'operator-sensitive' technique and on occasion a non-diagnostic sample is taken.

Ultrasound
Ultrasound is useful for distinguishing between solid and cystic lesions and may be used to guide biopsy needles to sample masses or aspirate collections. It is particularly useful in the investigation of salivary gland lesions as it can often distinguish between suspected inflammation and tumours. Ultrasound may also be able to distinguish whether a suspected tumour is benign or malignant.

Sialography
Sialography involves the injection of a radiopaque medium into salivary ducts which are then visualized with image intensification or plain films. It is a useful process in the investigation of neck swellings when stones, strictures, or intrinsic salivary gland pathology are suspected. Acute infection and iodine sensitivity are contraindications to sialography.

Examination under anaesthesia
This may be required to look for tumours of the upper aerodigestive tract, not visible by other means. It also allows for biopsy at difficult to reach sites (tongue base/supraglottic, etc.)

⑦ Lymphadenopathy

> *Lymphadenopathy in the neck (especially supraclavicular) can arise from disease both above and below the collar bones.*

Enlarged cervical lymph nodes (cervical lymphadenopathy), is the most common cause of a lump(s) in the neck. Lymphadenopathy in the neck (especially supraclavicular) can arise from disease both above and below the collar bones (e.g. bronchial/gastric malignancy). The two common causes of lymphadenopathy are infections and tumours.

Causes of enlarged lymph nodes

Local causes
- Local infection—dental, tonsillitis, skin sepsis
- TB neck nodes
- Neoplastic—lymphoma or metastatic (anywhere in head and neck)
- Intraparotid nodes (may occur with facial skin cancers)
- Supraclavicular lymph node (Virchow's node) can arise from disease both *above* and *below* the collar bones (e.g. bronchial/gastric malignancy).

Generalized causes
- URTI
- Infective mononucleosis
- Toxoplasma
- Cat scratch
- HIV
- Sarcoidosis
- Lymphomas (Hodgkin's disease, non-Hodgkin's lymphoma)
- Lymphatic leukaemia.

⑦ Infections causing lymphadenopathy

Acute infections are the commonest cause of lymph node enlargement in patients under 40. They are generally viral (colds, glandular fever, etc.) or bacterial (dental infections, tonsillitis, and scalp infections such as impetigo). TB is a chronic inflammatory cause that has seen an increase in incidence in recent years. TB lymph nodes tend to be firm and indurated and often give rise to sinuses. Clinically they may appear malignant.

Bacterial cervical adenitis
- Pathogens: most commonly group A streptococci and *Staphylococcus aureus.*
- Symptoms: tender, mobile lump, associated with constitutional symptoms (malaise, fever). Diagnosis is usually clinically but aspiration for culture and sensitivity may be required.
- Complications: untreated can rapidly progress to spreading infection, such as Ludwig's angina or generalized sepsis.
- Treatment: may require incision and drainage. All require antibiotics and treatment of the underlying cause (most commonly tooth/tonsil).

Atypical mycobacteria
- Pathogens: *Mycobacterium avium, M. scrofulaceum, M. intracellulare*. These are less virulent than *M. tuberculosis*. However they are also less responsive to antituberculosis medications.
- Common in children, immunocompromised, or those who travel abroad.
- Symptoms: unilateral cervical adenopathy (adherent to overlying skin with purplish discolouration). Induration and adherence are also features of malignancy and can cause diagnostic confusion.
- Diagnosis: clinical, culture requires 2–4 weeks, tuberculin testing is often negative.
- Treatment: these should be discussed with your local microbiologist. Often complete excision (avoid incision and drainage) is required in addition to antibiotics (may consider rifampin or macrolides for 3–6 months)

Non-specific lymphadenitis
This is a reactive adenitis, typically secondary to a nasopharyngeal or oropharyngeal infection, although it may also occur from any infection of the head and neck. The primary infection may have resolved leaving persistent, enlarged cervical lymph nodes. These may be confused with malignant lymph nodes (and vice versa) and therefore require a detailed clinical history and careful examination of the entire head and neck for primary infection or a tumour. FNA cytology may be required. Large nodes may be removed to enable a more precise diagnosis.

Cervical adenopathy in the patient with HIV
This carries a risk for lymphoma, atypical mycobacterium, carcinoma, and TB. Excision biopsy should be reserved for highly suspicious lesions.

Persistent generalized lymphadenopathy (PGL)
- Cervical adenopathy is the third most common lymphatic site (axillary and inguinal more common).
- Symptoms: typically asymptomatic adenopathy.
- Diagnosis: based on clinical history and exam. Neoplastic and infectious causes must be ruled out. Must have adenopathy of two or more sites for greater than 3 months
- Treatment: observation.

Cat-scratch disease
This is a self-limiting condition caused by the cat-scratch bacillus (bacillus angiomatosis). Symptoms include cutaneous lesions at primary site, tender cervical adenopathy, mild fever, and malaise. Diagnosis includes culture and cat-scratch antigen testing, together with a history of cat exposure. Treatment is generally supportive. Avoid incision and drainage to prevent sinus formation. If a specimen is required, consider aspiration.

⑦ Tumours causing lymphadenopathy
Primary: Hodgkin's disease and non-Hodgkin's lymphomas
- Lymphomas are malignant neoplasms of lymphoid tissue.
- Broadly divided into Hodgkin's and non-Hodgkin's type with further subdivisions on immunohistological criteria.

- Hodgkin's disease in 80% of cases involves cervical lymph nodes.
- Some patients present with systemic symptoms such as weight loss, fever, and night sweats (type B symptoms).
- Diagnosis is confirmed by biopsy (often excision biopsy is necessary after initial FNA cytology).

Secondary: metastatic disease
- Metastatic cervical lymph nodes, secondary to head and neck malignancy are quite common.
- In approximately 90% of cases spread to the cervical lymph nodes occurs in a predictable fashion (superior neck nodes being involved before inferior nodes).
- Pattern and extent of cervical lymph node involvement dictates the nature of treatment.
- Neck nodal involvement is the single most important prognostic factor in determining patients' survival.
- Factors of prognostic importance are the level, numbers, and size of nodal involvement and presence (or absence) of extracapsular spread.

Treat neck nodes seriously. Regard the solitary node as a malignancy until ruled out. Refer accordingly.

⑦ Thyroid/thyroglossal cyst/thymus

The enlarged thyroid gland
The thyroid gland lies in the midline of the lower third of the neck behind the pre-tracheal fascia. It consists of two pear-shaped lobes connected by an isthmus in the middle. A normal thyroid gland weighs approximately 20 g in adults. Posterior to the thyroid gland are superior and inferior parathyroid glands (calcium homeostasis).

Assessment of a thyroid lesion essentially involves answering the following questions:
- What is the patient's thyroid status—normal, over- or under-active?
- Is it a generalized enlargement of the gland or a solitary nodule?
- Can this be malignant? Both solitary and multinodular goitres can be benign or malignant.

⑦ Goitres
A goitre is an enlarged thyroid gland. The term goitre is generally used to refer to any enlargement without reference to the cause.

Different types of goitres
- Physiological (usually diffuse goitre): seen during pregnancy, at puberty and in conditions of iodine deficiency (now uncommon).
- Inflammatory (usually diffuse but can be multinodular): De Quervain's thyroiditis, Hashimoto's thyroiditis, Riedel's thyroiditis.
- Toxic (usually diffuse goitre): Graves' disease.
- Nodular: this is a simple benign enlargement of the thyroid gland. A nodular goitre can be a solitary nodule or multinodular. This only requires treatment if the patient is thyrotoxic, concerned with its appearance, or has symptoms of compression of adjacent structures (e.g. dysphagia or dyspnoea).

Key questions
- Rate of growth of goitre
- Pressure symptoms: hoarseness, pain, dysphagia
- Symptoms of hypo- or hyperthyroidism
- Radiation exposure, family history of thyroid disorders/cancers.

Investigations
- Thyroid function tests: TSH, free T4.
- FNA.
- Thyroid radionucleotide scintigraphy: to determine function, or identify ectopic thyroid tissue (retrosternal, lingual, and metastasis).
- Ultrasound: defines lumps from cysts and guides FNA.
- CT/MRI: evaluates substernal goitre, nodal involvement, airway and vascular displacement, tumour invasion.
- CXR: metastasis work-up, tracheal displacement.

Indications for thyroidectomy
- Excision may be required if there is suspicion of malignant change (rapid increase in size of goitre, lymph node enlargement, or hoarseness from recurrent laryngeal nerve involvement).
- Compression symptoms (airway compromise, dysphagia).
- Extension into the mediastinum (substernal goitre).
- Cosmesis.
- Failed medical management for Graves' disease or hyperthyroidism.

⑦ The solitary thyroid lump (nodule)
These have several causes:
- Cystic: this is usually a degenerative part of a nodular goitre although true cysts are also seen. Haemorrhage into the cyst is common and will present with pain and rapid enlargement.
- Adenoma: this may produce thyrotoxicosis if functioning. Subdivided histologically: papillary, follicular, embryonal, and hurtle cell.
- Carcinoma: 4–10% of solitary nodules can be malignant.

Different types of thyroid cancers
- Papillary adenocarcinoma: seen in younger age groups; low grade and rarely fatal.
- Follicular adenocarcinoma: a malignancy of middle age; bony metastases are common.
- Anaplastic carcinoma: an aggressive malignancy of the elderly; metastatic disease at presentation is common.
- Medullary carcinoma: seen in all age groups with equal sex incidence; moderate malignant potential spreading to lymph nodes.
- Malignant lymphoma: may occur in lymphatic tissue within the thyroid gland or as secondaries.
- Secondary: direct spread from adjacent malignancies or metastatic spread, most commonly from breast, renal, colon, and lung.

Risks factors for thyroid cancer
Extremes of age, nodule >5 cm, previous radiation therapy, autoimmune thyroiditis (develop lymphomas).

⑦ Thyroglossal duct cyst

Failure of complete obliteration of thyroglossal duct results in a midline painless neck mass. The cyst is attached to the hyoid bone so elevates with tongue protrusion. Patients may have dysphagia. Cysts can get infected. Malignant potential is rare. Refer for surgical excision

⑦ Thymic cysts

- Pathophysiology: remnant of third pharyngeal pouch between angle of mandible to midline neck.
- Symptoms: midline neck mass at lower neck.
- Diagnosis: biopsy, serum calcium (associated parathyroid disorders, DiGeorge's syndrome), CT, and MRI.
- Treatment is surgical excision.

⑦ Carotid body tumour

Carotid body tumours (chemodectomas) are rare, slow-growing lesions arising in the carotid bifurcation, distorting and encasing the carotid vessels. Chronic hypoxia has been reported as a causal factor (high incidence in high-altitude areas). A familial tendency in 10%, and 10% are bilateral. Left untreated about 5–10% will develop metastases within 10 years. May also become locally invasive.

Clinical features

- These usually present in patients over 50 years of age as solitary or bilateral lumps at the level of carotid bifurcation (Figure 5.5).
- They transmit the carotid pulse rather than being pulsatile itself.

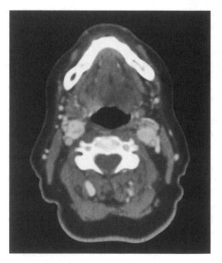

Figure 5.5 CT showing bilateral carotid body tumours.

- Most can be moved laterally (displacing the carotid pulse) but not vertically (Fontaine sign).
- Occasionally pressure on the carotid sinus by tumour may cause fainting attacks.

Management

Surgical excision is the management of choice in the young patient. In elderly, frail patients, follow-up only is required.

⑦ Branchial cysts/sinuses/fistulae

⑦ Branchial cyst

After the thyroglossal cyst, the branchial (lateral cervical) cyst is the second most common congenital swelling in the neck. It is thought that branchial cysts develop from remnants of the second branchial cleft. In some cases tracts are found running from the deep surface of the cyst to the pharyngeal wall. However, it has also been postulated that they are a result of cystic degeneration in cervical lymphatic tissue (Figure 5.6).

Clinical features

Most lesions present in the third decade of life. Patients complain of an enlarging mass arising along the junction of the upper and middle thirds of the SCM muscle. Frequently the cyst may appear as a swelling during an upper respiratory tract infection, which may be painful and persist after the infection has been treated. Recurrent infections can result in a firm, fixed mass adherent to surrounding structures such as the jugular vein, proving difficult to excise surgically.

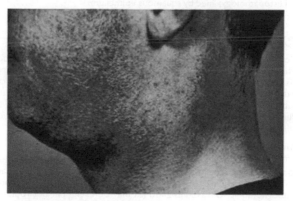

Figure 5.6 Branchial cyst.

Investigations
Diagnosis is usually made on the basis of the history and the site of the swelling. However, FNA biopsy can prove useful by producing an opalescent fluid containing cholesterol crystals or frank pus. CT or MRI helps define its size and depth.

Management
Surgical excision of the lesion is the treatment of choice following management of infections with appropriate antibiotics. All of the cyst lining should be removed as any remaining remnants may result in recurrence or a chronic discharging sinus from the wound.

⑦ Branchial sinus/branchial fistula
A branchial sinus is a small opening found over the anterior border of the SCM, which may discharge a mucous secretion. They are generally present at birth but may present in later life as a consequence of a ruptured, chronically infected branchial cyst. The sinus can extend superomedially between the internal and external carotid arteries to open onto the lateral wall of the pharynx forming a branchial fistula.

Summary of branchial cleft anomalies
- Pathophysiology: developmental alterations of the branchial apparatus results in cysts, sinuses (single opening to skin), or fistulas (opening to skin and digestive tract).
- Symptoms: neck mass in anterior neck (anterior to SCM), fistulas and sinuses may express mucoid discharge; secondary infections cause periodic fluctuation of size, tenderness, and purulent drainage.
- Diagnosis: CT with contrast (may consider injecting contrast into fistula), laryngoscopy to visualize internal opening.
- Histopathology: lined by squamous epithelium.

⑦ Plunging ranula

Congenital ranulas arise secondary to an imperforate salivary duct. These are very rare and spontaneously resolve. More commonly, ranulas arise from minor trauma to the sublingual gland, leading to mucus extravasation and formation of a pseudocyst. Partial obstruction of the sublingual duct leads to formation of an epithelial-lined retention cyst. Plunging ranulas can manifest as neck swellings usually in conjunction with swelling in the floor of the mouth.

Investigations
CT scan may show a unilocular hypodense lesion within the sublingual space. Plunging ranulas are occasionally noted on CT scanning to have a small tail extending into the sublingual space and this finding is almost pathognomonic. Ultrasound and MRI may be useful but not routinely necessary.

Treatment

Observation for spontaneous resolution of congenital ranulas is usually all that is required. Surgical treatment for acquired ranulas includes marsupialization or excision via the mouth or neck.

⑦ Dermoid cysts and teratomas

Dermoid cysts

These are considered the most common form of teratoma and are characterized by a predominance of ectodermal content. Most dermoids in the head and neck occur in the region of the floor of the mouth. They are believed to be caused by epithelial rests trapped during embryological development. Clinically, they manifest as slow-growing lesions that produce symptoms when their cystic lumens become filled with keratin debris. Sebaceous material may also be found in the cyst, alluding to its ectodermal origin.

Management

The management of these cysts is surgical excision.

⑦ Cervical teratomas

These are extremely uncommon lesions of the head and neck with prevalence of 1 in 16,000 births. In the neck, they most often occur in the midline and may manifest clinically with severe respiratory distress and dysphagia due to compression of the trachea and oesophagus. These lesions are known to often grow into a large size (as far as 12 cm) and histologically, may contain any combination of tissues from the three germ layers. They are sometimes classified in relation to proximity to the thyroid gland as follows: (1) teratomas of the thyroid gland, deriving its blood supply from thyroid arteries; (2) teratomas adjacent to the thyroid gland, in which a definitive blood supply cannot be identified; and (3) teratomas of the neck.

Management

Cervical teratomas are managed with surgical excision. Untreated cases risk possible malignant degeneration. The prognosis in non-neoplastic cases is excellent. The *ex utero* intrapartum treatment (EXIT) procedure is a technique that allow partial fetal delivery via Caesarean section, with establishment of a safe fetal airway. This may be necessary if there is fetal airway obstruction diagnosed by prenatal scanning.

When examining a salivary gland swelling, assess the following:
- Palpation (mobility, size, consistency)
- Bimanual palpation, with gland massage and inspection of any saliva expressed
- Tenderness (inflammatory process)
- Facial nerve dysfunction (suggests malignancy)
- Lingual and hypoglossal nerve dysfunction with submandibular gland tumours
- Parapharyngeal space (tonsil) displacement with parotid lumps
- Cervical lymphadenopathy.

The salivary glands

There are three pairs of major salivary glands and several hundred minor salivary glands distributed throughout the upper aerodigestive tract. The parotid is the largest gland and produces predominantly serous saliva. Submandibular and sublingual glands secrete mucoserous saliva. Salivary stones are more common in the submandibular gland because of its high mucinous content. Minor salivary glands are concentrated on palate, lips, and pharyngeal mucosa and secrete predominantly mucinous saliva which helps to keep mouth moist.

Swellings of the glands may present as a swelling in the neck, mouth, or side of the face. It is unusual for the sublingual gland to produce a true neck swelling except with a plunging ranula. *The causes of salivary gland swelling are in essence threefold: obstructive, infective, and neoplastic.* These may occur in isolation although they may coexist, e.g. a stone may result in infection.

ⓘ Obstruction

Obstruction of any part of the duct system may result in a build-up of salivary secretions and swelling. With recurrent bouts of obstruction, infection may supersede due to stagnation of secretions. The classic history is of swelling associated with meal times—the patient may report that the swelling settles a few hours after the end of eating (Figure 5.7).

Salivary calculi form as a result of calcium deposition around a nidus of organic material. 80% occur in the submandibular gland. Of the submandibular stones, 20% are radiolucent. In these cases sialography is indicated to locate them. Stones in the floor of the mouth may be removed through a local incision under local anaesthetic. However, recurrent damage to the gland may necessitate its removal.

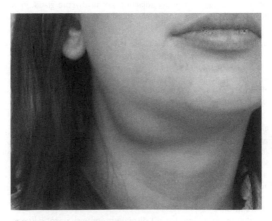

Figure 5.7 Acute submandibular obstruction.

Duct strictures can also form as a result of chronic trauma or iatrogenic injury or may be caused by ulceration around a salivary calculus. Fibrosis leads to duct stenosis and obstructive symptoms.

Neoplasia may occasionally present with obstructive symptoms.

① Infections

Infection in a major salivary gland usually presents with a painful, red, warm, tender swelling. The regional lymph nodes may be enlarged and tender, and pus may be seen to exude from the duct orifice on gently massaging the gland. Infection of the submandibular gland may present as a painful lump in the neck. Infection of the parotid gland tends to present as a painful swelling on the side of the face. Infections of the sublingual gland and minor salivary glands are generally rare and present with symptoms within the mouth.

Mumps

Both bilateral and unilateral painful parotid swelling is commonly due to a paramyxovirus infection. This is highly infectious, generally affecting children, with an incubation period of 21 days. Immunity is long-lasting after an attack. Treatment is symptomatic (analgesia and applying a warm or cool compress to help relieve pain). Complications of mumps include pancreatitis, meningitis, oophoritis, and orchitis (especially in adults).

Suppurative parotitis

This is seen in debilitated patients, particularly following major surgery, as a result of xerostomia secondary to dehydration. Oral flora ascends along the duct into the gland which becomes infected. Management includes rehydration and appropriate antibiotic therapy.

Chronic sialadenitis

Usually a complication of recurrent duct obstruction.

⑦ Tumours

70–80% of all salivary gland tumours arise in the parotid. Of these, approximately 80% are pleomorphic adenomas and 10–15% are malignant (Figure 5.8).

The classification of salivary gland tumours is complex. This includes (not an exhaustive list):

- Benign epithelial tumours (pleomorphic and monomorphic adenomas, myoepitheliomas, and Warthin's tumours)
- Malignant epithelial tumours (acinic cell, mucoepidermoid, and adenoid cystic carcinomas, salivary duct carcinomas)
- Soft tissue tumours (lymphangiomas, haemangiomas, and lymphomas)
- Metastatic tumours (skin cancers metastasizing to parotid nodes).

Lumps need urgent referral to a head and neck specialty (maxillofacial/ENT etc.). Imaging is usually required (CT/MRI or ultrasound). The role of FNA is controversial. Management is surgical removal.

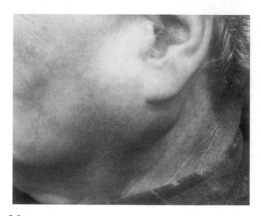

Figure 5.8 Parotid tumour.

⑦ Salivary gland dysfunction

Xerostomia (dry mouth)

There are many causes for this including primary salivary disorders (Sjögren's disease), medication induced (especially tricyclic antidepressants, antihistamines, antimuscarinic drugs, antiepileptic drugs, antipsychotics, beta-blockers, and diuretics), radiotherapy, dehydration, and mouth breathing from nasal obstruction. Treat with artificial saliva, sugar-free chewing gum, or pilocarpine. *Ask about dry/gritty eyes.* If present, this could be Sjögren's syndrome. Discuss with ophthalmology regarding ocular assessment.

Ptyalism (drooling)

True overproduction of saliva is very rare (causes include intraoral infections, foreign bodies such as new dentures, and mercury poisoning). More commonly patients just don't swallow normal amounts effectively. Causes include Parkinson's disease, epilepsy, and other swallowing disorders. It also occurs during pregnancy. Treatment includes scoline patches or in severe cases chorda tympani transection, ductal rerouting, ligation of Stenson's duct, or gland excision.

Some useful facts

- Mumps is the commonest cause of acute parotid swelling, whether it is unilateral or bilateral.
- Most parotid lumps are benign. Malignancy is more likely in submandibular/sublingual lumps.
- A lump associated with nerve dysfunction (facial, lingual, hypoglossal) suggests infiltrative pathology (i.e. tumour).
- Not all stones show up on plain X-rays.
- Ask about dry gritty eyes, joint symptoms, and rashes in anyone complaining of severe dry mouth or recurrent salivary symptoms.

- HIV can affect the salivary glands.
- Heerfordt's syndrome is sarcoidosis resulting in parotid enlargement, fever, anterior uveitis, and facial nerve palsy.
- Anxiety and medication are the commonest causes of a dry mouth.

⊙ Hoarse voice (dysphonia)/loss of voice

Dysphonia is a common condition and in most cases the underlying cause is benign and self-limiting. *However, persistence of symptoms requires careful evaluation: it can be an early sign of malignancy.*

Components of speech
- Respiration: source of energy from inhalation/exhalation
- Phonation: production of voice by vocal fold vibration
- Resonation: oral/nasal speech balance determined by velopharyngeal musculature and resonance of the sinuses, nasopharynx, nasal cavity, and oral cavity
- Articulation: speech sounds using muscles of lips, tongue, and jaw

Assessment of a patient with dysphonia (usually as an outpatient)

Character of dysphonia
Onset and duration, time course (acute vs chronic), periodicity (morning hoarseness with GORD and evening hoarseness with voice abuse).

Contributing factors
Voice abuse, recent URTI, fever, sore throat, cough, congestion; tobacco or alcohol abuse; PMH of neuromuscular disorders, hypothyroidism, psychological stressors, previous laryngeal trauma, surgery, or airway manipulation.

Associated symptoms
Dysphagia, aspiration, weight loss, hearing loss, heartburn.

Assess perceptual quality of voice
Abnormally high pitched or low pitched, abnormally loud or soft.

Examination
Indirect or direct laryngoscopy (mirror, flexible nasopharyngoscopy, videostroboscopy); assess vocal fold motion, examine laryngeal lesions and appearance of vocal folds, assess glottic competence. Neck masses, thyroid masses, neurological examination.

Videostroboscopy
Examines the vocal fold mucosa for general health, vocal fold anatomical defects, vocal fold disturbances, and mucosal wave dynamics.

Aerodynamic studies and laryngeal EMG
Measures airflow, pressures, and pattern of vibration of the vocal folds.

①Vocal cord palsy and other conditions

Unilateral vocal fold paralysis occurs from dysfunction of the recurrent laryngeal (RLN) or vagus nerve. Patients present with characteristic breathy voice often accompanied by swallowing difficulty, a weak cough, and the sensation of shortness of breath. Causes include iatrogenic injury to the vagus or recurrent laryngeal nerve (history of head, neck, and chest surgery). Recent URTI or recent intubation for any procedure can also result in a vocal cord palsy. Blunt trauma and malignant invasion of either the vagus or recurrent laryngeal nerve (skull base, thyroid cancer, lung/oesophageal cancer, and metastases to the mediastinum) are rare causes.

Investigations

These include chest radiography (Pancoast tumour, mediastinal mass, or massive cardiomegaly) and CT/MRI to visualize the path of the vagus/recurrent laryngeal nerve. A left cord palsy requires imaging from the base of skull to the mid chest (through the arch of the aorta) while a right cord palsy evaluation should extend from the base of the skull through the clavicle. EMG can be used to determine the prognosis of RLN recovery.

Management

Indications for treatment are usually when there is significant dysphonia or an ineffective cough in a patient at risk for aspiration. Medical therapy plays a very small role. When concomitant GORD and/or sinonasal allergic disease are present, medical therapy of these disorders may help. Voice therapy alone, or combined with surgical medialization of the paralysed vocal fold may help. Multiple surgical options are available. Temporary treatments involve endoscopic injection of a resorbable material (autologous fat, collagen, absorbable gelatin sponge, hyaluronic acid, etc.), into the affected vocal fold. The resultant medialization of the paralysed vocal fold improves glottal competence and may improve swallowing. Permanent treatment involves vocal fold injection or laryngeal framework surgery.

⑦Reinke's oedema

This is swelling of the vocal folds which results in polypoidal degeneration and a chronic hoarse voice with occasional stridor. Patients present with low-pitched, husky voices. Common causes include smoking, gastroesophageal reflux, hypothyroidism, and chronic voice abuse. Biopsy may be necessary to rule out underlying malignancy.

Management

This includes removal of precipitating factors and speech therapy. Surgery is usually ineffective in completely restoring the voice; however, stripping of the epithelium and letting the fluid to drain might help. CO_2 laser plays a role in debulking excessive polypoidal mucosa.

⑦ Vocal fold granulomas

Vocal cord granulomas are usually benign lesions found on the posterior third of the vocal fold corresponding to the vocal process of the arytenoid cartilage. They occur unilaterally or bilaterally. Granulomas of the larynx are classified under two groups: specific granulomas and non-specific granulomas. Specific granulomas are rare and include granulomas caused by TB and syphilis. Non-specific granulomas are benign and are histologically resemble pyogenic granulomas. Causes/contributing factors include:

- Contact granulomas as a result of voice abuse or misuse
- Granulomas of intubation
- Gastroesophageal reflux
- Smoking, allergy, infections, postnasal drip, and chronic throat clearing.

The differential diagnoses include carcinoma, granular cell tumour of the larynx, and sarcoid.

Presentation

Patients present with varying degrees of hoarseness and a low-pitched voice; cough; throat clearing; and a rough foreign body sensation. There may be a history of intubation, high-risk habits (smoking, caffeine), pulmonary symptoms (chronic cough, use of inhalers), etc. Untreated, these can result in airway obstruction, bleeding (usually minor), vocal fold fixation, and posterior laryngeal stenosis.

Management

Medical therapy includes cough suppressants, anti-reflux therapy, speech therapy, and topical/steroid injections (controversial). Surgical management has a high recurrence rate. Surgical is indicated for fibroepithelial polyps, airway compromise, or suspicion of cancer.

⑦ Muscle-tension disorders/functional voice disorders

Functional voice disorders (muscle tension dysphonia) may account for up to 40% of the cases of dysphonia. A recent URTI may precipitate an already stressed laryngeal system causing dysphonia. Other factors include medications, neurological disorders, laryngeal trauma, hypothyroidism, and psychiatric. All patients must undergo a complete ENT examination to rule out other causes.

⑦ Conversion dysphonia

The development of conversion dysphonia, also referred to as a psychogenic dysphonia, may result from a temporally psychological or emotionally traumatic event. The patient's vocal quality is usually hypofunctional or aphonic. Fibreoptic laryngoscopy may demonstrate a lack of vocal cord adduction during attempted phonation. However, coughing and throat clearing (vegetative phonation) demonstrate normal vocal cord adduction. Treatment is voice therapy.

⑦ Carotid artery disease

The common carotid artery divides into the internal carotid artery and the external carotid artery. The internal carotid artery supplies the brain. Like any large vessel it is at risk of vascular disease. Risk factors are similar to those for heart disease. They include:

- Age
- Smoking
- Hypertension
- Abnormal lipids or high cholesterol
- Diet high in saturated fats
- Diabetes
- Obesity
- Sedentary lifestyle
- Family history of atherosclerosis, either coronary artery disease or carotid artery disease.

⑦ Carotid stenosis

Atherosclerotic plaques can build up within the vessel wall, resulting in stenosis. These are common in the elderly and may remain stable and asymptomatic. However, they may also be a source of embolization. Fragments can break off and obstruct smaller arteries within the brain. The resulting ischaemia can be either temporary (TIA), or permanent (thromboembolic stroke).

Clinical features

TIAs by definition last <24 hours. They may present with:

- Weakness or loss of sensation of a limb or the trunk on one side
- Loss of sight (amaurosis fugax) in one eye
- Vertigo
- Tinnitus
- Difficulty speaking
- Confusion.

TIAs may be a warning sign, often followed by a stroke, a few days later. Symptoms of a stroke are similar to a TIA, the main difference being they are usually more severe and are permanent, with little recovery.

Carotid stenosis is usually diagnosed by colour flow duplex ultrasound of the neck. Occasionally CTA or MRA is required.

Management

This includes:

- Medication: antiplatelet drugs
- Carotid endarterectomy: surgical removal of the plaque and diseased portions of the artery.
- Carotid stenting: this is a newer treatment and less invasive.
  A catheter is threaded into the area of stenosis and dilated with a balloon. A stent is then placed to hold the vessel open.

In asymptomatic severe carotid artery stenosis, carotid endarterectomy reduces the risk of stroke in the next 5 years by around 50%. Patients with carotid stenosis should be referred for medication (antihypertensive drugs, anticlotting drugs, antiplatelet drugs, and statins). Clinical trials are still ongoing.

A TIA is a medical emergency because it is impossible to predict if it will progress into a major stroke. Immediate treatment may increase the chance of a full recovery.

☼ Carotid artery dissection

Carotid artery dissection is separation of the layers of the artery wall. It is a common cause of stroke in young adults. In addition to signs of a stroke, patients may also experience headache or neck pain and develop a Horner's syndrome (decreased pupil size with drooping of the upper eyelid). Spontaneous internal carotid artery dissection may have a history of stroke in their family or hereditary connective tissue disorders, such as Marfan's syndrome or Ehlers–Danlos syndrome.

Carotid artery dissection may also occur following severe trauma to the head or neck. This can also result in intimal dissections, pseudoaneurysms, thromboses, or fistulas.

Management

The aim of treatment is to prevent the onset or continuation of neurological deficits. Treatments include observation, anticoagulation, stenting, and carotid artery ligation.

① Coughing up blood (haemoptysis)

Haemoptysis needs to be differentiated from epistaxis and haematemesis. In children, lower respiratory tract infections and foreign body aspiration are common causes. In adults, bronchitis, bronchogenic carcinoma, and pneumonia are the major causes. Determine if the patient is coughing up clots, fresh blood, blood-stained sputum, or sputum with streaks of blood mixed in. Haemoptysis is classified as non-massive (<200 mL) or massive, based on the volume of blood loss daily. Bleeding from a high-pressure bronchial artery can be profuse. Consider the following:

- Upper airway (nasopharyngeal) bleeding
- GI bleeding
- Neoplasm (bronchogenic carcinoma)
- Bronchitis, bronchiectasis
- Airway trauma, foreign body, pulmonary embolism
- Lung abscess, pneumonia, TB, mycetoma
- Systemic coagulopathy/anticoagulants
- Goodpasture's syndrome, idiopathic pulmonary haemosiderosis, Wegener's granulomatosis
- Arteriovenous malformation, elevated pulmonary venous pressure (especially mitral stenosis), etc.

In up to a third of patients, no cause can be found. Blood from the lower bronchial tree typically induces cough, whereas a history of epistaxis or expectorating without cough would be consistent with an upper respiratory source. Examining the expectoration may help localize the source of bleeding.

Investigations
These include CXR, followed by fibreoptic bronchoscopy and high-resolution CT in cases when malignancy is suspected.

Management
This includes stopping bleeding, aspiration prevention, and treatment of the underlying cause.
- Haemoptysis >1000 mL per 24 hours carries a mortality rate. Airway maintenance is vital (death is more often due to asphyxiation). Give oxygen and commence fluid resuscitation. Call cardiothoracic/general surgeons urgently (local protocol).
- Mild haemoptysis often is caused by an infection and can be managed on an outpatient basis with close monitoring. If haemoptysis persists, refer urgently to a respiratory specialist.

:O: Foreign body ingestion

:O: Foreign body in the oesophagus
The most common foreign bodies in adults are fish bones, dentures, and meat. The most common objects in children are coins. 95% of oesophageal foreign bodies obstruct at the cricopharyngeus (narrowest part of adult GI tract). Patients present with dysphagia, drooling, chest pain, and later with a fever. *Left untreated, oesophageal perforation, mediastinitis, pneumomediastinum, pneumothorax, and aspiration can all occur.*

Investigations
CXR to identify object. *Always ask for soft tissue neck X-ray as well* (both anteroposterior and lateral views). CT may be required.

Management
- Obtain description of object (sharp objects like meat with bone or dentures needs retrieval).
- Conservative management—for food bolus without a bone.
- Consider admission for IV fluids, smooth muscle relaxants (hyoscine), sedation (diazepam), and observation.
- Rigid oesophagoscopy. This is indicated for foreign bodies that remain in the oesophagus for >2 days. *Large objects or batteries need immediate retrieval.*

:O: Caustic ingestion
- Alkaline ingestion (pH >12.5) causes liquefaction necrosis (and perforation of oesophagus). Common alkali agents include alkali batteries, bleaches, household ammonia, and hair straighteners.
- Acidic ingestion causes coagulation necrosis, rapid transit results in skip areas and more severe damage to the stomach.

- Liquids burn more distal; solids (powder) burn more proximal.
- Severity of external and oropharyngeal injury does not correlate with extent of oesophageal and gastric injury.

Patients present with drooling, mouth pain, stridor, dysphagia, chest or abdominal pain, and oral injury. Left untreated, stricture, pneumonia, tracheoesophageal fistulas, laryngeal oedema, mediastinitis, and perforation may occur.

Investigations
CXR. Direct laryngoscopy with oesophagoscopy.

Management
- Evaluate airway (may require an emergent surgical airway).
- Identify agent, determine pH, amount, and concentration (call toxicology information centre).
- Remove granules and powder with water, consider initial dose of corticosteroids, IV antibiotics, NBM, IV hydration, do not induce emesis, do not neutralize (this causes an exothermic reaction).
- Evaluate for complications: CXR (mediastinitis), abdominal series (gastric perforation), ABGs.

Miscellaneous conditions

⑦ Eagle syndrome (styloid–carotid artery syndrome)
This is a rare condition in which there is elongation of the styloid process, or calcification of the stylohyoid ligament. 'Classic' and 'vascular' forms are described. Patients are usually between 30 and 50 years old and can present with recurrent sore throat, dysphagia, neck pain, and otalgia. Blackouts and sudden death due to have also been reported and are due to mechanical pressure on the carotid. *Consider this when neurological symptoms occurs upon head rotation.* The tip of the styloid process may be palpable in the back of the throat. Plain films and CT confirm the diagnosis (the enlarged styloid may be visible on an OPT or a lateral soft tissue X-ray). In both types, treatment is surgical (partial styloidectomy).

Tracheostomy
Ideally this should be carried out in theatre settings. Tracheostomy tubes are placed through a small incision midway between the cricoid cartilage and suprasternal notch. Tissues are separated keeping to the midline of the neck. Meticulous haemostasis is essential at all times. Often the thyroid isthmus obstructs access to the trachea and needs to be retracted or securely ligated and divided. The thyroid is a highly vascular organ and carelessness in manipulation can result in profound bleeding postoperatively.

Once the anterior part of the trachea is defined, it is opened, the endotracheal tube withdrawn, and the tracheostomy tube inserted into the lumen. Several different access openings in the trachea have been described—a vertical slit, small hole, or the 'Bjork' flap (which is a U-shaped flap attached inferiorly). Each has its own merits and which is chosen is down to the operating surgeon. Once in place, the tube needs to be sutured to the skin and securely fastened around the neck with tapes and the wound closed.

Tracheostomy indications

- Bypass upper airway obstruction (e.g. sleep apnoea, tumour).
- Prevention of aspiration and airway protection (cuffed tube).
- Assist with tracheal-bronchial toileting (suctioning).
- Eliminate dead space and improve respiratory insufficiency (respiratory, cardiac, or neurological disease).
- Prevent complications from prolonged intubation (e.g. mucosal ulceration, laryngeal stenosis, granulomas).

Tracheotomy care

- Maintain airway: especially for first 48 hours to prevent accidental dislodgement of tube. Ensure the tracheostomy tube is sutured to the neck skin, clean the inner cannula daily. The first tracheostomy change may be considered after 3–5 days. This allows a tract to form.
- Humidification: prevents tracheal crusting and mucous plugs. *Patients with tracheostomies should never be without florid humidification.*
- Pulmonary toileting: tracheostomy tubes disrupt ciliary function, decrease subglottic pressure (causing ineffective cough), and increase risk of micro-aspiration; they may require regular suctioning for the first few days.
- Skin care: cuff dressings to prevent skin breakdown.
- Check cuff pressure: cuff pressure should be less than capillary perfusion pressure (<25 cmH$_2$O) to prevent pressure necrosis (and subsequent SGS, tracheal-innominate artery erosion, tracheomalacia).
- Feeding: it can be difficult for solid food ingestion when cuff is inflated; capping the tracheotomy tube facilitates swallowing.
- If patients are going to other departments in the hospital they should be accompanied by appropriately trained personnel at all times and should go with a mobile humidification system.

Although tracheostomy provides direct access to the lower respiratory tract for suctioning, many patients find it difficult to produce an effective 'explosive' cough, useful in clearing secretions from the lungs. However, they can be taught to expectorate, physiotherapists encouraging 'huffing' using the diaphragm. With a cooperative and well-humidified patient, very little suction is required; most patients can effectively clear their lungs on their own.

Decannulation

Tracheotomy tubes should be removed as soon as possible (especially in children) to prevent long-term sequelae such as tracheal ulceration, SGS, tracheomalacia. Prior to decannulation, patients may undergo tracheostomy tube downsizing and a trial of capping, but this is not always necessary. Flexible nasopharyngoscopy can evaluate airway patency. Once removed, place an airtight dressing to seal the stoma.

Tracheotomy complications

Tracheal stenosis, granulation tissue, tracheal-innominate artery erosion, SGS, vocal cord paralysis (the recurrent laryngeal nerve runs alongside the trachea), chest infection, tracheo-oesophageal fistula.

① Surgical (subcutaneous) emphysema

Subcutaneous emphysema occurs when air gets trapped in the tissues under the skin. It is usually seen in the chest wall or neck, but can occur in other parts of the body and is typically seen in trauma situations with penetrating injuries involving the airway. On palpation, a crackling sensation is felt under the skin as the gas is pushed through the tissue.

Aetiology

Air can enter the soft tissues from rupture of any gas-filled structure, or from the exterior. Causes therefore include:

- Ruptured lung (pneumothorax), often with rib fracture
- Ruptured bronchial tube
- Facial fractures
- Ruptured oesophagus
- Infection caused by gas-producing organisms (gas gangrene)
- Penetrating injuries
- Explosions.

This condition is rarely associated with breathing cocaine, corrosives or chemical burns of the oesophagus, forceful vomiting' (Boerhaave's syndrome), gunshot wounds, pertussis (whooping cough), and certain medical procedures (central venous line, intubation, and bronchoscopy). Massive emphysema has been reported following certain dental treatments (such as root canal treatment or surgical extraction of a tooth using an air-powered rotary drill).

Management

Treat the underlying cause and emphysema will spontaneously resolve. Rarely massive subcutaneous emphysema can cause significant discomfort and cause airway compromise or venous compression. This may require surgical drainage. When subcutaneous emphysema occurs due to pneumothorax, a chest tube is frequently necessary.

⑦ Mediastinal masses

Patients with mediastinal masses can present in different ways. It is often an incidental diagnosis during evaluation for an unrelated condition. Some patients present with complaints secondary to local mass effect on adjacent structures, such as respiratory symptoms or swelling due to compression of vascular structures or develop systemic symptoms resulting from the mediastinal mass. Both benign and malignant mediastinal masses can develop from structures that normally are in the mediastinum or present during development, as well as metastases of malignancies from elsewhere in the body.

Investigations
CXR, CT scan of the chest (and CT-guided needle biopsy), MRI of the chest, and mediastinoscopy with biopsy.

Management
The treatment used for mediastinal tumours depends on the type of tumour and its location. Thymic cancers require surgery, followed by radiation or chemotherapy. Lymphomas are treated with chemotherapy followed by radiation.

⑦ Globus

Globus is the feeling of a lump in the throat when actually there is no lump present. Usually it is idiopathic in nature (globus pharyngeus or globus hystericus), but occasionally may be secondary to identified pathology:
- Oesophageal spasm
- GORD
- Neuromuscular disorders such as myasthenia gravis, Parkinson's disease, and stroke
- Rarely, cancers of the upper GI tract.

The ear

Common presentations

- Abnormal sounds (tinnitus)
- Dizziness
- Fullness/discharge
- Injuries
- Itching
- Loss of hearing/deafness
- Pain (otalgia)
- Swellings.

Common problems and their causes

Abnormal sounds (tinnitus)

Common
- Wax impaction
- Glue ear
- Infections (otitis media)
- Perforated ear drum
- Noise induced
- Presbycusis
- TMJ disorders
- Ototoxic drugs
- Many patients have underlying depression and anxiety.

Uncommon
- Insects
- Otosclerosis
- Ménière's disease
- Trauma
- Acoustic neuroma
- AVMs and venous hums
- Glomus jugulare and carotid body tumours
- Patulous Eustachian tube and palatal myoclonus.

Dizziness

Common
- Otological causes:
  - Benign paroxysmal positional vertigo
  - Ménière's disease
  - Iatrogenic (middle ear/mastoid surgery)
  - Impacted wax
  - Ear infection (otitis media)
- Systemic causes:
  - Migraine
  - MS
  - Medications.

Uncommon
- Otological causes:
  - Cerebellopontine angle tumours
  - Perilymphatic fistulas
  - Trauma (temporal bone fracture)
  - Vestibular neuronitis/labyrinthitis
  - Oto syphilis
- Systemic causes:
  - Metabolic disorders (hypo/hyperthyroidism, diabetes)
  - Vascular cause (vertebrobasilar insufficiency, Eagle syndrome)
- Neurological disorders (stroke, seizures, Parkinsonism).

Fullness/discharge

Common
- Chronic suppurative otitis media (mucoid)
- Furunculosis or local abscess (purulent)
- Trauma (bloody/CSF)
- Eczema (watery)
- Acute otitis media (bloody)
- Eustachian tube dysfunction
- Wax.

Uncommon
- Nasopharyngeal malignancy (bloody)
- Cholesteatoma (foul smelling)
- Ménière's disease.

Injuries

Common
- Blunt/bruising
- Lacerations.

Uncommon
- Bites (animal/human)
- Avulsions/tears
- Barotrauma.

Itching

Common
- Otitis externa
- Contact dermatitis.

Uncommon
- Cholesteatoma.

Loss of hearing/deafness

Common
- Acute otitis media
- Acoustic trauma/trauma
- Eustachian tube dysfunction
- Wax impaction
- Presbycusis
- Idiopathic.

Uncommon
- Autoimmune, Ménière's, MS
- Infections (herpes, mumps, cytomegalovirus, toxoplasmosis, syphilis)
- Foreign body
- Otosclerosis
- Drugs
- Metabolic (diabetes/thyroid)
- Tumour.

Pain (otalgia)

Common
- Acute otitis externa
- Otitis media with effusion
- Referred pain
- Furuncles (infected hair follicles)
- Perichondritis.

Uncommon
- Malignant otitis externa
- Barotrauma
- Herpes zoster
- Tumours
- Mastoiditis.

Referred pain
- Tonsillitis and upper respiratory tract disease
- Eustachian tube dysfunction
- Dental pathology
- Disorders of the TMJ
- Parotid disease
- The oropharynx
- The larynx and pharynx
- Cervical spondylosis
- Malignancy of any of the above-listed (particularly the tongue base).

Swellings

Common
- Pinna haematoma (trauma)
- Perichondritis of the pinna.

Uncommon
- Seroma/pseudocyst of the pinna
- Erysipelas
- Gout
- Sebaceous cyst
- Herpes zoster.

Useful questions and what to look for

Abnormal sounds (tinnitus)

Ask about
- Character of tinnitus: unilateral or bilateral, high-pitched or low-pitched (roaring, buzzing), pulsatile, clicking
- Progression and frequency
- Severity: effect on sleep, daily life
- History of trauma
- Medications
- Underlying anxiety and depression.

Look for
- Look for retrotympanic masses
- Audible bruits
- TMJ dysfunction
- Similar work-up as evaluating hearing loss.

Dizziness

Ask about
- Describe dizziness: rotatory vertigo ('spinning', 'whirling', or 'turning' of patient or surroundings), disequilibrium ('off-balance'), lightheadedness (sense of impending faint), physiological dizziness (motion sickness)
- Duration: seconds to minutes (benign paroxysmal positional vertigo (BPPV), arrhythmia), hours (Ménière's, migraine), days (vestibular neuritis, labyrinthitis), or constant (central)
- Associated symptoms: hearing loss, aural fullness, tinnitus, sympathetic response (nausea, vomiting), central symptoms (numbness, weakness, diplopia, blurred vision)

- Contributing factors: medications (antihypertensives, ototoxic medications, sedatives); medical history (hypertension, cardiac arrhythmias, diabetes, vascular disease, otological disease, neurological disease, migraines).

Look for
- General exam: (pulse, BP: standing and lying, carotid bruits), with focus on neurological, cardiovascular, and peripheral vascular disorders
- Otoscopy: otitis media, glue ear, cholestatoma
- Neurological exam: for cranial nerve palsies, vestibulospinal reflexes (e.g. Romberg's test, gait, past pointing test), lateralizing signs (e.g. weakness, paraesthesia)
- Eye movements: check pursuit and for nystagmus
- Specific tests: Dix–Hallpike, head-shake, fistula test, caloric testing, tuning fork, and audiometry.

Fullness/discharge

Ask about
- Tinnitus
- Hearing disturbance
- Autophony (abnormal hearing of one's own voice and respiratory sounds)
- Nasal obstruction
- Otalgia
- Otorrhoea
- Rhinorrhoea
- Sore throat.

Look for
- Otoscopy for signs of infection, wax, discharge, etc.
- Examine the throat/nasopharynx for disease
- Nasal endoscopy
- Ask patient to perform the Valsalva manoeuvre.

Injuries

Ask about
- When it occurred?
- Mechanism of injury
- Loss of consciousness/neck, etc.
- Hearing loss
- Dizziness.

Look for
- Other injuries
- Facial nerve weakness
- Hearing loss (tuning forks if stable)
- Nystagmus

- Other neurological deficits and cranial nerve palsies
- CSF leak
- Haemotympanum
- External auditory canal lacerations
- Battle's sisgn (ecchymosis over the mastoid process).

Itching

Ask about
- Discharge from the ear
- Tenderness or pain
- Cough
- Fever and chills
- Headache
- Runny nose
- Sneezing
- Sore throat.

Look for
- Crusting or flaking skin
- Redness, warmth, or swelling.

Loss of hearing/deafness

Ask about
- Onset and duration, constant vs intermittent, progression, unilateral or bilateral, high or low tone loss, decreased speech intelligibility
- Contributing factors: recent infection; loud noise exposure
- Recent trauma: barotrauma, head injury; exacerbating factors for tinnitus (sleep, exercise, caffeine, alcohol)
- Previous otological surgery, infections
- Medications
- Systemic: history of autoimmune disease, hypertension, diabetes, vascular disorders, neurological disease (stroke), depression
- Family history of deafness
- Associated symptoms: aural fullness, fevers, vertigo, tinnitus, otalgia, otorrhoea, other neurological complaints.

Look for
- Malformations, auricular pits, scars, oedema, mastoid tenderness, tragal tenderness
- Otoscopy (wax, lesions, masses) and tympanic membrane (colour, thickness, presence of fluid, perforations)
- Pneumatic otoscopy: test mobility of tympanic membrane with positive and negative pressure
- Fistula test: positive pressure causes nystagmus which reverses with negative pressure (perilymph fistula and labyrinthitis)
- Neurological and vestibular exam, bruits
- Tuning fork tests.

Pain (otalgia)

Ask about
- Duration of symptoms
- Discharge
- Recent URTI
- Hearing loss
- Degree of pain and radiation (malignant otitis externa pain is often severe, post-auricular pain suggests mastoiditis)
- Previous episodes and treatment to date
- Previous ear surgery
- PMH (diabetes or other immune compromise)
- Injury to the mandible (fractured condyle).

Look for
- Swelling
- Discharge
- Furuncles
- Signs of injury
- CN VII weakness
- Systemic upset
- Tenderness over the mastoid prominence
- Otoscopy (bulging of the external auditory canal/tympanic membrane may appear red, perforated, and discharging).

Swellings

Ask about
- Any known aetiological factors
- History of trauma
- Any preceding otalgia (perichondritis can arise following otitis externa and trauma)
- Predisposing factors (e.g. immune compromise)
- Any painful (pseudocyst can present as a painless swelling).

Look for
- Confirm presence
- Discharge
- Otoscopy: inspection of ear drum and middle ear (otitis media, glue ear, cholesteatoma).

Examination of the ear

Applied anatomy

External ear

This comprises of pinna, external auditory meatus (EAM), external auditory canal, and tympanic membrane (ear drum). The skin on the outer part of the EAM is self-cleansing and contains hair follicles and wax-producing ceruminous glands. These are absent on the inner part. *Ears are normally self-cleansing and use of cotton buds should be discouraged*. If wax is dislodged into the deeper part of the canal it cannot be removed by this natural process.

Middle ear

This is an air-containing space allowing sound transfer to the cochlea. It contains three ossicles (malleus, incus, and stapes), two muscles (tensor tympani and stapedius), and part of the facial nerve (chorda tympani branch). Equalization of pressures occurs via the Eustachian tube. The mastoid air cells communicate with the middle ear space. This is closely related to the brain (middle cranial fossa), jugular bulb (posteriorly), and labyrinth (medially). *Infections in middle ear are potentially very serious* as they can extend into surrounding structures.

Inner ear

This comprises the cochlea, vestibule, and semicircular canals. The 'membranous' part is filled by endolymph and is surrounded by the bony labyrinth, which is filled with perilymph. The cochlea contains the organ of hearing (organ of Corti). The vestibule and semicircular canals are involved in balance.

Nerve supply to the ear

The ear is innervated by the V, IX, and X cranial nerves, and by the posterior roots of C2 and C3. Because of this, *pathology at sites of similar nerve distribution (TMJ, dental, oropharyngeal, laryngeal, and hypopharyngeal) can present with otalgia (referred pain)*.

Examination of the ear

Inspect the external ear first. Remove any discharge or wax. Look for obvious signs of abnormality:

- Size and shape of the pinna
- Extra cartilage tags/pre-auricular sinuses or pits
- Signs of trauma
- Skin lesions, e.g. neoplasia
- Skin condition of the pinna and external canal
- Infection/inflammation of the external ear canal, with discharge.

Then palpate for mastoid tenderness, tragal tenderness, and lymphadenopathy. Use an otoscope (auroscope) to inspect the external auditory canal and tympanic membrane. Grasp the pinna and gently pull it up and backwards. This helps straighten the canal for inspection (in infants, pull the pinna posteriorly). Note the condition of the canal skin and the presence of wax, foreign tissue, or discharge. Inspect the tympanic membrane for signs of injury, perforation, or discharge. The mobility of the eardrum can be evaluated using a pneumatic speculum, which attaches to the otoscope. Check facial nerve function.

Special manoeuvres include the following:

Dix–Hallpike manoeuvre
This is a positional test for BPPV. The patient sits upright with the legs extended. Their head is rotated by approximately 45 degrees. The clinician then helps the patient to quickly lie down backwards with the head held in approximately 20 degrees of extension. The patient's eyes are observed for nystagmus. If rotational nystagmus occurs then the test is considered positive for benign positional vertigo.

Head-shake nystagmus
Move the head in the horizontal plane for 20–30 seconds, then suddenly stop and evaluate for nystagmus.

Fistula test and pneumatic otoscopy
Positive pressure causes nystagmus which reverses with negative pressure (perilymph fistula and labyrinthitis). Test mobility of tympanic membrane with pressure changes.

Tuning fork tests

Rinne test
Use a 512 Hz tuning fork to compare air conduction (AC) and bone conduction (BC). Strike the tuning fork then place it within 1 cm of the EAM (AC) and then immediately place on the mastoid (BC).

Normal hearing
AC should be greater than BC and so the patient should be able to hear the tuning fork next to the pinna after they can no longer hear it when held against the mastoid.

Abnormal hearing
• If they are not able to hear the tuning fork after the mastoid, it means that BC is greater than AC. Something is inhibiting the passage of sound from the ear canal, through the middle ear apparatus and into the cochlea (i.e. there is a conductive hearing loss).
• In sensorineural hearing loss both BC and AC are equally diminished. Patients with sensorineural hearing loss can usually hear better on the mastoid process than air, but indicate the sound has stopped much earlier than conductive loss patients.

Weber test
Strike the tuning fork and place it in the centre of the forehead. The perceived sound should normally be heard centrally.

Remember that nasopharyngeal pathology can present with unilateral ear symptoms. Always look at the throat and nasopharynx, especially in adults presenting with unilateral glue ear—this can be a presenting symptom of a nasopharyngeal tumour.

Investigations

Laboratory tests

- FBC may show a raised WCC (neutrophils).
- Electrolytes: ototoxicity
- Glucose: screen for diabetes (associated with hearing loss)
- Coagulation and immunological profile: coagulopathies can be associated with hearing disorders
- ESR
- Treponemal studies: Lyme titres/TPHA/VDRL/FTA-ABS depending on where you work
- Lipid profile: atherosclerotic disease can be associated with sudden senorineural hearing loss
- Fluid analysis (beta-2 transferrin in suspected CSF leakage)
- Microbiology for any discharge.

Plain films

Mastoid X-rays: will show opacity of the air cells. These and other special views of the temporal bone (Schuller's, Stenvere's, Towne's views) have now largely been replaced by CT and MRI.

CT/MRI of temporal bones

These look for potential complications of suppurative ear disease, cholesteatoma, mastoiditis, temporal bone fracture, congenital disorder or neoplasm (especially acoustic neuroma).

MRI is often required for suspected cerebellopontine angle tumours, acoustic neuromas, meningiomas, and petrous apex lesions.

Audiometric tests

Audiometry tests are carried out in soundproofed rooms using precision equipment. Tests may be subjective (pure tone audiograms, speech audiometry), or objective (impedance audiometry, evoked response audiometry).

These tests are essential to define auditory function and to quantify the thresholds of AC/BC hearing for both ears. It distinguishes conductive loss from sensorineural hearing loss; cochlear versus neural dysfunction, and malingering (pseudohypacusis).

Different audiological tests:

- Pure tone audiometry: tests threshold of AC and BC.
- Tympanometry: checks middle ear pressure and impedance (indirect measure of Eustachian tube function).
- Auditory brainstem response (ABR): recording of the activity of the eighth nerve and central auditory pathway response to an auditory signal.
- Otoacoustic emissions (OAEs): tests objective sounds in external auditory canal emitted from outer hair cells (cochlear echo).
- ABR and OAE are objective tests and do not need the patient's cooperation and hence used identify malingerers and for medico-legal purposes.

① Injuries

Injuries localized to the external or middle ear include auricular hae-matoma, external auditory canal abrasion or laceration, tympanic membrane perforation, and ossicular chain dislocation. In addition, barotrauma, such as a slap to the ear or a blast injury, can cause a tym-panic membrane perforation or ossicular chain dislocation.

⚙ Temporal bone fractures

These represent roughly 20% of all skull fractures. Blunt trauma to the lateral surface of the skull (the squamous portion of the temporal bone) often results in a longitudinally orientated fracture. These follow the axis of the external auditory canal to the middle ear space. In a longitudinal fracture, the otic capsule is spared. In contrast, a blow to the occiput may go through the foramen magnum and result in a transverse fracture of the temporal bone. These course directly across the petrous bone, frac-turing the otic capsule and geniculate ganglion (facial nerve). Longitudinal fractures and transverse fractures represent 80% and 20% of temporal bone fractures respectively.
Symptoms and signs include:
- Hearing loss
- Nausea and vomiting
- Vertigo
- Battle's sign (post-auricular ecchymosis)
- External auditory canal laceration with bony debris within the canal
- Haemotympanum
- CSF otorrhoea.

CT of the head is usually performed due to the head trauma. High-resolution scanning of the temporal bone is valuable in delineating the extent of the fracture, but it is not required unless a complication is sus-pected (e.g. otic capsule fracture, facial nerve injury, or CSF leak). Tuning fork tests should always be performed on patients with a temporal bone fracture. The Weber tuning fork test radiates to the fractured ear if con-ductive hearing loss is present and radiates to the contralateral ear if sensorineural hearing loss is present. The presence or absence of facial nerve paralysis should be documented in all patients with temporal bone fractures. Complications of these fractures include:
- Conductive hearing loss
- Sensorineural hearing loss and vertigo
- Facial nerve injury
- CSF leak
- Perilymphatic fistula (fluctuating vertigo and sensorineural loss).

① CSF leak

There is usually clear otorrhoea or rhinorrhoea (CSF leak through Eustachian tube into the nasopharynx if ear drum is intact), and a salty taste. Look for the 'halo sign'. Fluid analysis (beta-2 transferrin) and CT usually confirm the diagnosis. Management is initially bed rest, head elevation, and diuretics (mannitol, acetazolamide, furosemide). If per-sistent, a lumbar drain or surgical exploration may be required. Refer urgently to ENT/neurosurgeons.

ⓘ *Dizziness following ear trauma*

This is usually self-limiting with mild inner ear injury (post-concussion syndrome). Injury to the vestibular labyrinth may cause a complete unilateral vestibular deficit. Rarely it can be due to perilymphatic fistulas. High-resolution CT of temporal bones may be required.

ⓘ Auricular haematoma

These occur following direct trauma (Figure 6.1). Bleeding occurs in the subperichondrial space superficial to the cartilage. This can result in cartilage necrosis and predispose to infection, especially if there is an overlying skin laceration. A haematoma presents as a painful, tender swelling with associated skin discolouration. Principles of treatment are evacuation of the haematoma, reapposition of perichondrium to the underlying cartilage, and removal of any 'dead space' to avoid infection or a 'cauliflower ear' deformity. Prompt wide-bore needle aspiration is often effective. Incision and drainage may be required in cases of recurrence or in late presentation. Gentle pressure can be applied by means of a pressure bandage, mattress suturing, or a silicone mould. *Do not put the bandage on too tight, this can result in cartilage necrosis.* Early review is required as haematoma can readily re accumulate.

ⓘ Seroma of the pinna

This is serous fluid that has collected between the perichondral layer of the pinna and the underlying cartilage. It can occur spontaneously or as the result of trauma. Treatment involves aspiration and a pressure dressing; however, there is a high propensity for recurrence.

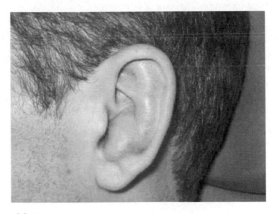

Figure 6.1 Auricular haematoma.

① Traumatic perichondritis

Trauma, with haematoma formation and subsequent infection, is the commonest cause. Other causes of perichondritis include malignant otitis externa, following ear piercing, or other sharp trauma which can introduce infection directly. It can also occur following mastoid surgery. Patients present with dull pain, erythema, and inflammation of the pinna. If left untreated, abscess formation and cartilage necrosis can occur. The most frequent microbe is *Pseudomonas aeruginosa*; others include *Staphylococcus aureus* and *Escherichia coli*. Treatment in the majority of cases is with IV antibiotics, with the addition of antimicrobial ear drops in cases of suspected otitis externa. Incision and drainage may be required where abscess formation is evident.

① Lacerations/tears and partial avulsions involving the EAM

Injuries to the external meatus/canal most commonly occur when a patient is trying to remove his or her own earwax with a cotton-tipped applicator or probe. The injury is usually a simple abrasion or laceration. Lacerations may also occur in association with fractures of the mandibular condyle. Treatment consists of using an antimicrobial drop to prevent bacterial or fungal infection. Patients with diabetes have a high risk of developing external otitis from this type of injury. These patients need to be followed up closely. Occasionally tears are associated with an underlying fracture. Meticulous repair is required to avoid trapping skin (causing implantation cholesteatoma) and canal stenosis.

① Barotrauma

A sudden pressure change in middle ear cleft can occur during diving or flying. Symptoms vary depending on the pressure gradient:
• Otalgia (pressure differential of 60 mmHg)
• Eustachian tube dysfunction (pressure differential of 90 mmHg)
• Tympanic membrane perforation (pressure differential of 100–500 mmHg).

Patients present with acute pain, haemotympanum, bloody otorrhoea, acute hearing loss, dizziness, and tinnitus.

Types of barotrauma
• Middle ear squeeze: on ascent, the Eustachian tube may close, failing to relieve pressure in the middle ear with decreasing pressure. This can cause an ear drum perforation or haemotympanum.
• Round window rupture may occur with an acute increase in CSF pressure transmitted through the perilymph.
• Inner ear decompression sickness (Caisson disease): with increased pressure (diving), nitrogen becomes more soluble and enters body fluids. If decompression occurs rapidly (rapid ascent), small gas emboli may form and occlude micro-blood circulation leading to end-organ damage causing blindness, deafness, paralysis, or death.

① Tympanic membrane perforation

This can occur following insertion of a cotton-tipped applicator, pin, or pencil, or following barotrauma (slap to the ear or a blast injury). Perforation is diagnosed by otoscopy. It is important to note how much of the tympanic membrane has been perforated. A central perforation does not involve the annulus of the eardrum, whereas a marginal perforation does. The Weber tuning fork test should be performed and the eyes checked for nystagmus. If the sound does not radiate to the affected ear and the patient has nystagmus, it is likely that an inner ear injury (perilymphatic fistula or stapes dislocation) has also occurred and requires urgent treatment. If no evidence of sensorineural hearing loss is found, no specific treatment is required. Traumatic tympanic membrane perforations, especially central perforations, typically heal spontaneously. Strict dry ear precautions should be followed to prevent water from getting into the ear. Instructions include no swimming and the placement of a cotton ball thoroughly coated with petrolatum (Vaseline®) in the affected ear during bathing. If the perforation has not healed by 3 months, a tympanoplasty may be needed.

① Ossicular chain dislocation

Ossicular chain dislocation with an intact eardrum manifests as a maximal (60 dB) conductive hearing loss. Ossicular chain dislocation with a perforated eardrum results in lesser degrees of hearing loss. Treatment is middle ear exploration and ossicular chain reconstruction, with tympanoplasty if needed.

① Infections of the external auditory meatus and pinna

① Acute otitis externa ('swimmer's ear')

This is often caused by a bacterial or fungal (lobomycosis, also known as Singapore ear) infection involving the skin of the external auditory canal. Predisposing factors include aggressive ear cleaning, lack of cerumen, digital trauma (e.g. cotton buds, fingernails) and retention of water (swimming). *Pseudomonas aeruginosa* is the most common pathogen, but others include Gram-negative bacilli, staphylococci, and fungi. *It is important to rule out malignant external otitis* (look for granulation tissue in the canal, cranial nerve involvement, and diabetic patients).

Patients present with severe ear pain, tragal tenderness, and pruritus. The EAM is swollen and oedematous with purulent discharge. There may be conductive hearing loss. In otomycosis, otoscopy reveals greyish white, thick debris with its characteristic 'wet blotting paper' appearance.

Management
- Thorough aural toileting with fine suction.
- Topical ear drops (acetic acid, antibiotic, or antibiotic/corticosteroid combination drops for 7–10 days).
- Consider placing a wick if the external auditory canal is too oedematous.
- Oral antibiotics are not required unless there are signs of periauricular cellulitis, or systemic illness.
- Avoid prescribing antibiotic and steroid drops in fungal otitis externa.
- Advise the patient to keep the ear dry and avoid self-cleaning of the ears.

① Chronic otitis externa

Thickening of the EAM skin can occur as a result of longstanding infection or inflammation. Often the patient's ear feels itchy and they scratch the canal prolonging irritation and symptoms.

① Eczematous otitis externa

This is a dermatological condition that affects the EAM (e.g. atopic dermatitis, contact dermatitis, psoriasis).

① Perichondritis

This is an infection of the perichondrium of the ear cartilage. It may arise from extension of inadequately treated otitis externa, periauricular cellulitis, or following exposure of the cartilage from trauma. It is also a known complication of surgery involving incisions within the cartilage (e.g. correction of bat ears). Clinically the pinna is tender, erythematous, and warm. *Pseudomonas aeruginosa, Staphylococcus aureus*, and *Streptococcus* are the common organisms involved. Treatment is with high-dose systemic antibiotics. There is a risk of cauliflower ear deformity if not treated quickly or aggressively enough.

① Infections of the middle ear

① Otitis media

Inflammation of the middle ear (otitis media) is a common condition, usually occurring bilaterally. It may be acute or chronic. Acute otitis media is commonly seen in children often following an upper respiratory tract infection. It may be viral or bacterial in origin. *Streptococcuc pneumoniae* and *Haemophilus influenzae* are common bacterial pathogens.

① Acute otitis media

Acute otitis media begins with mucosal inflammation and oedema, resulting in exudates in the middle ear. Oedema prevents drainage through the Eustachian tube and as pus accumulates, pressure builds up. This causes the ear drum to bulge. Untreated, the tympanic membrane eventually perforates. As the middle ear can now drain, the infection will slowly resolve.

Presentation

Patients complain of a throbbing ear ache (otalgia) which progresses in intensity until perforation of the drum relieves some of the pressure. A conductive deafness is usually present, possibly with tinnitus. Patients are often systemically unwell. The tympanic membrane ranges in appearance from the loss of the light reflex, to red and bulging, culminating in perforation with discharge. *Deafness in children is a treatable cause of developmental delay*—early detection and appropriate investigation and treatment are therefore imperative.

Management

- Antibiotics: penicillins are often the first line of treatment, but culture and sensitivities of known pathogens may alter this.
- Analgesics/antipyretics: paracetamol, NSAIDs
- If a bulging tympanic membrane persists, despite adequate antibiotic therapy, myringotomy under general anaesthetic enables the ear to drain.
- Patients who present with a discharging ear (perforation) should be started on broad-spectrum antibiotics after microbiology swabs have been sent for culture and sensitivities.
- If signs and symptoms do not resolve, consider altering the choice of antibiotic and consider underlying infection elsewhere (mastoid, nasopharynx, sinuses).

① Otitis media with effusion: 'glue ear'

This condition is said to affect 30–40% of children at some stage in their development and presents with deafness and a mild otalgia, occasionally associated with tinnitus. Otitis media with effusion is due to a build-up of fluid in the middle ear and although many cases will spontaneously resolve, a short course of antibiotics may prove useful if there is suspicion of underlying infection. *If pain or hearing loss persists for >10 weeks, surgery should be considered*. Myringotomy and grommet insertion is performed under general anaesthetic. A small incision is made in the tympanic membrane; a plastic grommet (drainage tube) is inserted. These often self-extrude after an average period of 6 months—repeated insertions may be necessary if the effusion persists. Adenoidectomy may be beneficial in the long-term treatment of 'glue ear'.

① Chronic suppurative otitis media

Chronic suppurative otitis media (CSOM) is a chronic inflammatory process affecting the middle ear and mastoid cavity. Patients can present with painless persistent or recurrent otorrhoea, with an associated tympanic membrane perforation. There is often some degree of conductive hearing loss. On auroscopic examination, the position of tympanic membrane perforation is important. Atticoantral perforations are more likely to be associated with cholesteatoma (described as 'unsafe' CSOM). 'Safe' CSOM is seen in those cases without evidence of cholesteatoma. There may also be evidence of granulation tissue in the external auditory canal. ENT referral is often required to carry out aural cleaning to allow effective administration of topical antibiotics.

Symptoms of otalgia, vertigo, systemic upset, or evidence of postauricular inflammation should prompt urgent referral to exclude intratemporal or intra-cranial involvement.

ⓘ Herpes zoster

A rare complication of varicella zoster virus (VZV) reactivation is herpes zoster oticus (Ramsay Hunt syndrome) which classically presents as a triad of lower motor neuron facial paralysis, otalgia, and vesicles in the auditory canal and auricle. Some patients may also present with tinnitus or hyperacusis and vertigo. Commonly patients are aged over 60 years but it can affect all ages. VZV reactivation in the geniculate ganglion can also spread to involve the eight cranial nerve. Cases have been reported in association with herpes simplex type 2. Diagnosis is based on clini-cal findings. Eye care and early treatment with steroids and antivirals is recommended, but there is little evidence of efficacy and complete recovery, especially of facial paralysis which is less likely compared to Bell's palsy.

Be careful prescribing steroids in VZV (and other viral) infections. If there is viraemia, the patient is at risk of developing viral encephalitis. Discuss the need for steroids with ENT (or follow local guidelines).

ⓘ Infections of the adjacent bones

ⓘ Osteomyelitis of the skull base (necrotizing or malignant external otitis)

This is an extension of infection from the EAM into the temporal bone, resulting in progressive osteomyelitis. It is usually caused by *Pseudomonas aeruginosa* and seen in immunocompromised patients (diabetics, HIV, radiation exposure). Patients present with *relentless severe otalgia* (out of proportion to patient's signs), granulation tissue in the EAM, and cranial nerve involvement. Diagnosis often requires CT of temporal bones, or technecium or gallium bone scans. It may also require biopsy and culture of the granulations. Untreated or late diagnosis can lead to cranial neu-ropathy, sinus thrombosis, septicaemia, and intracranial infections (men-ingitis), and carries mortality.

Management

This includes prolonged parenteral anti-*Pseudomonas* antibiotics (up to 6 months), antibiotic/corticosteroid ear drops (gentamicin with hydro-cortisone), meticulous cleaning, and debridement. Hyperbaric oxygen has been used in recalcitrant cases. Screen for diabetes.

ⓘ Mastoiditis

Mastoiditis is another potentially serious complication of acute otitis media. Infection passes into the mastoid air cells causing further suppura-tion and bone necrosis. Remember that infection can travel elsewhere—always consider other potential complications. These include:

- Intracranial (meningitis, brain abscess, extra and subdural abscess, Lateral sinus thrombosis)
- Extracranial (labyrinthitis, facial nerve paralysis, mastoiditis).

Presentation
Patients complain of a persistent and throbbing pain with increasing deafness. Discharge is present which is usually creamy and may be profuse. They are pyrexic and tachycardic. There is usually tenderness over the mastoid prominence, often with a postauricular swelling that pushes the pinna forwards. Otoscopy may show bulging of the roof or posterior wall of the external auditory canal. The tympanic membrane is usually red, perforated, and discharging.

Investigation
Mastoid X-rays may show opacity of the air cells. CT scans will give far more information but are not always indicated.

Management
- Patients often need admission for IV antibiotics and pain relief. If the causative organism is unknown then broad-spectrum antibiotics are given, e.g. amoxicillin and metronidazole.
- In the absence of a rapid or complete response to antibiotics or if a subperiosteal abscess is present, surgery may be indicated. A cortical mastoidectomy is performed. Here the mastoid air cells are opened to remove any necrotic debris whilst leaving the middle ear intact.

⊙ Otalgia ('earache') and otorrhoea

Otalgia is a common symptom and is usually due to local disease. *But pain may also be referred. If the ear looks normal, check distant sites (TMJ, oropharynx, nasopharynx, larynx, teeth, etc.).*

Local causes
- Acute otitis externa—a short course of antibiotic/steroid drops or dressing may be required
- Furuncles (infected hair follicles)—drain and prescribe antibiotics
- Acute and 'malignant' otitis externa
- Perichondritis—the pinna is swollen and tender due to infection of the cartilage
- Barotrauma
- Herpes zoster
- Tumours.

Facial palsy, disproportionately severe pain, and progressive deafness are worrying features and warrant careful consideration.

Distant causes (referred pain)
Due to its varied innervation, pain can also arise secondarily from the following sites:
- Tonsillitis and upper respiratory tract disease
- Eustachian tube dysfunction
- Dental pathology
- Disorders of the TMJ
- Parotid disease
- The oropharynx and nasopharynx

- The larynx and pharynx
- Cervical spondylosis
- Malignancy of any of the above-listed, but particularly the tongue base.

Never forget tumours of the upper aerodigestive tract as possible causes of earache in adults.

⊙ Otorrhoea

Discharge from the ear may arise from several causes. The commonest is due to middle ear infections. The nature of the discharge may give a clue to its cause:
- Watery: CSF or eczema
- Mucoid: chronic suppurative otitis media
- Purulent: furunculosis or local abscess
- Bloody: trauma/acute otitis media/malignancy
- Foul smelling: cholesteatoma.

⊙ Deafness

Hearing loss is extremely common and has a wide spectrum ranging from a nearly undetectable degree of disability, to a profound loss. It can present at any age. Nearly 10% of the adult population has some hearing loss and around one-third of individuals over the age of 65 have loss sufficient to require a hearing aid. Hearing loss can result from disorders of the auricle, external auditory canal, middle ear, inner ear, or central auditory pathways. In general, lesions in the auricle, external auditory canal, or middle ear cause conductive hearing loss. Sensorineural hearing loss results from lesions in the inner ear or eighth cranial nerve (Table 6.1). Sensorineural hearing loss may result from damage to the hair cells caused by intense noise, viral infections, fractures of the temporal bone, meningitis, cochlear otosclerosis, Ménière's disease, and ageing. Many drugs can produce sensorineural hearing loss (e.g. salicylates, quinine, aminoglycosides, loop diuretics, and some chemotherapeutic agents).

Classification of hearing loss

Sensorineural
Nerve impulses are prevented from reaching the brain by a defect of either the auditory nerve (CN VIII) itself or the functioning of the cochlea.

Conductive
Sound is prevented from reaching the cochlea apparatus by some form of mechanical obstruction in the outer or middle ear.

Mixed deafness
A combination of sensorineural and conductive deafness in the same ear.

Table 6.1 Aetiology of sensorineural hearing loss

Aetiology	Diagnosis
Developmental and hereditary	
Syndromic	Alport syndrome, Usher syndrome
Non-syndromic	Large vestibular aqueduct syndrome
Infectious	Otitis media, viral, syphilis
Pharmacological toxicity	Aminoglycosides, loop diuretics
Trauma	Head injury, noise-induced, barotrauma
Neurological disorders	MS
Bone disorders	Paget disease
Neoplasms	Acoustic neuroma, meningioma
Unknown aetiology	Presbycusis, Ménière's disease

Assessment

A simple clinical assessment may be made by an examiner repeating certain words at different intensities and at different distances to each ear in turn. By convention this is recorded as (for example) WV @ 200 cm (whispered voice at 200 cm).

Tuning fork tests
- Rinne's test: a 512hz tuning fork is struck and held close to the ear; it is then placed firmly on the ipsilateral mastoid process. The patient is asked to say whether the tuning fork is heard better by BC or AC.
- AC >BC Rinne +ve (middle/outer ear functioning normally).
- BC >AC Rinne –ve (defective middle/outer ear).
- Weber's test: a struck tuning fork is held on the vertex of the patient's head. They are then asked to say whether the sound is heard centrally or more to one ear than the other.
- Conductive deafness: sound heard in deafer ear.
- Sensorineural deafness: sound heard in better hearing ear.
- Audiometry specialist tests are carried out in soundproofed rooms.

Causes of hearing loss in children

Deafness in children is a treatable cause of developmental delay – early detection and appropriate investigation and treatment are therefore imperative.

Otitis media with effusion ('glue ear')
This is the commonest cause of deafness in children with around 60% of cases going undetected in the first year. Commonly presenting with hearing loss and otalgia there is a higher incidence in children with Down's syndrome or cleft palate. Treatment in the short term involves antibiotics and decongestants, progressing to surgery if symptoms persist (myringotomy and grommets). *Otitis media with effusion is rare in adults and so further investigation must be undertaken to exclude a neoplastic growth. Progressive unilateral sensorineural deafness must raise the suspicion of an acoustic neuroma.*

Congenital and genetic causes of hearing loss
Congenital malformations of the inner ear cause hearing loss in some adults. Genetic predisposition alone or combined with environmental factors may also be responsible. More than 200 syndromes are known to be associated with hearing loss.

Causes of hearing loss in adults

The main causes of deafness in the adult population are wax impaction and ageing (presbycusis in the over 60s).

⑦ *Otosclerosis*

This is the formation of new bone occurring within the inner ear resulting in immobility of the auditory ossicles and conductive deafness.

⑦ *Drug induced*

Drugs that are renal toxic are commonly ototoxic, e.g. cytotoxics, systemic aminoglycosides. Many other drugs are also ototoxic.

⑦ *Presbycusis*

This is the gradual onset of (usually) bilateral sensorineural hearing loss that occurs as with ageing. It is most pronounced at higher frequencies, with difficulty hearing in noisy environments. The aetiology is multifactorial. Risk factors include previous noise exposure, ototoxic medications, and family history. In the UK, approximately 50% of those over 55 years of age have some degree of hearing impairment. It is a diagnosis of exclusion. In mild cases, reassurance and advice (e.g. face-to-face communication can help). In more severe cases, hearing aids can be of benefit.

⑦ *Noise-induced hearing loss*

Noise-induced hearing loss results from recreational as well as occupational activities and often begins in adolescence. High-risk activities require that the user wears hearing protection.

Sudden onset of sensorineural hearing loss

Sudden onset of unilateral hearing loss, with or without tinnitus, may represent an inner ear viral infection or a vascular accident. Patients usually complain of reduced hearing, poor sound localization, and difficulty hearing clearly with background noise.

Gradual loss of hearing

Gradual progression in a hearing deficit is common with otosclerosis, noise-induced hearing loss, acoustic neuromas, and Ménière's disease. In addition to hearing loss, Ménière's disease may be associated with episodic vertigo, tinnitus, and aural fullness. Hearing loss with otorrhoea is most likely due to chronic otitis media or cholesteatoma.

Mixed hearing loss

Mixed hearing losses are due to pathology that can affect the middle and inner ear simultaneously; causes include otosclerosis involving the ossicles and the cochlea, transverse and longitudinal temporal bone fractures, head trauma, chronic otitis media, cholesteatoma, and middle ear tumours.

Management of hearing loss
- Hearing aids: these vary in size, site configuration, and strength.
- Cochlear implants: cochlear implants convert sound energy to electrical signals and can be used to stimulate the auditory division of the eighth nerve directly. A microphone picks up acoustic information that is sent to an external speech processor (located on the body or at ear level). This processor converts the mechanical acoustic wave into an electric signal that is transmitted via the surgically implanted electrode in the cochlea to the auditory nerve. With the current generation of multichannel cochlear implants, almost 75% of the patients with these implants are able to converse on the telephone.

① Dizziness/'vertigo'

Vertigo is defined as the sensation of movement, even though the patient is motionless. However, patients with an injury to the vestibular system usually complain of 'dizziness'. Dysfunction of the peripheral or central vestibular system causes asymmetry in signal input into the vestibular centres, resulting in vertigo, nystagmus, vomiting, and a sense of falling toward the side of the injury. Duration of symptoms and loss of hearing are useful diagnostic clues (Table 6.2). Disorders of the middle and inner ear can also cause these symptoms. They include:
- Impacted wax
- Acute otitis media
- Otitis media with effusion
- Chronic suppurative otitis media
- Trauma (temporal bone fracture)
- Labyrinthitis and vestibular neuronitis
- Ménière's disease (endolymphatic hydrops)
- Otosclerosis/otosclerotic drugs
- BPPV

Table 6.2 Differential diagnosis of vertigo based on its duration and the presence of hearing loss

Time	No associated hearing loss	Hearing loss present
Seconds	Benign positional paroxysmal vertigo	Perilymphatic fistula Cholesteatoma
Minutes	Vertebral basilar insufficiency Migraines	
Hours	Vestibulopathy	Ménière's disease
Days	Vestibular neuronitis	Labyrinthitis
Weeks	CNS disorders Lyme disease MS	Acoustic neuroma Autoimmune Psychogenic

- Iatrogenic (middle ear/mastoid surgery)
- Cerebellopontine angle tumours
- Perilymphatic fistulas
- Oto syphilis.

Remember non-auricular causes as well (cardiac, cervical, neurological, etc.). In elderly patients, vertigo is often multifactorial with many systemic diseases affecting balance.

What to ask for in the history for vertigo
- Duration
- Periodicity
- Circumstance of the vertigo
- Presence of other neurological signs or symptoms
- Hearing loss
- Otalgia.

What to look for
- Head and neck examination, including cranial nerves
- Spontaneous and gaze-evoked nystagmus
- Positional testing—Dix-Hallpike test
- Cerebellar tests— rapid alternating movements (e.g. finger to nose)
- Posture—Romberg, tandem walking and gait
- Head thrust and headshake—check for nystagmus
- Dynamic visual activity—look at Snellen chart with head shake (worsening by >2 lines on chart)
- Ocular examination—range of eye movement, pupil size, and symmetry
- Corneal reflex, trigeminal anaesthesia.

Management of patients with dizziness
- Precautions: avoid heights, driving, and operating heavy machinery when symptomatic.
- Acute vestibular suppressants: these are indicated for intolerable symptoms but only in the short term. Prolonged use can delay central compensatory mechanisms; common medications include prochlorperazine, phenothiazine, meclizine, cinnarizine, diazepam, and antiemetics.
- Vestibular rehabilitation: (exercise and physiotherapy) indicated for chronic complaints, involve positional tasks, head movements, and oculomotor exercises to facilitate central compensation.
- Surgical treatment: may be indicated for specific diagnoses (intratympanic gentamycin for Ménière's disease).

⊙ Labyrinthitis and vestibular neuritis
- Vestibular neuritis is inflammation of the vestibular nerve.
- Labyrinthitis is inflammation of the labyrinth in the inner ear, although the vestibular nerve may also be involved.

The causes and symptoms of both these conditions are similar and it is often impossible to tell which one is present. If there is hearing loss, labyrinthitis is more likely (because the cochlea may also be inflamed). Vestibular neuritis may be associated with nystagmus. Both conditions result in unilateral vestibular dysfunction. This can result in loss of balance, vertigo, hearing loss, and tinnitus. The underlying cause is believed to be a viral infection (as symptoms usually follow a URTI), but it can also occur from bacterial infection, head injury, or from taking certain drugs. Some cases of vestibular neuritis are thought to be caused by an infection of the vestibular ganglion by herpes simplex virus type 1. Infective labyrinthitis can cause permanent hearing loss.

Signs and symptoms

One of the main symptoms is severe vertigo. Nausea, anxiety, and a general feeling of being unwell are also common. Examination will demonstrate nystagmus.

Management

Prochlorperazine or cinnarizine is commonly prescribed to help alleviate vertigo and nausea. Some authorities suggest that viral labyrinthitis should be treated early with steroids and antiviral medication. Vestibular rehabilitation therapy may help reduce any residual dizziness from labyrinthitis. This works by challenging the vestibular system and stimulating adaption.

ⓘ Ménière's disease (endolymphatic hydrops)

Ménière's disease is an idiopathic inner ear disorder characterized by attacks of vertigo, fluctuating hearing loss, tinnitus, and aural fullness. Patients typically present in the fifth decade of life. The cause of Ménière's disease is unknown. Anatomical, infectious, immunological, and allergic factors have all been suggested. The endolymphatic sac may also be defective. This is important in inner ear metabolism.

Presentation

Episodic attacks last for hours. The main symptoms and signs include
- Unilateral, fluctuating sensorineural hearing loss (often low frequency)
- Vertigo that lasts minutes to hours
- Increasing tinnitus typically before or during the vertiginous attack
- Aural fullness.

The acute attack is also associated with nausea and vomiting, and afterwards patients feel exhausted for a few days.

Investigations

Ménière's disease is a clinical diagnosis. Electrophysiological studies and imaging are obtained as needed but there is no diagnostic test specifically for Ménière's disease. Audiology shows a low-frequency sensorineural hearing loss. Electrocochleography and electronystagmography (ENG) may be needed in atypical presentation or if ablative therapy is considered. ENG with caloric testing shows peripheral vestibular dysfunction.

Management
- Dietary modifications (sodium-restricted diet, dietary restrictions on caffeine, nicotine, alcohol, and foods containing theophylline, e.g. chocolate).

- Acute attacks are managed with vestibular suppressants (e.g. meclizine and diazepam) and antiemetic medications (e.g. prochlorperazine).
- Aminoglycoside therapy: medically refractory patients may benefit from intratympanic gentamicin therapy.
- Steroid therapy: acute exacerbation of Ménière's disease may respond to a short burst of oral steroids. Intratympanic steroids have also been used to treat active disease and avoid the systemic complications associated with oral steroids.
- Surgical measures: patients who have failed medical and gentamicin treatment may require surgical intervention. Endolymphatic sac surgery and vestibular nerve sections preserve hearing while labyrinthectomy ablates hearing.
- ENT follow-up advised.

ⓘ Benign paroxysmal positional vertigo

BPPV is one of the most common types of peripheral vertigo, arising as a result of debris in the posterior semicircular canal. It can affect any age but more commonly affects those over 50 years of age. Patients complain of vertigo lasting seconds, with no associated hearing loss and when in certain positions. Nearly 20% of patients seen at vertigo clinics have BPPV; 20% have a preceding history of vestibular neuronitis; and another 20% have a history of head trauma.

BPPV occurs because a semicircular canal has debris either attached to the cupula or free floating in the endolymph. The semicircular canal becomes stimulated by the movement of these particles in response to gravity. Movement of the debris within the endolymph stimulates the hairs lining the canal which in turn connect to the vestibular nerve. The resultant conflicting signals from the side affected in comparison to the unaffected side cause the vertigo sensation.

Presentation

Patients usually complain of a sudden onset of vertigo that lasts 10–20 seconds with certain head positions (rolling over in bed, getting out of bed, looking up, and bending over). This occurs as the calcium crystals (otoliths) in the labyrinth move. Audiogram and tympanogram should be normal. *Asymmetric hearing loss calls into question the diagnosis of BPPV* and further evaluation is required.

Management

- Particle repositioning manoeuvres (such as Epley's).
- A bone vibrator may also be placed on the mastoid bone during the manoeuvres to loosen the debris. 80% of patients are cured by a single repositioning manoeuvre. If the symptoms persist or if patients have recurrent symptoms, it may be repeated.
- Generally symptoms are resistant to medical management.
- Surgical treatment is rarely indicated but includes posterior semicircular canal occlusion or singular neurectomy.

Epley's manoeuvre (modifications exist)
Only perform this if you have been shown how to do so and if there are no contraindications.

- Sit the patient upright, with the legs fully extended and the head rotated 45 degrees towards the affected side.
- The patient is then quickly and passively forced down backwards into a supine position with the head held approximately in a 30 degree neck extension (Dix–Hallpike position). The affected ear faces the ground.
- Observes the patient's eyes for nystagmus for approximately 1–2 minutes.
- The patient's head is then turned 90 degrees to the opposite side so that the affected ear faces up, while maintaining the 30 degree neck extension. Remain in this position for approximately 1–2 minutes.
- Keeping the head and neck fixed relative to the body, the patient rolls onto their shoulder, rotating the head with the body. The patient should now be looking downwards at a 45-degree angle.
- Observe the eyes for nystagmus for approximately 1–2 minutes.
- Finally, the patient is slowly brought up to an upright sitting posture, while maintaining the 45-degree rotation of the head. The patient holds this position for up to 30 seconds.

This may be repeated two more times. Post treatment the patient may wear a soft collar during the day to avoid any head positions that may precipitate symptoms. They are advised to be careful bending, lying backwards, moving the head up and down, or tilting it to either side.

Contraindications to Epley's manoeuvre
- Severe carotid stenosis
- Unstable heart disease
- Severe neck disease
- Advanced rheumatoid arthritis.

ⓘ Tinnitus (ringing/buzzing in the ear)

Tinnitus can affect up to one in five of the general population with a high prevalence after noise exposure. Tinnitus can be classified as subjective and objective. Subjective tinnitus is the perception of sound in the absence of any acoustic or external stimuli. Objective tinnitus is perception of sound caused by an internal body sound or vibration (bruit, hum, palatal myoclonus). Subjective tinnitus is more common and is typically associated with high-frequency hearing loss in old age. The pathophysiology of subjective tinnitus is largely unknown although it may involve the subcortical auditory pathways. *If tinnitus is unilateral and accompanied by unilateral sensory neural hearing loss, this may indicate acoustic neuroma. Persistent pulsatile tinnitus may warrant imaging to rule out paragangliomas or aberrant vascular anomalies in the middle ear cleft.*

Noise can also arise from many causes, including conditions of the TMJ, Eustachian tube, and carotid artery. Causes include:

- Wax impaction
- Insects
- Otosclerosis
- Glue ear
- Noise induced
- Presbycusis
- Ménière's disease
- Trauma/tympanic membrane perforation
- Ototoxic drugs
- Labyrinthitis
- Acoustic neuroma
- AVMs
- TMJ disorders
- Glomus jugulare
- Carotid body tumours
- Patulous Eustachian tube and palatal myoclonus.

Management

- Hearing aids: for tinnitus associated with hearing loss. This reduces tinnitus by amplifying ambient sound to mask it.
- Maskers: these utilize a band of white noise centred around the tinnitus; indicated for intractable tinnitus.
- Tinnitus retraining therapy and tinnitus counselling by hearing therapists/relaxation techniques.
- Drug therapy: benzodiazepines, tricyclic antidepressants, and carbamazepine; may result in some improvement.
- Refer to a tinnitus support group.
- For further information, see http://www.tinnitus.org.uk.

⑦ Wax impaction

This is a common cause of tinnitus and conductive hearing loss. It is readily identified by auroscope examination where the tympanic membrane is often obscured. Can be compounded by repeated attempts by the patient to try to remove with cotton buds. Best removed by means of aural micro-suction, which is often carried out in a nurse-led clinic and facilitated by an ENT referral.

① Foreign body/insects

Often there is no clear history of insertion and therefore it is important to remember that foreign bodies can present with ear ache or discharge. If the foreign body has been present for a period of time visualization can be obscured by wax build-up on auroscope examination. If the patient is cooperative it may be possible to attempt removal. If there are no suitable instruments, or the patient is uncooperative, this will need ENT referral for examination and removal. Insects in the ear can be very distressing and can present with significant excoriation or swelling of the EAM.

Removing a foreign body
- Calm and reassure the person (usually a child).
- If the object is sticking out and easy to remove, do so with forceps.
- Objects within the canal can sometimes be retrieved with an aural hook. If the patient is cooperative and the object smooth, a small drop of superglue on the tip of an applicator may help.
- If you think the object is lodged deep within the ear, or you cannot see it, *do not* reach inside the ear canal with tweezers. This may do more harm than good. Turn the patient's head to the affected side and let gravity help. Shake the head gently.
- If the object doesn't come out, refer.

Removing an insect
- Do not let the patient put a finger in the ear. This may cause the insect to bite or sting.
- Turn the patient's head so that the affected ear is up. Wait and see if the insect flies or crawls out.
- If this doesn't work, slowly pour mineral oil, olive oil, or baby oil into the ear, gently pulling the ear lobe backward and upward (adult), or backward (child). Water will not work, as insects can trap air and therefore do not drown. Oil should drown or dislodge most creepy-crawlies which will then float out.
- Discuss with ENT even if this is successful, as small insect remains can irritate the EAM.

⑦ Otosclerosis

This is caused by abnormal bone remodelling within the middle ear, primarily affecting the stapes bone. It usually begins in one ear but will eventually affect both with a variable course. Typically it leads to a conductive hearing loss but if progressive, the cochlear nerves can be affected. This results in deafness which commonly presents below the age of 30. The EAM and tympanic membrane appear normal on examination. Audiometry is required to quantify the degree of hearing loss.

Causes
Most cases are genetic in nature and can be inherited. Certain drugs may cause this as a side effect. Paget's disease and measles have also been associated.

Management
- Hearing aids are usually very effective in the early stages of the disease
- Surgery. Stapedectomy (or stapedotomy) may be required for definitive treatment.

① Tympanic membrane perforations

Rarely patients present with tympanic membrane perforation as an emergency. Often these are of infectious or traumatic aetiology. Symptoms include hearing loss and tinnitus. Pain may precede perforation if there has been a middle ear infection. There may also be a discharge. Diagnosis is confirmed by otoscopic examination and audiography.

Causes of ear drum perforation
- Acute/chronic suppurative otitis media (most common cause)
- Persistent perforation after extrusion of a grommet
- Trauma (blow to the ear, barotrauma, diving, water skiing, explosion, forceful irrigation)
- Iatrogenic
- Cholesteatoma (associated with marginal perforations).

Types of perforation
- Central: perforation does not involve the annulus, typically infectious
- Marginal: involves the annulus. There is a higher association with cholesteatomas
- Subtotal: large defect with an intact annulus.

Management
This involves keeping the ear dry and ear drops if infected. Send an ear swab if there is persistent discharge. Refer to ENT. Tympanoplasty may be required for a persistent perforation.

⑦ Eustachian tube problems

⑦ Eustachian tube dysfunction
This is a condition in which the Eustachian tube fails to provide adequate ventilation to the middle ear. The resultant decreased air pressure in the middle ear places the tympanic membrane under tension. It then fails to vibrate correctly in response to sound waves. This results in muffled or dull hearing. Temporary dysfunction is commonly experienced by many people during take-off and landing when travelling by air. Symptoms can last from a few hours to several weeks depending on the cause. Any cause of tube blockage, tube inflammation or failure of the tube to open can cause Eustachian tube dysfunction. Common precipitants include URTI, glue ear, allergies, or enlarged adenoids. More rarely, especially if presenting in older patients, *tumours in the nasopharyngeal region should be excluded*. Often symptoms are short-lived and no cause is identified. Nasal decongestants can help in cases where allergy is suspected. Where symptoms persist, ENT opinion should be sought.

⑦ Patulous Eustachian tube
This is a benign condition in which the Eustachian tube fails to close normally, remaining patent most of the time. It doesn't typically lead to ear problems or otitis media. However, patients can report autophony (hearing one's own voice and breathing) or muffled sounds, due to variations in pressure associated with respiration being transmitted to the middle ear. Patulous Eustachian tube can be associated with weight loss, mucosal scarring secondary to surgery, inflammation, or radiation, and neuromuscular disorders causing muscle atrophy such as MS or following a stroke. *PET can be misdiagnosed and treated as congestion*, however decongestants and steroids spray are ineffective. Diagnosis is based on clinical evaluation that can be confirmed by nasendoscopy and audiology and tympanogram studies. Mild cases may only require reassurance; potassium iodide treatment can have a role in thickening secretions, in more moderate cases, with surgical management reserved for failure of medical management.

Miscellaneous conditions

⑦ Chondrodermatitis nodularis helicis

These are painful, tender, erythematous paulonodules localized to the pinna with occasional scale or crust. The superior part of the helix is most frequently affected but lesions have been reported all around the pinna. Despite the lesion being only a few millimetres wide, it results in exquisite tenderness. The condition most commonly affects men from the age of 40 and above. Trauma, pressure (headphones, pillows), and cold are thought to be pathogenic factors. The patient is advised to avoid pressure to the affected area. Treatments include intralesional steroids, cryotherapy, or surgical removal of the inflamed cartilage.

⑦ Arteriovenous malformation and venous hum

A form of pulsatile tinnitus defined as the perception of sound heard with a regular rhythm corresponding to the heart beat. It typically is described as a 'whooshing' noise, rather than a 'ringing' and can be positional with the sound intensity influenced by head movement. When examining it is important to auscultate for an audible bruit in the neck, as pulse synchronous tinnitus that can be heard on auscultation is referred to as objective pulsatile tinnitus and suggests a vascular aetiology. There are several potential vascular causes such as AVM, usually involving branches of the external carotid artery. These patients should be referred.

⑦ Glomus jugulare tumours

Glomus jugulare tumours, also known as jugulotympanic paragangliomas are vascular, commonly benign paragangliomas. They can arise either from the promontory of the middle ear or the adventitia of the jugular bulb. As these tumours grow, they can fill the middle ear, resulting in pulsatile tinnitus with or without conductive hearing loss. As they enlarge further they can also erode bone, especially inferiorly, placing cranial nerves at risk. Tumours may also impinge on the ossicles and the tympanic membrane, impairing the motility of either or both. Patients can present with hearing loss or lower cranial nerve defects. A bluish pulsatile mass may be visible on auroscope examination. CT is usually required with arteriography for large tumours. Traditionally treated by surgical removal, there is an increasing role for the use of stereotactic radiation therapy.

⑦ Palatal myoclonus

A rare condition in which rapid spasm of either the levator or tensor veli palatini muscles causes a sensation of 'clicking' or 'popping' in the ears or tinnitus. It is most often secondary to a brainstem or cerebellar lesion such as pontine infarct but can occur in the absence of any structural abnormality. When associated with eye movements, it is known as oculopalatal myoclonus.

⑦ Gout

Gout tophi (uric acid deposits under the skin), can occur typically in the pinna, in association with chronic tophaceous gout. On examination they can have a white or yellowish appearance and are not usually tender or painful. Other sites of deposition include the olecranon bursa and proximal and distal interphalangeal joints of the fingers. It would be rare for the appearance of tophi to be the presenting symptom in a patient with gout. Small deposits can resolve on uric acid-lowering medication, larger deposits may require surgery to remove.

⑦ Aural fullness

This is the sensation of 'ear fullness', or 'ear pressure' often associated with tinnitus, hearing disturbance, autophony, nasal obstruction, and sore throat. It is often reported in the early stages of Ménière's disease and idiopathic sensorineural hearing loss. Ear fullness can be caused by Eustachian tube dysfunction, otitis media with effusion, and chronic otitis media. The underlying mechanisms may involve any part of the ear, from the external auditory canal to the inner ear. However, in around 10% of patients no cause can be found. *Rarely this can be a symptom of nasopharyngeal carcinoma.*

⑦ Ear itching

Itching can be a symptom of ear infection, commonly otitis externa. Other possible causes include insect bites, contact allergies, and trauma. Chickenpox is accompanied by red, oozing blisters that cause intense itching. Eczema, contact dermatitis, scabies, and ringworm are other sources of itching.

⑦ Perilymphatic fistulas

This is a pathological defect between the air-filled middle ear and the fluid-filled inner ear, in either the round window or oval window membranes. The result is leakage of perilymph fluid from the semi-circular canals into the middle ear with changes in middle ear pressure transmitted directly to the inner ear. Symptoms include sensorineural hearing loss, which can be sudden or progressive, vertigo, and tinnitus. It can be a congenital condition, the consequence of middle ear disease such as cholesteatoma, secondary to trauma or rapid pressure changes that can occur in SCUBA diving or following middle ear surgery. Definitive diagnosis is by means of surgery with direct visualization of the fistula. Symptoms can resolve with bed rest, with surgery reserved for those with persistent symptoms.

The nose and naso-orbitoethmoid region

Common presentations

Common presentations for the nose/nasoethmoid region:
- Blocked nose
- Crusty nose
- Epistaxis
- Injuries
- Irritation/itchiness
- Loss of smell (anosmia)
- Offensive smell (cacosmia)
- Pain
- Runny nose
- Sneezing
- Swelling.

Common problems and their causes

Blocked nose

Common
- Rhinitis (allergic, vasomotor)
- URTI
- Sinusitis
- Trauma
- Anatomical variations (e.g. septal deviation, concha bullosa).

Uncommon
- Nasal polyps
- Side effect of medication
- Rhinitis medicamentosa
- Hormonal changes (e.g. pregnancy, puberty, hormone replacement therapy, hypothyroidism).

Rare
- Severe GORD, empty nose syndrome
- Tumour (nasal or sinus)/Wegener's granulomatosis
- Nasal myiasis.

Crusty nose

Common
- Dry environment
- Atrophic rhinitis
- Staphylococcal infection.

Uncommon
- Tumour
- Previous nasal surgery
- Ciliary disease, e.g. cystic fibrosis

- Chronic nose picking
- Basal cell carcinoma
- Vestibulitis
- Perforated nasal septum.

Epistaxis

Common
- Trauma
- Sinusitis
- Foreign body
- Anticoagulant therapy
- Chronic nose picking.

Uncommon
- High altitude
- Hypertension
- Nasal surgery
- Bleeding disorders.

Rare
- Leukaemia/lymphoma
- Nasal/sinus tumours/Wegener's granulomatosis
- Septal perforation.

Injuries

Common
- Fractures
- Septal haematoma
- Minor injuries
- Foreign bodies (especially in children)
- Lacerations.

Uncommon
- Bites.

Irritation/itchiness

Common
- Allergic rhinitis
- Asthma.

Uncommon
- Fungal infection
- Chronic nose picking
- Tumour (nasal or sinus)
- Nasal myiasis.

Loss of smell (anosmia)

Common
- Trauma (skull base)
- Post viral.

Uncommon
- Nasal/sinus tumours
- Nasal polyps
- Post surgery.

Offensive smell (cacosmia)

Common
- Atrophic rhinitis
- Sinus infection.

Uncommon
- Fungal infection
- Dental infection
- Tumours
- Psychological.

Pain

Common
- Trauma
- Infection (abscess)
- Foreign body
- Facial pain.

Uncommon
- Sinusitis
- Relapsing polychondritis
- Tumour (nasal or sinus)/Wegener's granulomatosis
- Nasal myiasis.

Runny nose

Common
- Rhinitis (allergic, vasomotor)
- URTI
- Sinusitis
- Nasal polyps
- Foreign body (especially in children).

Uncommon
- CSF
- Hormonal changes (e.g. pregnancy, puberty, hormone replacement therapy, hypothyroidism)
- Migraines/cluster headaches

- Recreational drug use
- Tumour (nasal or sinus).

Rare
- Churg–Strauss syndrome
- Wegener's granulomatosis.

Sneezing

Common
- Rhinitis (allergic, vasomotor)
- URTI
- Environmental irritants.

Uncommon
- Rhinitis medicamentosa
- Trauma
- Opiate withdrawal.

Swelling

Common
- Abscess
- Sinusitis
- Trauma
- Septal haematoma.

Uncommon
- Nasal polyps
- Tumour (nasal or sinus)
- Nasal glioma
- Dermoid cyst
- Dentoalveolar cyst
- Rhinophyma.

Useful questions and what to look for

Blocked nose

Ask about
- Pain, bleeding, foul smell
- Onset: sudden or gradual
- Progression
- Previous episodes
- Unilateral or bilateral
- History of trauma/travel abroad
- Childhood history

- Previous treatment: ?perennial problem
- Medications applied.

Look for
- Foreign body/infestation
- Nasal deviation
- Septal deviation
- Septal haematoma
- Obstruction: nasal polyps, turbinate hypertrophy, congested middle meatus
- Discharge
- Inflamed mucosa.

Crusty nose

Ask about
- Pain
- Progression
- Unilateral or bilateral
- Previous episodes
- History of trauma
- History of nose picking
- History of previous treatment
- Medications applied.

Look for
- Whether crustiness is dry or moist
- Signs of infection
- Adjacent tissues (? basal cell carcinoma/squamous cell carcinoma)
- Foreign body: unilateral nasal vestibulitis ± discharge in children is almost diagnostic of a foreign body.

Epistaxis

Ask about
- Previous episodes
- History of trauma
- How much blood has been lost
- Unilateral or bilateral
- Nose picking
- Medications.

Look for
- Check BP
- One or both sides
- Any foreign body, polyps, intranasal tumours
- Signs of infection
- Signs of septal perforation.

Injuries

Ask about
- When it occurred
- Mechanism of injury
- Neck/head injury
- Progression of symptoms since time of injury
- Other injuries.

Look for
- Other injuries
- CSF leakage
- Intercanthal distance
- Vision, diplopia
- Nasal deviation, septal haematoma
- Lacerations.

Irritation/itchiness

Ask about
- Known precipitants, travel abroad
- Any discharge
- Unilateral or bilateral
- Previous episodes
- Concurrent symptoms (sneezing, irritation, itchy eyes)—rhinitis
- Medications applied.

Look for
- Signs of congestion
- Foreign body/infestation
- Nasal polyps.

Loss of smell (anosmia)/offensive smell (cacosmia)

Ask about
- Constant or intermittent
- Sudden or gradual
- History of trauma
- Headaches
- Nasal discharge/bleeding
- Obstruction.

Look for
- Discharge
- Foreign bodies
- Nasal polyps
- Intranasal tumours
- Basal skull trauma.

Pain

Ask about
- Type/site of pain
- History of trauma
- Swelling
- Discharge
- Loss of smell.

Look for
- Signs of injury
- Infection (skin, septum, sinuses).

Running nose

Ask about
- Watery or thick
- Clear or coloured (blood, mucus, pus)
- Unilateral or bilateral
- Previous episodes, seasonal, diurnal variation
- Concurrent symptoms (sneezing, irritation, itchy eyes)—rhinitis
- History of trauma
- Other symptoms (sneezing, irritation, itchy eyes)
- PMH of atopy, asthma, previous treatments, medications.

Look for
- Confirm present
- Signs of congestion
- Foreign body
- Nasal polyps
- Mucous retention cysts
- Intranasal tumours.

Sneezing

Ask about
- Known precipitants
- Discharge
- Previous episodes, number of bouts per day
- Other symptoms (irritation, itchy eyes)
- Medications applied.

Look for
- Signs of congestion
- Foreign bodies
- Nasal polyps
- Conjunctivitis.

Swelling

Ask about
- How long/progression
- History of trauma
- Painful/painless
- Discharge
- Loss of smell.

Look for
- Signs of injury, septal haematoma
- Internal/external component
- Solid/cystic
- Surface characteristics (normal mucosa/haemorrhagic/pus)
- Abscess.

Examination of the nose

The structure of the nose is related to its function: the large surface area of mucosa over the turbinates humidifies, warms, and filters particles from the air. The roof of the nose contains specialized neuroepithelium to provide the sense of smell. Normal air flow fluctuates slightly through each nostril (nasal cycle).

Thorough examination of the nose requires special equipment:
- Headlamp.
- Nasal mirror and tongue spatula: it may be necessary to anaesthetize the oropharynx with topical anaesthesia prior to examining the postnasal space.
- Thudichum's speculum: this is useful to view the anterior–inferior nasal septum including Little's area.

Position the patient in a chair slightly higher than your own. Ask the patient to remove any glasses.

External nose
- Examine the skin for lesions or scarring.
- Note any redness, discharge, crusting, or offensive smell.
- Palpate the nasal bones and lateral cartilages, looking for asymmetry, mobility, or other abnormality.
- Have the patient tilt their head back to allow you to inspect the columella and alar cartilages.

Internal nose
- Examine the appearance of the nasal mucosa, including colour, texture, and hydration.
- Check for inflammation, position of the septum, and presence of polyps (insensitive to touch).
- A foreign body, usually accompanied by an offensive unilateral discharge, may be seen inside the nose of a child. Infestation is rare.

- Check nasal airway patency by occluding each nostril in turn and asking the patient to sniff in. Check for alar collapse during this time. Alternatively, check for misting on a nasal mirror.
- Inspect the postnasal space using a nasal mirror. Try to visualize posterior choanae, inferior turbinates, and any adenoidal tissue

Cottle's test

This is performed to assess the patency of the nasal valve. Place your thumb in the nasolabial furrow and push the cheek outward. If the airway improves, the test is positive. The valve will need mechanical support (a graft).

Some swellings around the base of the nose may be secondary to dental pathology. Often there is bony swelling in the labial sulcus. If the teeth are not managed correctly the cyst will recur. Request an OPT and refer to maxillofacial surgeons for advice.

Examination of the nasoethmoid region

(See ➔ 'Naso-orbitoethmoid fractures', pp. 221–2.)

- Examine nose as detailed earlier in this section; note displacement
- Check intercanthal distance
- Check for CSF leaks/signs of head/neck injury
- Check for ocular injury.

These are potentially serious injuries.

Useful investigations

Laboratory tests

- FBC and coagulation screen to rule out bleeding disorder as the cause of epistaxis.
- Beta-2-transferrin in rhinorrhoea fluid. This is a high specificity test for CSF which has superseded other diagnostic techniques including glucose and tau-protein testing.
- Electron microscopy of nasal brushings can be used to test for ciliary disease.

Plain films

Occipitomental views may be of use if sinus disease or nasal/sinus fractures are suspected. Opacity of the sinuses may be secondary to infection, a fluid level or polyposis. Also look for bony expansion or erosion, suggestive of neoplasm. Generally speaking, plain films of the nose are no longer taken to diagnose a fracture. This is made on clinical grounds.

CT/MRI scanning

CT is indicated for patients with complex nasal/facial trauma, skull base trauma, CSF rhinorrhoea, or suspected malignancy. It is not always indicated for soft tissue pathology (e.g. polyps), but it can demonstrate intrasinus mucosal thickening which would be missed on plain radiographs. MRI is useful in the assessment of possible tumours.

Allergy testing

Nearly all patients with seasonal allergic rhinitis show positive skin prick tests. However, these tests can be used to help isolate specific allergens in cases of perennial allergic rhinitis. RAST (radio-allergo-absorbent test) blood tests are also used to detect the presence of circulating immunoglobulins.

Air flow measurement

Usually nasal obstruction is easily assessed clinically. However, peak inspiratory nasal air flow can be measured with a modified peak flow meter.

ⓘ Epistaxis (non-traumatic)

Patients should have their pulse and BP checked and if bleeding has been severe, should be investigated for bleeding disorders. *Elderly patients in particular are affected more by blood loss and may develop postural hypotension or syncope.* Occasionally IV fluids may be required. Patients who have had major nose bleeds should be admitted for observation, bed rest, and IV fluids. Following trauma, although these are technically open (compound) fractures, nasal fractures associated with epistaxis generally do not require antibiotic cover.

ⓘ Minor bleeding

This usually settles on its own, or requires only simple first-aid measures (sitting forward and pinching the cartilaginous part of the nose for at least 20 minutes). If the bleeding stops advise the patient against picking, blowing, or sniffing for 24 hours.

   If bleeding continues, the vestibule and septum should be examined for bleeding points. These may be cauterized using silver nitrate sticks or needle diathermy under topical anaesthesia. *Be careful if cauterizing the septum—extensive cautery or bilateral cautery carries a risk of septal perforation.* Cocaine paste causes vasoconstriction and may also help to control bleeding. However, care is required as too much is toxic. Xylocaine with adrenaline (epinephrine) spray can be used instead. Where the bleeding source cannot be seen, the nose can be packed using ribbon gauze impregnated with petroleum jelly or bismuth iodoform paraffin paste (BIPP).

☀ Major bleeding

More secure packing involves using specially designed packs (such as Mercoel® or Rapid Rhino®). If these are not available a soft Foley catheter may be used. However, this can be very difficult in the awake patient. The catheter is inserted (deflated) through the nose until visible at the back of the throat. The balloon is then inflated and gentle traction applied, 'wedging' the balloon between the soft palate and nasopharynx. Ribbon gauze can then be packed anteriorly, being careful not to allow it to slip out of place into the nasopharynx (risk of aspiration). Packs are generally retained for around 48 hours following control of haemorrhage. Antibiotics are usually required.

In rare instances where haemorrhage cannot be controlled by packing, urgent surgical intervention or interventional radiology may be required. Call for help, secure IV access, and check the patient's clotting status. Take blood for cross-match. Surgical ligation can be achieved endoscopically through the nose. External carotid artery and anterior ethmoidal artery ligation are now rarely undertaken. The anterior ethmoidal artery passes through the orbit and is exposed via a transorbital approaches. These are rare procedures, but may be required in those cases of continuing major bleeding resistant to all other treatments.

⊙ Nasal fractures

This usually refers to disruption of either the bony or cartilaginous skeleton of the nose (usually both) (Figure 7.1). The nose is the most commonly fractured bone in the face. *Diagnosis is clinical not radiological.* The type and severity of injury depends on the magnitude and direction of the force applied (lateral or frontal direction).

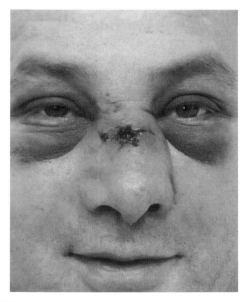

Figure 7.1 Nasal fracture.

Reproduced from *Atlas of Operative Maxillofacial Trauma Surgery: Primary Repair of Facial Injuries*, 'Nasal Fractures', 2014, Figure 10.37a, eds M. Perry and S. Holmes, Copyright © 2014, Springer-Verlag London. With permission of Springer Nature.

Three levels of injury are often described:
- Injuries involve the cartilaginous nasal skeleton only
- Injuries limited to the external nose and do not cross the orbital rims
- Injuries extend beyond the nose and involve orbit walls and possibly the cranium—these are termed nasoethmoidal fractures.

Patients present with a history of trauma to the nose, together with nasal deformity, epistaxis, and an obstructed nasal airway.

① Septal haematoma

This forms as a result of bleeding between the septal cartilage and its perichondrium. It must be ruled out in every injury and appears as a dark swelling on the septum with narrowing of the nasal airway. This requires urgent incision and drainage. *If missed, it can result in a septal abscess (and intracranial complications), or a delayed 'saddle nose' following necrosis and cartilage loss.*

Management

Urgent measures
- Anterior nasal packing may be required if there is any nasal bleeding. For more serious bleeding, post-nasal packs may be required. For haemorrhage uncontrollable by packing, surgery or embolization may be necessary.
- Septal haematoma may be aspirated or drained under local anaesthetic.

Non-urgent measures
- No treatment is indicated if there is no significant deformity, airway obstruction, or haemorrhage. Antibiotics are not required.
- Ice packs may be applied if the injury is very recent.
- Closed manipulation (manipulation under anaesthetic) is carried out to correct simple deformity. If undertaken very early (sports field), it often requires no anaesthesia. Cases must be selected carefully, as manipulation may start bleeding. Otherwise manipulation requires general anaesthesia.
- With more extensive injuries (extensive lacerations/nasoethmoidal fractures), surgical repair may be required. Refer urgently and if possible keep the patient fasted. Start antibiotics.

Beware nasal fractures with associated black eyes—these may be nasoethmoid injuries or associated with skull base fractures.

① Naso-orbitoethmoid fractures

This refers to injuries which extend beyond the nose to involve the orbits and ethmoid sinuses. Fractures of this region are often complex and comminuted. The drainage pathways of the frontal sinus may also be blocked, predisposing to long-term complications (mucocoele formation). NOE fractures occur following a direct blow to the bridge of the nose. The ethmoid sinuses act as a crumple zone absorbing the impact.

This results in a 'pushed-in' look to the bridge of the nose, sometimes referred to as a 'Miss Piggy nose'. Clinically there can be:
• Severely comminuted nasal fractures ± soft tissue lacerations
• Separation of the medial canthi (telecanthus)
• Fracture of the anterior cranial fossa with CSF leakage
• Fracture of the frontal sinus.

An upturned nose and/or separation of the canthi are highly suggestive of NOE fractures. The 'bow-string' test assesses for canthal detachment. The lateral canthus is pulled laterally, if there is detachment medially the medial canthus will also move laterally. Consider also possible injuries to the:
• Head/neck
• Eye
• Nasolacrimal apparatus.

Severity of the injury may vary considerably in this region. The degree of bone displacement and comminution is difficult to visualize on plain radiographs and CT is necessary. This also facilitates assessment for skull base fractures. Usually there is extensive comminution of the involved bones with associated soft tissue injuries.

Management
These are high-impact injuries. Initially follow ATLS® guidelines.

Urgent measures
Anterior nasal packing may be required. For more serious bleeding, post-nasal packs may be required. Care is required (be aware of the potential for skull base fractures). Any septal haematoma may be aspirated but may require open drainage under local or general anaesthesia.

Non-urgent measures
Surgical repair is indicated in the majority of cases. Non-operative treatment may be appropriate where the fracture is undisplaced or the general condition of the patient prevents surgery. Simple closed reduction of the nasal bones may be undertaken with minimal displacement. More complex fractures may require open reduction and internal fixation. Accurate repositioning of the canthal ligaments is required for a good cosmetic result. Correct management of the frontal sinus is also essential. An open approach (usually via a bicoronal flap) is indicated for complex fractures or when frontal sinus treatment is required. In general, the best cosmetic result is obtained when repair is carried out early.

ⓘ Foreign bodies and infestation

ⓘ Foreign bodies
This is a common problem in children. Patients present with a unilateral foul-smelling discharge, obstruction, and vestibulitis, as well as epistaxis in some cases. If cooperative, the foreign body can be removed by asking the patient to blow their nose and attempting retrieval. Hard items can be removed by passing a wax hook or Jobson–Horne probe past the

foreign body and gently pulling it outwards. Alternatively, a small drop of 'superglue' on the end of a narrow wooden or plastic applicator lightly held against the foreign body will hopefully stick enough to provide traction. It is not advisable to use tweezers as this may push the item back. Soft foreign bodies (such as chips) may be retrieved with suction.

'Mummy's kiss'

This technique may work if there is total obstruction of the nostril. The child is positioned on the parent's lap (usually the mother) with the 'intention' of receiving a 'big kiss'. The parent then places their own lips over the mouth of the child, ensuring an air tight seal. The opposite patient nostril is occluded by the parent and a forceful exhalation given to deliver a short puff of air into the child's mouth. This positive pressure may be enough to blow out the foreign body. In theory, such positive pressure techniques carry a risk of causing barotrauma to the airway, lungs, or tympanic membranes. However, these complications have not been reported and are minimized with small volumes of exhaled air.

If the patient is uncooperative or if retrieval otherwise fails, a referral should be made to ENT. A foreign body which is not removed can accumulate a calcareous deposit over time and present years later as a rhinolith—a foetid, stony mass. If large these can be difficult to remove and can cause erosion of the lateral wall and floor of the nose.

① Infestation

Nasal myiasis is a parasitic infestation of the nose by fly larvae (maggots), commonly from the botfly. It is rare and therefore easily overlooked. Consider this in anyone who has travelled abroad/works with animals and where no foreign body is obvious. Infestation usually occurs in countries where livestock (particularly sheep, cattle, and goats), are kept under hot, wet conditions. It is therefore commonly seen in Africa, Australia, and New Zealand but it can occur worldwide. Patients present with symptoms similar to a foreign body, i.e. nasal obstruction and discharge. They also complain of severe irritation in the nose. In some cases facial oedema and fever can develop. Death has also been reported. Larvae can usually be removed with forceps. Discuss the need for antibiotics with microbiology. Larvae can also grow in other sites, so enquire about other sites of swelling/irritation anywhere on the body.

⑦ Rhinitis

Rhinitis is a common condition in which there is inflammation of the nasal lining. It can occur in isolation or in association with sinusitis (rhinosinusitis). Symptoms include a blocked nose, runny nose, postnasal drip, chronic or nocturnal coughing, sneezing, and lacrimation. A patient can be diagnosed with rhinitis if they suffer two or more of these symptoms for over an hour every day for 2 weeks.

Rhinitis is commonly allergic or infective in nature. However, there are other, rarer causes, and it can be part of a systemic disease (see Table 7.1). It is therefore important to take a good history. This includes asking about any past history of atopy or asthma and any seasonal or

Table 7.1 Classification and causes of rhinitis

| Common | | Rare | |
Allergic	Infective	Other	Systemic disease
Seasonal	Acute	Idiopathic	Primary mucus defect
Perennial	Chronic	NARES (non-allergic rhinitis with eosinophilia)	Cystic fibrosis
Occupational			Young's disease
			Primary ciliary dyskinesis
		Drug induced: beta-blockers, oral contraceptives, aspirin, NSAIDs, local decongestants	Kartagener's syndrome
			Immunological
			SLE
			Rheumatoid arthritis
		Autonomic	AIDS
		Atrophic	Antibody deficiency
			Granulomatous disease
			Wegener's/sarcoidosis
			Hormonal
			Hypothyroidism
			Pregnancy
			Old man's drip

diurnal variation. The patient's main symptom will help direct choice of treatment. Document what medications are being used and the effectiveness of any previous treatment. Smoking is also a common contributor.

⑦ Simple acute infective rhinitis

This is a self-limiting condition usually caused by the common cold, it is of viral origin and spread by droplet transmission.

⑦ Allergic rhinitis

Sensitization of the nasal lining to allergens causes a hypersensitivity reaction, resulting in congestion, oedema, rhinorrhoea, and irritation. Seasonal allergic rhinitis such as hayfever is where allergens are present at a particular time of year (e.g. grass pollens in summer or autumnal fungal spores), and is usually accompanied by itchy or watery eyes. Perennial allergic rhinitis is where allergens are present year-round (e.g. dust mites). Such patients will often have oedematous nasal turbinates prone to hypertrophy if the allergy is long-standing.

⑦ Vasomotor rhinitis

This has similar symptoms to allergic rhinitis but without positive allergen tests. Some patients give a history of symptoms relating to positional or temperature changes. Management is as for allergic rhinitis.

⑦ Rhinitis medicamentosa

This is an acquired sensitivity of the nasal lining due to prolonged use of nasal decongestants. This is caused by a cycle of nasal congestion, treatment, and rebound vasodilatation caused by cessation of the decongestants. This results in turbinate hypertrophy and nasal obstruction.

⑦ Atrophic rhinitis

There is loss of cilia and atrophy of the nasal lining associated with abnormal patency of the nostril. This leads to the build-up of large crusts with an unpleasant odour and frequent bleeding. It usually occurs as a result of nasal surgery. Chronic atrophic rhinitis is chronic inflammation together with atrophy of the nasal mucosa, glands, turbinate bones, and the nerve supply. Chronic atrophic rhinitis may be primary and secondary.

Assessment

This is tailored according to the probable cause

- Anterior rhinoscopy: look for enlarged turbinates, bluish mucosa, nasal polyps.
- Nasal endoscopy to check for mucus or polyps around the middle meatus.
- Skin prick allergy tests or RAST tests for allergies.
- Peak flow as asthma is often a contributor.

Medical management

Treatment is based on the aetiology and severity of symptoms:

- Allergen avoidance and advice.
- Steroid sprays/drops.
- Oral steroids: effective but systemic effects long term.
- Antihistamines: non-sedating antihistamines are effective against sneezing, itching, and watery rhinorrhoea but not for blockage.
- Nasal decongestants: useful in the short term, but prolonged used can result in rhinitis medicaments, and turbinate hyperplasia.
- Ipratropium bromide: used as an intranasal spray, can be effective against watery/vasomotor rhinitis.
- Sodium cromoglycate: this is a mast cell stabilizer useful for allergic rhinitis.

Surgical management

This has a limited role in rhinitis and is considered only after medical treatments have failed. Preoperative CT of the paranasal sinuses may be required to review the need for sinus surgery. Procedures include

- Turbinate reduction: turbinate hypertrophy is common especially in allergic rhinitis.
- Septal surgery: correction of any deviated septum.
- Functional endoscopic sinus surgery: aimed at removing any blockage of the osteomeatal complex to restore functional drainage of the sinuses.

⑦ Septal problems

⑦ Septal deviation

Congenital septal deviation can occur following birth trauma or from the variations in growth from the skull. Traumatic septal deviation can also occur from a broken nose. Most often a deviated septum is asymptomatic; however, impaired airflow can bother patients. Assessment includes anterior rhinoscopy to exclude other causes of obstruction, Cottle's test to exclude valve collapse, and nasendoscopy to exclude sinusitis. Treatment is initially by intranasal steroids for 3 months. Surgery is often required. Refer to ENT/plastics or oral and maxillofacial surgery depending on local protocol.

⑦ Septal perforation

Patients with a perforation may complain of whistling, bleeding, or crusting at the site of perforation. Causes include trauma (including nose picking), previous surgery, granulomatous disease, or inhaled recreational drug use. Treatment is to keep the area moist with petroleum jelly, use of a septal obturator button (which may be intolerable for some patients), or surgical repair.

⑦ Granulomatous conditions

These conditions may also affect the nose:

- Wegener's granulomatosis: a multisystem disease which causes perivascular granuloma formation usually causing renal and respiratory problems.
- Sarcoidosis.
- Syphilis: this may also affect the nose.

Patients may present with both systemic and nasal symptoms but may also have isolated nasal symptoms, e.g. septal perforation or crusting. Investigations include blood tests (FBC, U&Es, ESR, syphilis serology, antineutrophil cytoplasmic antibodies (ANCA)), CXR, and biopsy. Treatment should involve medical specialists and may require immunosuppression.

Other anatomical abnormalities

Congenital atresia of one posterior choana may not present until adult life. A total unilateral obstruction may cause surprisingly little trouble to a patient. However, if symptoms are marked, the atresia can be treated surgically with removal of the bony obstruction.

⑦ Concha bullosa

This is a pneumatized cavity within one of the turbinates. It is a common normal anatomical variant. If large enough it may obstruct the opening of the adjacent sinus, resulting in recurrent sinusitis. In such cases the turbinate can be reduced in size (turbinectomy). The nasal septum is often deviated towards the opposite side and may require repositioning also.

ⓘ Tumours of the nose

Intranasal malignancy is rare and may present with:
- Nasal obstruction
- 'Polyps'
- Epistaxis/nasal discharge
- Cacosmia
- Anosmia
- Cranial nerve palsies
- Proptosis.

Maxillary tumours may encroach into the nose (as well as the orbit or oral cavity). Ethmoid tumours may cause diplopia, headache, and unilateral obstruction. Common types of malignancy affecting the nose are squamous cell carcinoma, adenoid cystic carcinoma, adenocarcinoma, malignant melanoma and olfactory neuroblastoma. Investigations include CT/MRI imaging, biopsy, and if necessary, angiography. Treatment may involve surgical resection and/or chemoradiotherapy.

ⓘ Nasopharynx carcinoma

This is the most common cancer originating in the nasopharynx, usually within the lateral nasopharyngeal recess (fossa of Rosenmüller). It occurs in both children and adults. Nasopharynx carcinoma differs significantly from other cancers of the head and neck in its occurrence, causes, clinical behaviour, and treatment. Viral (notably Epstein–Barr virus), dietary, and genetic factors have been implicated in its causation. Histologically this is a squamous cell carcinoma. Cervical lymphadenopathy is often the initial presentation in many patients. Other symptoms include trismus, pain, otitis media, nasal regurgitation, hearing loss, and cranial nerve palsies. Large tumours may produce nasal obstruction or bleeding. Nasopharyngeal carcinoma may be treated by surgery, chemotherapy, or by radiotherapy.

ⓘ Olfactory esthesioneuroblastomas

This arises from the olfactory epithelium superior to the middle turbinate. Olfactory esthesioneuroblastomas are initially unilateral and can grow into the adjacent sinuses and the contralateral nasal cavity. They can also spread into the orbit and the brain. Patients are best treated with combined-modality therapy. Surgical resection may involve either local resection or craniofacial resection with postoperative radiation therapy.

Miscellaneous conditions

⑦ Nasal glioma

A benign polypoid swelling attached to the septum which presents in infants and children. A CT scan is needed to exclude (rare) intracranial attachment, and biopsy is required to confirm the diagnosis.

⑦ Dermoid

A cystic swelling often just above the medial canthus, sometimes with a sinus. As there may be extension of the cyst deep to the nasal bones or orbit, CT is often required.

⑦ Nasoalveolar cyst

This causes external flattening of the nasolabial fold and flaring of the alae nasi. In the anterior nares the cyst extends into the floor of the nose and displaces the inferior turbinate upwards. Be careful these are not dental in origin. Request an OPT. Management is surgical.

⑦ Rhinophyma

Here, the skin becomes thickened and vascular and may produce gross deformity. Shaving/lasering the excess skin without skin grafting is possible. Irregular areas of epithelium should be sent for histology since basal or squamous cell carcinoma may occur within a rhinophyma.

⑦ Vestibulitis

Eczema of the vestibular skin can result from nasal discharge and skin infection. It can affect both nostrils. This may cause crusting, irritation in the anterior nares, and nasal obstruction. Causes include nose picking, overly vigilant cleaning, and inhaled recreational drug. Treatment includes antibiotic and corticosteroid ointments.

⑦ Relapsing polychondritis (atrophic polychondritis/ systemic chondromalacia)

This is a presumed autoimmune disease characterized by inflammation and destruction of cartilage. Although the disease usually causes pain and deformity if unrecognized and untreated, it can be life-threatening when the respiratory tract, heart valves, or blood vessels are affected. It commonly presents in patients in their late 40s to early 50s although children and young adults may also be affected. Any cartilage may be affected, although in many cases the disease affects several sites, while sparing others. Common sites include the nose, ears, joints, and rib cage. Tracheomalacia and vasculitis can also occur. One sign to look for is a painful, red, and swollen ear. There is no specific test for relapsing polychondritis although inflammatory markers (such as ESR or CRP) may be high. Biopsy may help with the diagnosis. Treatment is often systemic steroids sometimes with azathioprine or cyclophosphamide.

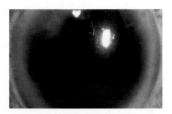

Plate 1 Hyphaema. Note some blood is in suspension and obscuring the view of iris and pupil. (See also Figure 10.1.)

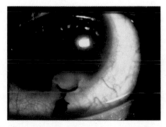

Plate 2 Penetrating eye injury. Note jagged corneal laceration with shreds of iris prolapsing. (See also Figure 10.2.)

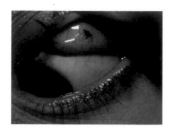

Plate 3 Eversion of upper lids showing foreign body. (See also Figure 10.4.)

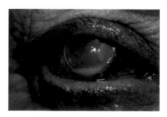

Plate 4 Corneal ulcer with hypopyon. (See also Figure 10.5.)

⊙ Anosmia (loss of sense of smell)

Reduction in the sense of smell (hyposmia) is relatively common and temporary. However, total and permanent anosmia is rare and has many causes. Some people may be anosmic for one particular odour—'specific anosmia'. Very often no cause for anosmia can be found. Nevertheless this can be an early indication of serious pathology.

Commoner causes

- URTI (e.g. sinusitis or the common cold)
- Nasal polyps
- Head trauma, damage to the ethmoid bone
- Tumours of the frontal lobe
- MS
- Asthma/hayfever
- COPD
- Long-term alcoholism
- Cushing's syndrome
- Stroke
- Epilepsy
- Radiation therapy to the head and neck
- Liver or kidney disease
- Parkinson's disease
- Alzheimer's disease
- Primary ciliary dyskinesia
- Olfactory esthesioneuroblastoma
- Intranasal drug use
- Smoking
- Pernicious anaemia
- Zinc deficiency
- Sarcoidosis
- Chronic atrophic rhinitis
- Paget's disease of bone
- Wegener's granulomatosis
- Primary amoebic meningoencephalitis.

Presentation

Patients with anosmia may find food less appetising. It can also be potentially dangerous because it hinders the detection of gas leaks, fires, etc. Occasionally losing an associated sentimental smell memory has been reported to cause feelings of depression. Rarely loss of olfaction may lead to the loss of libido.

Investigations

This can be confirmed using commercially available 'smell testing kits'. Imaging studies (CT/MRI) may be required.

Management

This is to treat the underlying cause.

⑦ Rhinorrhoea: 'runny nose'

This is a condition in which the nasal cavity is filled with a significant amount of clear fluid. It is a common symptom seen in allergies and URTIs. It also occurs following exposure to cold air/cocaine or withdrawal from opiate drugs. Additional symptoms include sneezing, nosebleeds, anosmia, and nasal discharge.

Causes

- Exposure to cold air
- Infection (especially common cold and influenza)
- Allergies (especially pollen, dust, and animals)
- Lacrimation
- Head trauma (CSF rhinorrhoea)
- Opioid withdrawal
- Cystic fibrosis
- Whooping cough
- Nasal tumours
- Cluster headaches
- Primary ciliary dyskinesia.

Management

In most cases treatment is not necessary. Saline nasal sprays and vasoconstrictor nasal sprays may be used, but prolonged use causes rhinitis medicamentosa. Any identified underlying cause should be managed accordingly.

⑦ Nasal congestion

This is not to be confused with the nasal cycle, which is a normal (and usually unnoticeable) cycle of alternating partial congestion and decongestion of the nasal cavity, often affecting one side and then the other. This is physiological congestion.

Pathological nasal congestion has many causes and can vary significantly. *Nasal congestion in an infant can interfere with breastfeeding and cause respiratory distress. This is because they are obligate nasal breathers.*

Causes

- Common cold or influenza
- Deviated septum
- Hayfever/allergic reaction
- Rhinitis medicamentosa
- Sinusitis
- Nasal polyps
- Empty nose syndrome
- GORD.

The treatment of nasal congestion frequently depends on the underlying cause. Antihistamines and decongestants may be used.

① Ethmoid sinusitis

This usually occurs with other sinus infections (see ● Chapter 3 and ● Chapter 9). Patients complain of deep-seated throbbing pain, deep to the bridge of the nose, between the eyes. *The medial orbital walls are paper thin, so orbital cellulitis can rapidly develop. Infection can also ascend into the frontal sinus.* Chronic sinus disease in the ethmoid sinuses can predispose to polyps.

Clinical features
- Headache/facial pain.
- Sensation of dull, constant pressure over the affected sinus.
- Symptoms are usually localized over the involved sinus and are often made worse on bending, straining or lying down.
- Nasal discharge.
- Halitosis.
- Post-nasal drip.

Management of sinusitis
Antibiotics and, in some cases, sinus washout with opening of the draining channels, using functional endoscopic sinus surgery. Ephedrine nasal drops and menthol inhalations may help reduce congestion and improve sinus drainage.

The throat

Common presentations

Common presentations in the throat:
- Acid regurgitation
- Difficulty swallowing (dysphagia)
- Foreign body
- Painful swallowing (odynophagia)
- Snoring
- Sore throat
- Swellings/lumps in the throat.

Common problems and their causes

Acid regurgitation

Common
- Hiatus hernia
- GORD
- Medications, spicy foods, acid/alcoholic drinks.

Uncommon
- Paterson–Kelly syndrome
- Zenker's diverticulum
- Achalasia
- Oesophageal diverticula
- Oesophageal cancer
- Eosinophilic oesophagitis.

Difficulty swallowing (dysphagia)

Common
- Diffuse oesophageal spasm
- Hiatus hernia
- GORD.

Uncommon
- Paterson–Kelly syndrome
- Zenker's diverticulum
- Benign strictures
- Retrosternal goitre
- Achalasia
- Oesophageal diverticula
- Scleroderma
- Webs and rings
- Oesophageal cancer
- Eosinophilic oesophagitis
- Motor disorders.

Foreign body

Common
- Fish/rabbit bone.

Uncommon
- Meat/bread
- Coins/sharp objects.

Painful swallowing (odynophagia)

Common
- Very hot/cold food or drink
- Drugs
- Ulcers
- URTIs/quinsy
- Foreign body (especially fish bones).

Uncommon
- Immune disorders
- Epiglottitis
- Tumours
- Motor disorders.

Snoring

Common
- Physiological (obesity)
- Obstructive sleep apnoea
- Sedative drugs/alcohol
- Enlarged tonsils/adenoids
- Retruded mandible.

Uncommon
- Nasal polyps
- Tumours.

Sore throat

Common
- Tonsillitis
- Pharyngitis
- Dental infections
- Foreign body (fish bones).

Uncommon
- Acid regurgitation
- Snoring
- Tumour.

Swelling/lump in the throat

Common
- Tonsillar enlargement ± tonsilloliths
- Swollen uvula
- Foreign body (fish bones).

Uncommon
- Deep neck space abscess
- Papilloma/leucoplakia
- Tumour
- Globus/psychogenic.

Useful questions and what to look for

Acid regurgitation

Ask about
- Describe symptoms/treatments
- Globus sensation or burning sensation in throat
- Dysphagia and frequent throat clearing
- Early morning hoarseness and nocturnal cough
- Postnasal drip
- Atypical chest pain (may mimic heart attack)
- Predisposing factors (obesity, pregnancy, alcohol, smoking)
- Medications (steroids, NSAIDs, antacids)
- Dietary history (spicy foods, acid drinks, caffeine).

Look for
- Posterior pharyngeal wall erythema
- Congestion and granular changes
- Indirect laryngoscopy if possible.

Difficulty swallowing (dysphagia)

Ask about
- Onset
- Where obstruction is felt
- Intermittent or progressive
- Solids or liquids or both
- Weight loss
- Vomiting/regurgitation
- Symptoms of aspiration (cough etc.).

Look for
- Swollen/displaced tonsil
- Lymphadenopathy
- Ulceration

- Tumour
- Anaemia/cachexia
- Examine chest
- Cranial nerve exam
- Indirect laryngeal exam or nasopharyngeal scope.

Foreign body

Ask about
- Description of object
- Dysphagia, gagging, choking.

Look for
- Airway patency
- Locate object.

Painful swallowing (odynophagia)

Ask about
- Onset
- Intermittent or progressive
- Weight loss
- Vomiting
- Symptoms of aspiration.

Look for
- Lymphadenopathy
- Ulceration
- Tumour
- Anaemia/cachexia
- Examine chest.

Snoring

Ask about
- Onset
- Intermittent or progressive
- Sleep deprivation, effect on work
- Daytime drowsiness
- Irritability
- Lack of focus
- Decreased libido (if appropriate).

Look for
- Enlarged/displaced tonsils
- Enlarged uvula
- Collar size
- Obesity
- Retruded mandible
- Check BP.

Sore throat

Ask about
- Onset
- Known precipitant
- Unilateral or bilateral
- Symptoms of URTI
- Discomfort when swallowing
- Contact with other people with similar symptoms
- Fever/chills/headache/photophobia
- Neck stiffness.

Look for
- Swollen/displaced tonsil
- Ulceration
- Pus/quinsy
- Lymphadenopathy/rash
- Pyrexia
- Neck stiffness, photophobia, Kernig's sign.

Swelling/lump in the throat

Ask about
- Onset
- Known precipitant
- Unilateral or bilateral
- Symptoms of URTI
- Difficulty when swallowing.

Look for
- Swollen/displaced tonsil or uvula
- Tonsilloliths
- Lymphadenopathy
- Tumour
- Enlarged thyroid/parotid gland.

Examination of the throat

Thorough clinical examination of the pharynx requires good lighting, a tongue depressor, and mirror. Ideally it also includes flexible fibreoptic laryngoscopy. Detailed examination is often carried out by otolaryngologists. In the emergency department, head light examination using a tongue depressor and mirror may also reveal useful signs. Clinically the throat needs to be regarded as more than just the back of the mouth.

Nasopharynx

Applied anatomy

The nasopharynx (nasal part of the pharynx) is the uppermost part of the pharynx. It extends from the base of the skull to the upper surface of the soft palate. It differs from the rest of the pharynx in that its cavity is always patent. Anteriorly it communicates through the choanae with the nasal cavities. Laterally the Eustachian tubes open into it. Behind this opening is a deep recess, the pharyngeal recess (fossa of Rosenmüller)— a common site for nasopharyngeal malignancy. Posteriorly lies the pharyngeal tonsil.

The location of the nasopharynx makes it very difficult to access and examine easily. If endoscopy is not available the only way to examine the nasopharynx is posterior rhinoscopy. A small, angled mirror is placed at the back of the pharynx. A strong light is then directed towards the mirror. This is reflected upwards, showing the posterior nasal cavity. Unfortunately both the tongue and uvula can hamper the view. Endoscopic techniques have now considerably improved visualization. Nasopharyngeal endoscopy may be performed transorally or transnasally and will provide detailed views of the region.

Oropharynx

Applied anatomy

The oropharynx opens into the mouth. Its lateral walls are composed of the two palatine arches between which is the palatine tonsil. Most structures of the oropharynx can be visualized during the examination of the oral cavity. The palatine tonsils are assessed for symmetry, mobility, and for the presence of any coatings or ulceration.

Tonsilloliths may be visible in the crypts and crevasses of the tonsils. They are usually yellow/white in colour and seen as pale spots. A laryngeal mirror or laryngoscope may be used to examine the tongue base and the lateral walls of the oropharynx. *If possible, palpate the tongue base/tonsillar region for induration if symptoms raise suspicion of a tumour.*

Hypopharynx

Applied anatomy

The hypopharynx (laryngopharynx) lies inferior to the epiglottis, passing down to diverge into the larynx and oesophagus. The oesophagus lies posteriorly. The hypopharynx is divided into three areas (piriform sinus, postcricoid area, and the posterior pharyngeal wall). Clinical examination of the hypopharynx (mirror examination, endoscopy) is performed along with examination of the larynx.

Waldeyer's ring

This refers to a ring-like arrangement of lymphoid tissue in the naso- and oropharynx. It consists of:
- Pharyngeal tonsils (or adenoids)
- Tubal tonsil (where each Eustachian tube opens into the nasopharynx)
- Palatine tonsils (tonsils)
- Lingual tonsils (on the posterior tongue).

Lymphoid tissue in Waldeyer's ring gradually increases in size from birth and attains a relatively larger size when the child is around 4 years of age.

Oesophagus

In experienced hands, the oesophagus can be examined by means of flexible or rigid endoscopy. Flexible oesophagoscopy can be performed under local anaesthesia. It is generally well tolerated and allows for concomitant examination of the stomach and duodenum. Rigid oesophagoscopy is performed under general anaesthesia and indicated when looking for foreign bodies, or visualizing the pyriform fossa and postcricoid region.

Steps in examination

- Ask the patient to remove any dentures.
- If appropriate, examine trunk for rash—a scarlet fever rash generally starts on the chest and spreads to the neck and face. The rash associated with infectious mononucleosis tends to be generalized.
- Examine the neck for cervical lymphadenopathy. Note any trismus.
- Inspect the tongue and throat. In streptococcal disease there may be a 'strawberry tongue'. In cases of infectious mononucleosis there may be petechiae on the palate.
- Examine the back of tongue and tonsils (press down on the tongue with a tongue depressor).
- If there is any discharge or loosely adherent plaques/slough, gently try to wipe off for microbiology/pathology.
- Palpate the base of the tongue (feeling for tumours).
- Look at the uvula and palate.
- Examine the nasopharynx and larynx with a mirror or flexible fibreoptic nasendoscope.

Remember—examination of the mouth and throat is not just a case of looking. If possible (without causing excessive gagging) always palpate suspicious areas. Tumours can easily be missed if this is not routinely undertaken. If one of the tonsils is displaced medially, examine the associated parotid—tumours of the deep lobe can displace the tonsil. Not all tumours are obvious to the naked eye.

Useful investigations

Laboratory tests

- Complete blood count including differential count is required for infective conditions.
- Monospot or Paul–Bunnell test if glandular fever is suspected
- Liver function test if glandular fever is suspected
- Serum biochemistry and renal functions if dehydrated
- Serum ferritin levels and iron profile if Plummer–Vinson syndrome suspected
- Specific tests for gonococci, syphilis, chlamydia, diphtheria, etc.
- Throat swab for a rapid strep test if streptococcal sore throat is suspected
- Throat swab for culture if no clinical response to first-line antibiotics
- Tests for *Helicobacter pylori* infection (which can predispose to acid reflux and GORD).

Plain films

Conventional radiographs have become largely obsolete in the investigation of diseases of the pharynx. However, a contrast swallow is still a useful tool in the investigation of some oesophageal disorders (diverticula, tumours, stenoses, and disorders of motility). Various contrast media can be used (e.g. barium, sodium amidotrizoate, iopromide, iotrolan), depending on the nature of the investigation and any pre-existing disorders. If there is a risk or suspicion of a perforation or aspiration, barium should not be used.

CT/MRI

Cross-sectional imaging with CT and MRI is useful in the diagnosis of pharyngeal tumours/masses and in some inflammatory processes (abscess).

Videofluoroscopy

This is used mainly to assess swallowing disorders using high-speed cineradiography. This technique evaluates the different phases of swallowing with high-speed image resolution (approximately 50 images per second). Modified barium swallow is a videofluoroscopic study that visualizes oral and pharyngeal phases of swallowing.

Manometry

This measures duration, amplitude, and velocity of peristaltic waves.

Laryngoscopy and oesophagoscopy

Indicated if suspect malignancy, to remove foreign bodies, and to biopsy a mass or lesion.

Functional (fibreoptic) endoscopic evaluation of swallowing

This allows bedside evaluation of swallowing function.

ⓘ The infected throat

Most infected throats are minor infections which will settle quickly with supportive measures or following a short cause of antibiotics.

However, some sore throats are caused by organisms which can result in serious consequences if overlooked or inadequately treated.

Some causes of the infected throat and important sequelae
- Non-specific viral pharyngitis
- Mumps
- Herpangina
- Influenza
- Bacterial pharyngitis (strep throat)
- Scarlet fever
- Rheumatic fever
- Post-streptococcal glomerulonephritis
- Tonsillitis
- Quinsy

- Infective mononucleosis (glandular fever)
- Epiglottitis
- Uvulitis
- Diphtheria
- Gonorrhoea
- Chlamydia
- HIV (candidiasis)
- Dental infections
- Deep neck infections.

Usually the diagnosis can be made following a careful history and examination. Salient points include:
- Contact history (including sexual contact if suspected sexually transmitted disease)
- Any known epidemic
- Symptoms of meningism
- Joint pains
- Cardiac symptoms
- Neurological symptoms (Sydenham's chorea/St. Vitus' dance)
- Airway compromise
- Very high fever
- Lethargy
- Presence of a rash
- Skin nodules
- Pericardial rub
- Appearances of the throat
- Drooling
- Haematuria.

The presence (or absence) of these features should help you identify the more serious infections from the more common, minor ones.

① Pharyngeal infections

① Acute pharyngitis

This is a common condition. It is mostly viral in aetiology but can develop a secondary bacterial infection. Pathogens include adenovirus, rhinovirus, and enterovirus with secondary bacterial infection from *Streptococcus, Pneumococcus*, and *Haemophilus influenzae*. Patients present with sore throat, odynophagia, malaise, and fever. On examination, there is diffuse erythema and a granular appearance of the posterior pharyngeal wall. There is also cervical lymphadenopathy. Treatment is generally supportive (hydration, lozenges, antipyretics). Gargling aspirin or applying benzydamine (Difflam®) spray may sooth symptoms. Antibiotics are rarely indicated (as most infections are viral). *Take a throat swab if suspicious of bacterial infection and consider the more serious infections in your differential diagnosis (discussed later).*

Non-infective pharyngitis can also occur secondary to sinonasal disease, acid reflux, air pollution, or chronic allergy. Symptoms are similar although the patient is usually systemically well.

⑦ Chronic pharyngitis

This is often associated with postnasal drip (chronic rhinosinusitis), irritants (dust, dry heat, chemicals, smoking, alcohol), acid reflux, chronic mouth breathing (adenoid hypertrophy), allergy, and granulomatous diseases. There is frequent throat clearing with a dry throat, thickened and granular pharyngeal wall, and pharyngeal crusting

Treatment is supportive, but it is important to address underlying aetiology and avoid contributing factors.

⑦ Chronic adenoiditis

Typically a polymicrobial infection, this may be related to GORD, especially in children. It may be difficult to distinguish from sinusitis. Patients present with persistent nasal discharge, malodorous breath, and nasal obstruction (snoring). Consider the possibility of a foreign body in the nose in children. Treatment is initially conservative but if symptoms persist, refer to ENT for consideration of adenoidectomy.

① Infectious mononucleosis (glandular fever)

The Epstein–Barr virus causes an acute pharyngitis as a part of the infectious mononucleosis syndrome. This is common in children and young adults and is transmitted by oral contact (hence its other name—'kisser's disease'). Patients present with fever, generalized malaise, lymphadenopathy, hepatosplenomegaly, and pharyngitis. On examination there are massively enlarged tonsils and nasopharyngeal lymphoid tissue, covered with greyish-white exudates and petechiae at the junction of the soft and hard palates.

Investigations include a complete blood count. This may show lymphocytosis with atypical lymphocytes (activated T cells) on peripheral smear. The monospot test or Paul–Bunnell test are often diagnostic but non-specific (heterophile antibody test). They can be negative in 10–15% of patients in the first week of illness. Treatment is largely supportive. Antibiotics may be indicated to treat or prevent super-added bacterial infection. *Avoid ampicillin—this can cause skin rashes in patients with glandular fever.*

☼ Diphtheria

Despite widespread use of universal childhood immunization, several hundred cases of pharyngeal infection with *Corynebacterium diphtheriae* are seen annually, even in the developed countries. These occur mostly in non-immunized persons. Diphtheriae is characterized by a grey, firmly adherent pseudo-membrane covering the pharynx and tonsils. When scraped (with difficulty), the underlying surface usually bleeds. Usually the disease is localized to the pharynx but rarely may spread to the larynx causing potential airway compromise. Some bacterial strains can produce a lethal exotoxin. Toxins can result in cardiac arrhythmias, myocarditis, and peripheral nerve palsies. The disease should be immediately reported and treatment commenced even before confirmation with culture. Treatment includes antitoxin therapy (administered within 48 hours of the onset of symptoms) and high-dose penicillin. Diphtheria is a notifiable disease (see http://www.hpa.org.uk/Topics/InfectiousDiseases/InfectionsAZ/NotificationsOfInfectiousDiseases/ListOfNotifiableDiseases).

ⓘ Tonsil (adenotonsil) infections

In most cases, tonsillitis is a 'strep throat' caused by a streptococcal infection. The oropharynx is normally colonized by *Staphylococcus*, *Streptococcus*, *Lactobacillus*, *Bacteroides*, and *Actinomyces* (plus many other organisms). Viral tonsillitis presents with fever and oropharyngeal erythema without a tonsillar exudate and is usually self-limiting. It requires only symptomatic treatment.

ⓘ Acute streptococcal tonsillitis

Group A beta-haemolytic *Streptococcus* is the most common pathogen causing acute bacterial pharyngotonsillitis. It is commonly seen in children and is characterized by fever, sore throat, cervical lymphadenopathy, dysphagia, and odynophagia. Examination reveals tonsillar and pharyngeal erythema which is covered with purulent exudates. The tongue may also be involved ('strawberry tongue'). Take a swab.

The main consideration in treating group A beta-haemolytic *Streptococcus* is preventing its complications (notably acute rheumatic fever and post-streptococcal glomerulonephritis). The primary antibiotic of choice is penicillin. Consider second-line therapy with co-amoxiclav (ideally following discussion with a microbiologist), if no response is evident within 48 hours. Consider antibiotic therapy for at least 7–10 days to decrease the recurrence rates.

ⓘ Recurrent acute tonsillitis

In most cases, an episode of acute tonsillitis is followed by complete recovery. However, the tonsils with their numerous crypts and crevices, can harbour bacteria and persistent or recurrent infection may occur. Aggressive medical therapy for recurrent acute tonsillitis may not always prevent these infections. Many otolaryngologists and primary care physicians agree that tonsillectomy is indicated in recurrent acute tonsillitis. Therefore refer to ENT.

Current NICE and SIGN guidelines recommend surgery if there are more than six or seven episodes of acute tonsillitis in 1 year, five episodes/year for 2 consecutive years, or three episodes/year for 3 consecutive years.

Complications of acute tonsillitis

ⓘ *Scarlet fever*

This typically presents with fever, severe dysphagia, exudates covering the tonsils and pharynx, a diffuse erythematous rash, red inflamed tongue ('strawberry tongue'), facial flush, and petechial rashes. The eruptions are followed by desquamation caused by erythrogenic exotoxin which is pathognomonic. Treatment is with penicillin and supportive care. Scarlet fever is a notifiable disease.

⦂Ȍ: *Acute rheumatic fever*

Acute rheumatic fever occurs 2–3 weeks after infection with group A beta-haemolytic *Streptococcus*. This infection produces cross-reactive antibodies, leading to damage of the heart tissues with subsequent endocarditis, myocarditis, or pericarditis. Preventing rheumatic fever requires eradication of *Streptococcus* from the throat which may include long term antibiotics and tonsillectomy. You may need to discuss this with ENT and/or cardiology.

① *Post-streptococcal glomerulonephritis*

Post-streptococcal glomerulonephritis usually occurs as an acute nephritic syndrome around 10 days after a pharyngotonsillar infection (10–25% incidence) by group A beta-haemolytic *Streptococcus*. The disease is now on the decline in developed countries, while it continues to occur in developing countries. Pathogenesis involves deposition of immune complexes and circulating autoantibodies in the glomeruli. Antibiotic treatment has not been shown to affect the incidence of the disease.

① *Peritonsillar abscess (quinsy)*

This is caused by the spread of infection beyond the tonsillar capsule into the peritonsillar space. Patients usually present with a relentless sore throat, unilateral otalgia, dysphagia, and odynophagia. They may be dehydrated. On examination there is a unilateral tonsillar/peritonsillar bulge with uvular deviation. Patients often have trismus, restricting access for incision and drainage. *Untreated, this can lead to potential airway compromise, parapharyngeal or retropharyngeal abscess, aspiration pneumonia or sepsis.* Urgent CT may be required if a para-pharyngeal abscess is suspected. Management includes needle aspiration or (preferably) incision and drainage under local anaesthesia if not too extensive. Antibiotics and analgesics are prescribed. Drainage can often be performed in the emergency department, or alternatively patients can be referred urgently to ENT. Some patients may need admission for IV fluids and antibiotics if oral intake is poor. 'Quinsy tonsillectomy' (tonsillectomy at time of infection) may be considered for younger children or unresponsive cases.

☼ Deep neck infections

(See also ➜ Chapter 5.) Deep neck infections can occur as a complication of any bacterial tonsillitis or pharyngitis. However, with widespread antibiotics usage, the incidence of these complications has dramatically decreased. Para-pharyngeal abscesses may present with asymmetric pharyngeal wall swelling, extending inferiorly into the hypopharynx. Definitive diagnosis requires a CT scan of the neck. Management includes control of the airway, IV antibiotics and fluids, and urgent surgical drainage of the abscess. Refer urgently as patients can rapidly deteriorate.

Other types of throat infections

ⓘ Coxsackievirus (herpangina)

This presents as ulcerative vesicles over the tonsils, pharynx, and palate. It is often seen in children and presents with generalized symptoms of headache, fever, anorexia, and odynophagia. Treatment is mostly supportive, but antibiotics may be needed if bacterial super-infection.

ⓘ Sexually transmitted disease infection

Patients with exposure to sexually transmitted diseases can develop tonsillar infections with *Neisseria gonorrhoeae* (gonococcal), *Chlamydia*, or *Treponema pallidum* (syphilis). Gonococcal infections present as exudative tonsillitis and pharyngitis. Chlamydial infections can infect the eyes (conjunctivitis) and throat following unprotected oral sex. Infection in the throat is less common and usually causes minimal symptoms. Syphilitic infections result in oral chancres (with primary infections) and exudative lesions (with secondary syphilis).

⚙ Epiglottitis (supraglottitis)

Acute epiglottitis is a potentially life-threatening disorder due to the risk of laryngospasm and loss of the airway. It is characterized by inflammatory oedema of the arytenoids, aryepiglottic folds, and the epiglottis. Acute epiglottitis can occur at any age. It is typically caused by *Haemophilus influenzae* type B, but infection with group A beta-haemolytic *Streptococcus* has become more frequent after the widespread use of *Haemophilus influenzae* vaccination. Non-infectious causes of epiglottitis include trauma, inhalation injury, and chemical burns. It can also be associated with systemic disease. Typical presentation includes:

- Acute high fever/malaise
- Severe sore throat
- Difficulty in swallowing
- Patients often sit up and lean forward in order to improve airflow (tripod sign).

The most common differential diagnosis in the paediatric age group is croup and a foreign body in the airway (see ➲ Chapter 5). Croup has a more gradual onset than acute epiglottitis, and is commonly associated with low-grade fever, barking cough, and absence of drooling and dysphagia. In acute epiglottitis, a radiological 'thumb sign' is indicative of severe inflammation of the epiglottis. Confirmation is by flexible fibreoptic laryngoscopy in a controlled clinical setting.

Because of the risk of inducing laryngeal spasm and/or total airway obstruction, examination should only be attempted by experienced clinicians and in an area with adequate equipment and staff prepared to intervene should upper airway obstruction develop, ideally, in the operating room.

Patients with signs of an advancing upper airway obstruction from acute epiglottitis should be treated as a medical emergency and as an airway emergency. Tracheal intubation is potentially difficult and the team should have a surgeon capable of performing an immediate tracheotomy if necessary. Muscle relaxants are avoided and spontaneous ventilation should be maintained during inhalational induction.

Do not send a child with suspected epiglottitis for X-ray alone and do not perform examination in uncontrolled setting due to the risk of inducing laryngospasm. Try not to distress the child

⑦ Tonsilloliths

Food and secretions may stagnate in deep tonsillar crypts (usually in the upper pole of the tonsil), leading to bacterial overgrowth and localized infection. Some patients may have a foreign body sensation in the throat, halitosis, and express out white debris from the tonsils (tonsilloliths). Treatment is initially conservative (aggressive mouth care, which includes irrigation or cleaning with cotton swab, hydrogen peroxide gargles, antiseptic mouth rinse, etc.). Tonsillectomy may be considered in recalcitrant cases.

⑦ Fungal infections

Fungal infection in the throat is a serious condition that is more commonly seen in immunocompromised individuals. Candidiasis (oral thrush) is relatively common (see ➲ Chapter 13); however, extension of the infection into the throat is more worrying. At-risk groups include:

- Newborn babies (especially premature)
- Immune deficiency (diabetes and AIDS)
- Patients on long-term antibiotics, chemotherapy, or steroids
- Self-neglect (alcoholics, drug abuse)
- Malnourished.

Treatment for a candidal throat infection is more intense than for oral thrush. Any predisposing cause should be managed. An intense course of topical and systemic antifungal drugs is required and should be discussed with a microbiologist. Infections in patients with AIDS are difficult to eradicate, due to their compromised immunity and the high chance of recurrence. Certain home remedies (eating garlic) are reported to reduce further infection. Intestinal candidiasis and systemic candidiasis are rare but serious complications. Patients with fungal throat infections should be screened for high-risk groups. HIV testing may be necessary (see http://www.bashh.org/documents/1838.pdf).

① Tuberculosis

TB more commonly infects the lungs, but it can infect the throat as well. Patients may present with hoarseness, if the organism involves the vocal cords. TB is a notifiable disease.

⑦ Chronic adenotonsillar hypertrophy

Chronic adenotonsillar hypertrophy is the most common cause of sleep-disordered breathing in children, with symptoms ranging from upper airway obstruction to obstructive sleep apnoea syndrome (OSAS). Hypertrophy of the lymphoid tissue occurs in response to colonization with normal flora or pathogenic microorganisms. Nasal obstruction, rhinorrhoea, and a hypo-nasal voice are the usual presenting symptoms of adenoid hypertrophy, whereas tonsillar enlargement can cause snoring, dysphagia, and muffled voice. Upper airway obstruction can manifest as loud snoring, chronic mouth breathing, and secondary nocturnal enure-sis (bedwetting). A history of apnoeic episodes, hyper-somnolence, fre-quent night-time awakenings, poor school performance, and a general failure to thrive are common manifestations of OSAS. Severe cases of OSAS can lead to pulmonary hypertension, cor pulmonale, and alveo-lar hypoventilation resulting in chronic CO_2 retention. Adenotonsillar hypertrophy and chronic mouth breathing are associated with craniofa-cial growth abnormalities with subsequent malocclusion (adenoid facies).

Diagnosis of adenotonsillar hypertrophy is based on the clinical history and physical examination. Flexible endoscopy is helpful in diagnosing ade-noid hypertrophy, adenoid infections, and velopharyngeal insufficiency, as well as ruling out other causes of nasal obstruction. Lateral neck soft tissue radiography is rarely indicated.

Management
- For acute upper airway obstruction, consider corticosteroids and antibiotics.
- Medical treatment includes intranasal corticosteroid sprays for adenoid hyperplasia.
- Tonsillectomy and adenoidectomy may be required as definitive therapy.

Beware of unilateral tonsillar hyperplasia—it is important to consider the possibility of neoplasms (carcinoma, lymphoma) or unusual infections (Mycobacterium tuberculosis, atypical mycobacteria, actinomycosis and fungal).

Hypopharyngeal/upper oesophageal-related problems

⑦ Candidiasis (thrush)
This is discussed in 'Other types of throat infections', pp. 246–7.

⑦ Plummer–Vinson syndrome (Patterson–Kelly syndrome)
This may be secondary to nutritional deficiency (iron). It typically pres-ents in middle-aged women. Symptoms include dysphagia, microcytic hypochromic anaemia (iron deficiency), cervical (pharyngoesophageal) webs, angular cheilitis, hypothyroidism, hiatus hernia, splenomegaly, and koilonychia of the nails. Investigations include blood tests (iron levels, FBC) and oesophagram or flexible endoscopy. These patients have a higher risk for upper oesophageal and hypopharyngeal carcinoma and hence careful monitoring is warranted. Treat any iron deficiency.

⑦ Diffuse oesophageal spasm (beware cardiac ischaemia)
This is caused by non-peristaltic contraction in oesophageal smooth muscle. Patients present with sudden-onset, severe odynophagia and dysphagia to solids and liquids. They may also present with chest

pain, mimicking cardiac pain. Both cardiac and oesophageal pain may be relieved with glyceryl trinitrate, adding to any diagnostic confusion. *Consider ECG/troponin levels if in doubt.* The pain from oesophageal spasm is sometimes relieved by eructation (belching/burping). Diagnosis may also be confirmed by oesophagram and manometry. Treatment is medical (nitrates, calcium channel blockers, anticholinergics). Refractory cases may be considered for dilation and myotomy.

⑦ Gastroesophageal reflux disease

GORD is caused by incompetence of the lower oesophageal sphincter or its transient relaxation. There is also delayed oesophageal clearance and delayed gastric emptying. Predisposing factors include obesity, alcohol abuse, hiatus hernias, and pregnancy. Typically patients present with heartburn, choking spells at night, regurgitation, hoarseness (worse in the morning), globus, a nocturnal cough, and chronic throat clearing. Diagnosis is often made on the history and response to empirical anti-reflux treatment. Untreated cases can lead to complications such as Barrett's oesophagus (gastric metaplasia of the distal oesophagus which predisposes to malignancy), oesophageal strictures, gastric and oesophageal ulcerations, aspiration pneumonitis, laryngeal granulomas, etc. In infants, GORD can cause failure to thrive and sudden infant death syndrome. Diagnosis is usually made by careful history. Although an anti-reflux regimen may be prescribed based on the history, consider referral for testing if symptoms don't resolve, recur, or complications develop.

Investigations
- Nasopharyngoscopy
- Barium swallow
- Oesophagoscopy: this evaluates for oesophagitis and oesophageal strictures and allows histological confirmation of Barrett's oesophagus.

Management
- Dietary changes and smoking cessation; elevate head of bed at night; avoid tight fitting clothing; avoid overeating, abstain from caffeine, fatty foods, alcohol and chocolates; avoid aspirin, nitrates, and calcium channel blockers. Medication includes:
  - Liquid antacids (calcium carbonate, hydroxides of aluminium and magnesium, sodium bicarbonate). Be careful—overuse may result in acid–base and other metabolic disturbances.
  - H2-blockers (cimetidine, famotidine, ranitidine, nizatidine): considered for uncomplicated GORD; side effects include constipation, diarrhoea, confusion, and elevated liver enzymes.
  - Proton pump inhibitors (omeprazole, lansoprazole): highly effective, first-line agents for complicated GORD or failed first-line regimens.
  - Prokinetic agents (cisapride, metoclopramide): indicated for delayed gastric emptying, increases lower oesophageal sphincter pressure; side effects include tardive dyskinesia and confusion.
- Surgical management is indicated for failed medical regimen; fundoplication increases tone of the distal oesophagus.

⑦ Oesophagitis

Various forms exist:

- Reflux oesophagitis.
- Candidal oesophagitis
- Herpes oesophagitis. Multiple ulcerations, most commonly seen in immunocompromised patients.
- Drug-induced oesophagitis. Typically punctate ulcerations; causative drugs include tetracycline, quinidine, aspirin, and clindamycin.
- Radiation oesophagitis. May be acute (during therapy) or chronic (scarring and stenosis 6–18 months after radiation therapy).
- Eosinophilic oesophagitis. This is an allergic inflammatory condition of the oesophagus, sometimes called allergic oesophagitis. Symptoms include swallowing difficulty, food impaction, and heartburn. *It should be considered if gastroesophageal reflux does not respond to high-dose proton-pump inhibitors or if pH studies rules out GORD.* Biopsy may be required. Treatment includes corticosteroids and other anti-inflammatories. Mechanical dilatation may be considered with strictures.

⑦ Oesophageal diverticulum (pharyngeal pouch)

A pharyngeal pouch is created by herniation of mucosa through the muscular wall. There are three areas of natural weakness in the upper oesophageal/hypopharyngeal segment:

- Killian's triangle: inferior to the cricopharyngeal muscle and superior to the cricothyroid muscles
- Killian–Jamieson space: laterally, between cricopharyngeal and oesophagus muscle
- Laimer–Haeckermann space: between cricopharyngeus superiorly and circular fibres inferiorly
- Several types of diverticulum exist.

⑦ Oesophageal neoplasms

Benign tumours and cysts

These are rare and are less common than malignant tumours. Patients present with dysphagia, pressure behind the sternum, bleeding, and weight loss. Diagnosis is by barium swallow and endoscopy (with biopsy), CT/MRI. Treatment requires endoscopic or open excision.

Malignant tumours

These typically present in elderly males with a history of tobacco and alcohol abuse. They are also seen in association with caustic burns, radiation, oesophageal webs, Plummer–Vinson disease, achalasia, pernicious anaemia, nutritional deficiencies, oesophagitis, and GORD. Tumours may initially result in painless dysphagia which develops later into odynophagia. There may also be haemoptysis, a cough, hoarseness, and weight loss. Investigations include barium swallow, endoscopy and biopsy and CT/MRI. Management is multimodal therapy (surgery, radiation/chemotherapy). Overall there is a poor prognosis.

⑦ Oesophageal webs and rings

Webs are asymmetric, thin, membranous projection into the lumen, composed of mucosa and submucosa only. Rings are thicker, composed of mucosa, submucosa, and muscularis mucosa. Upper cervical webs may be associated with Plummer–Vinson syndrome. Diagnosis is confirmed with oesophagrams or oesophagoscopy. Treatment options include dilation and endoscopic laser excision.

☼ Oesophageal rupture and perforation

Aetiology includes iatrogenic instrumentation (most common cause), blunt and penetrating trauma, neoplasms, inflammation, and increased abdominal pressure:

- Mallory–Weiss syndrome: incomplete tear of oesophageal mucosa from increased abdominal pressure (vomiting in alcoholics), presents as an upper GI bleed.
- Boerhaave syndrome: increased abdominal pressure results in a full-thickness tear of the lower oesophagus. Symptoms include bloodstained vomiting, chest pain, dyspnoea, and hypovolaemia.

Examination may reveal tachycardia, fever, respiratory distress, dysphagia, subcutaneous emphysema, Hammer's sign (crunching sound over heart from subcutaneous emphysema). Investigations include CXR (mediastinal widening, pneumothorax) and oesophagram (sodium amidotrizoate). Untreated cases can lead to complications including chemical mediastinitis and septic shock. Usually need early surgical repair and drainage, antibiotics and anti-reflux medication.

⑦ Globus

Globus is a feeling of a lump in the throat when actually there is no lump present. It is often associated with anxiety. Usually it is idiopathic in nature (globus pharyngeus or globus hystericus), but occasionally may be secondary to identified pathology:

- Oesophageal spasm
- GORD
- Neuromuscular disorders such as myasthenia gravis, Parkinson's disease and stroke
- Rarely, cancers of the upper GI tract.

Miscellaneous conditions involving the throat

⑦ Aphthous ulcers

These most commonly occur in the oral cavity but can also present in oropharynx. They are mostly idiopathic, but can be immunological, hormonal, stress induced, traumatic, or nutritional related.

- Minor aphthous ulcers are the most common. There is burning and tingling before ulcer formation. Ulcers are <1.0 cm in diameter and painful.

- Major aphthous ulcer. These are more painful and larger (1–3 cm in diameter), multiple (1–10), and carry a risk of scar formation.
- Herpetiform. These form numerous small ulcers 1–3 mm in diameter.

Treatment includes observation (self-limiting), consider anti-inflammatory agents, oral and topical corticosteroids. Screen for haematinic deficiencies.

① Swollen uvula (Quincke's disease or sign)

An acutely swollen uvula can present with foreign body sensation or fullness in the throat, muffled voice, and gagging. Examination reveals the uvula is swollen, pale, and translucent. It may be seen resting on the tongue, moving in and out with respiration. There may also be an associated rash, history of exposure to allergens, or a recurrent seasonal incidence. Consider foods, drugs, physical agents, inhalants, insect bites, and hereditary angio-oedema. Initial treatment includes parenteral antihistamines. More severe cases may need nebulized adrenaline (epinephrine) and parenteral corticosteroids. If there is a history of recurrent episodes or family history, consider checking for C4 complement level or C1 esterase inhibitor levels to screen for hereditary angio-oedema. All patients should be observed for an adequate period of time to insure that there is either improvement or no further worsening.

② Eagle syndrome (styloid–carotid artery syndrome)

This is a rare condition in which there is elongation of the styloid process, or calcification of the stylohyoid ligament. 'Classic' and 'vascular' forms are described. Patients are usually aged between 30 and 50 years and can present with recurrent sore throat, dysphagia, neck pain, and otalgia. Blackouts and sudden death due have also been reported and are due to mechanical pressure on the carotid. *Consider this when neurological symptoms occurs upon head rotation.* The tip of the styloid process may be palpable in the back of the throat. Plain films and CT confirm the diagnosis (the enlarged styloid may be visible on an OPT or a lateral soft tissue X-ray). In both types, treatment is surgical (partial styloidectomy).

② Leucoplakia and erythroplakia

(See also ⮕ Chapter 13.) These can also occur in the pharynx. Leucoplakia anywhere in the oral cavity and pharynx carries a small risk of malignant change. However, the risk is often site dependent (notably floor of mouth) and particularly related to smoking and alcohol abuse. Erythroplakia has a higher risk of malignancy. All chronic leucoplakia or ulcerative lesions that fail to heal after 3–6 weeks should be referred.

② Snoring and obstructive sleep apnoea

Snoring occurs as a result of vibration of the upper respiratory structures (usually the uvula and soft palate) secondary to partial obstruction of air movement while sleeping. Intensity and loudness can vary considerably. Associated causes include:

- Intrinsic muscular weakness, causing the throat to relax during sleep
- Retruded mandible jaw
- Enlarged tonsils/adenoids
- Large collar size/obesity

- Obstruction in the nasal passageway
- Obstructive sleep apnoea
- Muscle relaxants including alcohol or drugs
- Sleeping on one's back, which may result in the tongue dropping to the back of the mouth.

Snoring may be an early sign of obstructive sleep apnoea (OSA). This condition is known to cause sleep deprivation resulting in daytime drowsiness, irritability, lack of concentration, and decreased libido. The Epworth sleepiness score is a tool often used to assist with diagnosing the condition and monitoring its management. The history from a partner can be also very useful (do they stop breathing, sleep in another room, how does it affect lives, etc.)

More recently, studies have shown an increased risk of myocardial infarction, hypertension (both systemic and pulmonary), and stroke.

Treatment includes management of reversible causes (avoid alcohol, lose weight, etc.). In some units, respiratory physicians run OSA clinics and patients may need to be referred there (either directly or from their own doctor) for assessment. After attending to modifiable factors nocturnal nasal continuous positive airway pressure may be tried. Mandibular advancement devices are also useful. They posture the jaw forward to prevent the tongue falling into the hypopharynx. In other cases tonsillectomy or uvulectomy may increase the airway diameter. Positive pressure ventilation and jaw advancement surgery are occasionally required in severe cases. Tracheostomy is now rarely performed. Jaw advancement surgery is effective but carries risk due to co-morbidities.

⑦ Dysphagia and aspiration

Dysphagia is an important symptom, which may signify significant or sinister pathology. It therefore requires careful assessment and often urgent referral. On average, people swallow once or twice every minute. It takes approximately 1 second. Aspiration is the intrusion of food or liquid into the unprotected airway below the level of the vocal folds. This can lead to infections of the respiratory system, pneumonitis, and pneumonia.

⑦ Odynophagia

This is painful swallowing, either in the throat (oropharynx) or oesophagus. It can occur with or without dysphagia. If persistent, it results in weight loss. Odynophagia can be caused by many conditions

Causes of dysphagia
- Xerostomia (irradiation, salivary glands disease, or drugs)
- Poor head posture
- Ineffective lip seal
- Restricted tongue movement
- Cleft palate or reduced velopharyngeal seal
- Delayed or absent swallow reflex due to postoperative swelling or cranial nerve injury

- Restricted laryngeal elevation results in unsatisfactory closure of the larynx and aspiration
- Vocal fold paralysis following cranial nerve injury
- Reduced pharyngeal motility
- Pharyngeal/oesophageal pathology (notably strictures and tumours)
- Stroke and other neurological disorders
- The presence of a tracheostomy tube can restrict laryngeal elevation
- Ineffective peristalsis hinders the passage of food to the stomach.
- Incomplete or constricted cricopharyngeal and cardiac sphincters hinder passage of food to stomach.
- Ingestion of very hot or cold food or drink
- Drugs
- Mucosal ulcers
- URTIs
- Immune disorders
- Epiglottitis
- Tumours
- Motor disorders.

Useful clues in assessment
- Character of dysphagia: solid dysphagia (obstructive) vs liquid dysphagia (neurological)
- Progressive (tumour, achalasia)
- Odynophagia (suggests acute process, foreign body, pharyngitis, laryngitis)
- Regurgitation (nasal or gastric regurgitation, timing of regurgitation), type of regurgitated food (digested or undigested)
- Aspiration (cough after ingestion, recurrent pneumonia, choking)
- Contributing factors: history of GORD, history of foreign body ingestion or trauma
- Indicators for potential malignancy (weight loss, family history of cancer, hoarseness, smoking, alcohol abuse)
- History of neurological, connective tissue, or autoimmune disorders.

Assessment of dysphagia

The history and examination may provide important clues to the underlying cause.

Signs of aspiration
Acute
- Distress
- Coughing, choking, and gasping
- Respiratory difficulty—wheezing or gurgling
- Loss of voice or gurgling 'wet' sounding voice
- Change of colour (greyness)
- Tachycardia and sweating.

Chronic
- Respiratory problems/chest infections
- Coughing and choking
- Excess oral secretions
- Loss of weight
- Hunger
- Refusal to eat.

Silent aspiration
Patients with loss of sensation in the larynx may aspirate without coughing and without awareness of the problem. Nasogastric tubes may also be easily passed into the trachea without obvious signs.

Investigations
These are tailored according to the suspected pathology:
- Modified barium swallow.
- Manometry: measures duration, amplitude, and velocity of peristaltic waves.
- CXR: reveals pneumonitis, pneumonia, masses, or a displaced airway.
- Laryngoscopy and oesophagoscopy: indicated if suspect malignancy, to remove foreign bodies, and to biopsy a mass or lesion.
- Functional (fibreoptic) endoscopic evaluation of swallowing: outpatient evaluation of swallowing function.
- Videostroboscopy: evaluates vocal fold motion, pooled secretions, and anatomical defects (masses, glottal chinks, etc.).
- CT/MRI: may be considered to evaluate masses.

Management of dysphagia
Medical management of dysphagia
- Address underlying cause (e.g. iron supplementation for Plummer–Vinson, pyridostigmine for myasthenia gravis, benztropine for Parkinson's disease, antibiotics for acute bacterial pharyngitis).
- Utilize an alternative temporary route of nutrition (nasogastric tube feeds, parenteral nutrition).
- Anti-reflux regimen for GORD.
- Address aspiration pneumonia if any (hold oral feeds, antibiotic regimen, and aggressive pulmonary toilet).
- Botulinum toxin injections: considered for cricopharyngeal spasms.
- Refer to speech and language therapy for swallowing rehabilitation.

Surgical management of dysphagia
- Oesophageal dilation: may be considered for pharyngeal or oesophageal strictures, webs, postoperative scarring, and post-radiation strictures.
- Cricopharyngeal myotomy: may be considered for cricopharyngeal spasms.
- Gastric or jejunal feeding tube: temporary or permanent enteric feeding.

- Tracheostomy (cuffed): indicated for severe pulmonary complications, prevents aspiration pneumonia by allowing easier pulmonary toilet and preventing gross aspiration (but does not prevent micro-aspiration).
- Laryngeal suspension: indicated for severe aspiration from supraglottic and pharyngeal dysfunction; suspends larynx anteriorly by positioning thyroid cartilage under mandible, may improve voicing and swallowing.
- Laryngeal diversion or separation: indicated for severe aspiration, creates a permanent tracheostomy with proximal tracheal segment diverted back to the oesophagus.
- Laryngectomy: rarely indicated. It is undertaken for life-threatening complications.
- Bilateral submandibular excision and parotid duct ligation: may be considered in patients who aspirate saliva.

! Cancers of the throat

This is a non-specific term. It generally refers to a varied group of cancers including cancers of the:
- Tonsil
- Upper oesophagus
- Nasopharynx
- Posterior oropharynx
- Larynx.

These are described in the relevant anatomical chapters.

! Tonsil tumours

Malignancy of the tonsils is an uncommon entity. More than 70% of malignancies are squamous cell carcinoma followed by lymphomas. Squamous cell carcinomas are about three to four times more common in men than in women, and seen typically in advanced age. Other more uncommon malignancies include minor salivary gland tumours and metastatic lesions. Risk factors include smoking and ethanol abuse and more recently association with human papilloma virus (HPV). Recent studies have identified HPV presence in approximately 60% of tonsillar carcinomas. Typically they present with unilateral tonsillar enlargement with or without cervical lymphadenopathy. Treatment is mutimodal (surgery and or radiotherapy), depending on the type and stage of the tumour.

! Squamous cell carcinoma

Squamous cell carcinoma is more commonly seen in the oropharynx (see
➔ Chapter 13). Posterior oropharyngeal tumours can extend pass the fauces and involve the throat. The usual presentation is that of a painless ulcer and trismus. Patients are usually emaciated. It is commonly seen in smokers and alcoholics. Prognosis is generally poor.

Any ulcer that has been present for >3 weeks, without an obvious cause, should be referred urgently as a possible cancer.

The cheek and orbit

Common presentations

Some common periorbital problems:
- Double vision
- Infections
- Injuries
- Pain (see also ➲ Chapter 10)
- Proptosis
- Swelling.

Common problems and their causes

Double vision

Common
- Alcohol intoxication
- Fractures to the zygoma/orbit
- CN III, IV, VI injury
- Orbital swelling/bruising.

Uncommon
- Fractures to the NOE/skull
- Orbital myositis
- Tumours
- Migraine
- Neurological disease (MS)
- Sinusitis
- Orbital abscess
- Graves' disease
- Strabismus
- Globe disorders.

Infections

Common
- Eyelid infections (see ➲ Chapter 10)
- Skin infections
- Dental infections
- Sinusitis.

Uncommon
- Orbital cellulitis.

Injuries

Common
- Fractures (zygoma or isolated orbital)
- Lacerations (eyebrows, eyelids)
- Foreign body injuries.

Uncommon
- Chemical injury to eyes (see ⊋ Chapter 10)
- Penetrating eye injuries (see ⊋ Chapter 10).

Pain
(See also ⊋ Chapter 10.)

Common
- Trauma
- Eyelid/sinus infections
- Migraine/cluster headaches
- Eye strain.

Uncommon
- Orbital cellulitis
- Tumour/pseudotumour
- Thyroid eye disease
- Temporal arteritis
- Herpes zoster.

Proptosis and swelling

Common
- Trauma
- Eyelid/sinus infections
- Thyroid eye disease
- High myopia (short-sightedness).

Uncommon
- Retrobulbar haemorrhage (RBH)
- Tumour
- Orbital cellulitis
- Orbital inflammatory disease
- Dermoid/epidermoid cysts/haemangioma
- Carotid cavernous fistula.

Useful questions and what to look for

Double vision

Ask about
- Onset
- Static or progression
- One or both eyes
- Diplopia looking in one direction or all directions
- Recent injury

- Is the double vision worse at the end of the day or when tired?
- Any deterioration in vision
- Any other symptoms (swelling/headaches).

Look for
- Obvious squint
- Signs of injury
- Proptosis
- Numbness of cheek and forehead (and CN examination)
- Examine the eye/eye movements.

Infections

Ask about
- Duration/previous episodes
- Recent skin infections or trauma
- Pain, erythema, and swelling
- Changes in visual field, blurred vision, diplopia
- Systemic symptoms
- Impaired mental status
- Discharge from nose or eye
- Headaches
- Medications taken.

Look for
- Site and extension (confined to eyelids or spreading into surrounding tissues)
- Skin erythema swelling and any fluctuant swelling
- Systemic involvement (pyrexia, sweating, lethargy)
- Assess cranial nerves
- Assess the eye (see ➲ Chapter 10)
- Numbness of the cheek and forehead.

Injuries

Ask about
- Mechanism of injury
- Any other injuries
- Possibility of foreign body
- Associated neurological deficit—numbness or change in vision, visual field, diplopia
- Pain and discharge from eye or wounds
- Alcohol or medications taken
- Chemical exposure to eye.

Look for
- Assess GCS/C-spine
- Assess visual acuity
- Lacerations or foreign bodies

- Assess bones of orbit, maxilla, forehead, and mandible
- Intercanthal distance >40 mm
- Assess eye movements in all directions/diplopia
- Assess cranial nerves
- Numbness of cheek and forehead.

Pain

Ask about
- Onset
- Static or progression
- Recent injury
- Pain in the eye, behind the eye, or around the eye
- Headache and associated symptoms
- Photophobia
- Blurred vision/diplopia.

Look for
- Assess visual acuity
- Eye movements/diplopia
- Signs of injury
- Signs of infection
- Proptosis
- Numbness of cheek and forehead
- Neck stiffness/photophobia
- Tenderness in the temple (temporal arteritis).

Proptosis and swelling

Ask about
- Recent skin/upper dental infections or facial trauma
- Duration—hours, days, or weeks
- One vs both sides
- Painful/painless
- Change in vision/ocular symptoms
- Systemic symptoms
- Headaches.

Look for
- Assess visual acuity
- Eye movements/diplopia
- Signs of injury
- Is swelling around the orbit or behind the eye?
- Is proptosis pulsatile?
- Numbness of cheek and forehead
- Systemic involvement (pyrexia/malaise/thyroid status).

Examination of the cheek and orbit

Examination of the cheek and orbit is not complete without an examination of the eye itself. This latter part of the examination is discussed in detail in Chapter 10 on the eye but is noted briefly here.

Applied anatomy

The cheek

The 'cheek bone' is formed predominantly by the zygomatic bone. This has a superior process, which fuses with the frontal bone at the fron-tozygomatic suture just at the lateral aspect of the eyebrow. *This is a key site in examination; tenderness and step deformity suggest a fracture of the cheek.* Medially, the zygoma joins with the maxilla approximately two-thirds of the way along the infraorbital rim. This provides support for the lower eyelid. Lower down anteriorly, the cheek bone fuses with the anterior wall of the maxilla, passing medially to form the piriform (nasal) aperture. The lower lateral aspect of this bony complex (often referred to as the 'buttresses') can be palpated from within the mouth, just above the roots of the upper premolar and molar teeth. *Tenderness and step deformity of this buttress suggest a fracture of the cheek.* Bruising may also be visible.

The body of the zygoma forms the prominence of the cheek. Together with the supraorbital ridge it provides a degree of protection to the globe. The bones in this region also provide support to the soft tissues, notably the lower eyelid and the medial and lateral canthal tendons. Displacement of the bones results in obvious asymmetry and a vertical drop in the position of the lateral canthus, sometimes termed an 'anti-mongoloid slant'. There may also be hypoglobus. The zygomatic arch is a key 'strut' in maintaining the forward projection of the cheek. Its importance can be overlooked when assessing facial X-rays.

The orbit

This is a pyramidal-shaped structure enclosed by four bony walls—the roof, floor, medial, and lateral walls. These converge at the orbital apex. The globe is a round ball approximately 24 mm in diameter which occupies only about a quarter of the orbital volume. The remainder is made up of the lacrimal apparatus, muscles, fat, blood vessels, and nerves. The cornea of the globe is bathed in tears which originate from the lacrimal gland (upper lateral aspect of the orbit) and pass across the cornea in a medial direction towards the punctae. From there they pass through the canaliculi and lacrimal sac, which sits in a bony recess, the lacrimal fossa, before passing into the nose.

The walls of the orbit are of varying thickness and strengths. The medial orbital wall is particularly thin and perforated by numerous valve-less blood vessels and nerves through a number of defects (Zuckerkandl dehiscences). *This allows for easy communication of infectious material between the ethmoidal air cells and orbital soft tissues.* The vessels here can bleed profusely into the orbit following trauma, which can result in a retrobulbar haematoma. Sensation to the cheek and lateral nose comes from the infraorbital nerve which passes along the orbital floor. Sensation to the forehead is from the supraorbital and supratrochlear nerves, both arising from the ophthalmic division of the trigeminal nerve. All these nerves are at risk of injury following either trauma to the orbit or from other intra-orbital pathology.

The upper part of the orbit is also part of the frontal bone. Significant force is required to fracture this bone. *Injuries to this area may therefore be associated with dural tears, CSF leakage, and brain or cervical injury.* The lateral wall of the orbit is composed of the zygoma and greater wing of the sphenoid (part of the middle cranial fossa). The most common injury in this region is fracture of the zygomatic bone.

Where the infra-orbital nerve passes along the floor of the orbit, the bone is especially weak. Isolated fractures of the orbital floor, or those associated with fractures of the zygoma, usually pass along this canal. *Numbness of the cheek and upper lip is therefore an important sign that could indicate an underlying fracture.* Occasionally the orbital contents herniate out following fracture of the orbital floor or medial wall. This is mostly periorbital fat but occasionally the extraocular muscles herniate. Entrapment prevents the coordinated action of the ocular muscles and may result in restricted eye movements and double vision (diplopia).

There are six striated muscles responsible for moving the eye: the four recti muscles (medial, lateral, superior, and inferior) and the superior and inferior oblique muscles. The nerves supplying these are the oculomotor, trochlear, and abducens nerves—'SO4(LR6)3' indicates the individual muscle innervations. The recti muscles have a common point of origin along the tendinous ring at the orbital apex. From there they pass forwards forming a muscular cone before inserting into the sclera. This cone can act as a closed compartment and contain blood following surgery or trauma (RBH).

The optic nerve runs from the back of the globe to the orbital apex and enters the cranial cavity via the optic foramen. Running in the opposite direction within this foramen is the ophthalmic artery which is a branch of internal carotid artery. The remaining blood vessels and nerves to the orbital contents gain access to the orbit via the superior orbital fissure.

Anteriorly the orbit is enclosed and protected by the eyelids. The upper eyelid is the most mobile and is elevated by the combined actions of a smooth muscle and a striated muscle (Müller's muscle and levator palpebrae superioris respectively). The orbital septum is a layer of fascia extending vertically from the peripheral periosteum of the orbital rim into the levator aponeurosis in the upper eyelid and the inferior border of the tarsal plate in the lower eyelid. This is important as infection that passes deep to the septum can enter the orbit, resulting in orbital cellulitis. *Eyelid and periorbital swellings therefore require prompt diagnosis and management.*

Examination

(See also ➲ Chapter 10.) The face should be inspected from the front and side of the patient. It should also be viewed from above, looking down over the brow. *With all orbital-related conditions, early assessment of the eye is essential as management initially takes priority.* If the eyelids are closed due to painful swelling, gently pressing on the eyelids (not the globe) for a few minutes can often reduce swelling sufficiently to assess the eye. However, be careful if the swelling is thought to be due to cellulitis or an abscess. If necessary, a Desmarres retractor, lid speculum, or even a bent sterile paper clip can be used to gently retract the eyelids, while avoiding pressure on the globe. If necessary, apply topical anaesthetic (either tetracaine or proparacaine drops) to decrease discomfort. When there is significant swelling, assessment of the eye can be limited. As a minimum, make sure you assess visual acuity, pupils, extraocular motility, and visual fields. *Never allow a patient with orbital pathology to go home if you have been unable to assess the eye. Inability to open the eyelids is not an acceptable reason. If you cannot assess the eye, discuss with ophthalmology.* Gross examination of the eyelids, conjunctiva, sclera, cornea, and anterior chamber may reveal lacerations, anatomic disruption, haemorrhage, or foreign bodies. Contact lenses and superficial foreign bodies should also be removed. *If a penetrating injury to the eye is suspected, pressure should be avoided.*

External examination

The eyelids and periocular region should be inspected, taking note of asymmetry, oedema, ecchymosis, lacerations, foreign bodies, or abnormal eyelid position. *Any 'black eye' with a sharply defined border should be regarded as a sign of an underlying fracture* (Figure 9.1).

Ptosis (drooping of the upper eyelid) is common following injury and is typically the result of oedema. Other causes include third nerve palsy, levator muscle injury, or traumatic Horner's syndrome. Medial eyelid lacerations should raise the suspicion of canalicular injury. *The presence of fatty tissue within a lid laceration indicates perforation of the orbital septum and should raise suspicion for an orbital injury, globe injury, and a foreign body.* The orbital rims should be palpated for bony steps and tenderness. Any sensory loss in the cheek and forehead should be noted and compared to the other side. Periorbital *surgical emphysema* is highly suggestive of a fracture involving the cheek, orbital floor, or medial orbital wall. When the nose is blown, air normally contained within the sinuses

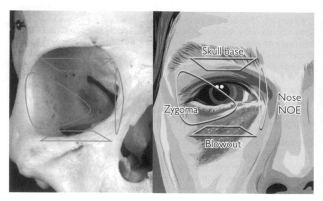

Figure 9.1 Fractures resulting in a 'black eye'.

escapes into the soft tissue. It can also occur in some infections or any erosive pathology that destroys bone. The intercanthal distance has a wide range; in Caucasians, for example, it is about 28–35 mm. Increased intercanthal distance >40 mm (approximately the width of the patient's eye) suggests displacement of the medial canthal tendon. These patients require CT imaging (see ➲ Chapter 7).

Visual acuity

This should be determined independently in each eye using a Snellen chart, with the patient wearing their spectacles or using a pinhole. Topical anaesthetics may help if the patient has acute pain or blepharospasm. If unable to visualize print, record counting fingers at a specified distance, hand motion, light perception, or no perception.

Pupil examination

Pupil size and reactivity are important determinants of globes status, particularly in the unconscious. The size, shape, symmetry, and reaction to light should be noted. Patients should also be assessed for a relative afferent pupillary defect (RAPD).

Globe position and ocular motility

The presence of proptosis and dystopia should be noted. This may indicate haemorrhage, infection, inflammation, or tumour. Looking at the orbits from above (bird's-eye view) or below (worm's-eye view) assists in determining the degree of proptosis. Reflection of light off the patient's corneas should be in the same position in both eyes. This means that the globes are level and looking in the same direction. If one eye appears lower than the other this is called hypoglobus, or vertical ocular dystopia. This may be seen in zygomatic or orbital floor fractures, or space-occupying lesions or swellings. If the eye appears 'sunken in' this is likely to be enophthalmos, indicating an orbital fracture. *Be careful, the globe may also appear sunken in if it is ruptured or is a prosthesis.* Proptosis (exophthalmos) is common, but usually mild following injury. Remember non-traumatic causes as well.

The patient should be able to painlessly move their eyes in all directions. Limited motility has many causes (notably fractures, muscle injury, entrapment, cranial nerve injury, or orbital oedema and blood). When assessing eye movements, move the object slowly—otherwise subtle restriction may be overlooked. Look closely as they look up. If there is entrapment the axis of rotation shifts and sometimes the eye can be seen to rotate into the orbit. This is called a 'retraction sign'.

It is important to distinguish whether diplopia is monocular or binocular. *Diplopia that persists when the opposite eye is covered is monocular and suggests an abnormality of the globe, such as corneal irregularity, lens abnormality or iridodialysis.* Diplopia that resolves when covering either eye is a defect in the coordinated eye movement. Diplopia on upward gaze is a clinical sign of orbital floor entrapment whereas in downward gaze it can be associated with dysfunction of the inferior rectus from simple bruising.

Visual field testing
Visual field testing can detect a number of disorders. Confrontational (face-to-face) visual field assessments are measured one eye at a time and can be performed by comparing the patient's fields to the examiner's own field (assuming that the examiner has normal visual fields). At a normal conversational distance, a target (e.g. fingers or cotton-tipped applicators) can be placed at the periphery of the visual field equidistant between the examiner and patient. Care must be taken to ensure that the unexamined eye of the patient is completely covered.

Intraocular pressure measurement
Elevated intraocular pressure (IOP) can result from numerous conditions, including hyphaema, glaucoma, RBH, tumours, thyroid eye disease, or carotid-cavernous fistula. Decreased IOP can result from open-globe injury, uveitis, cyclodialysis (separation of the ciliary body from the sclera), or retinal detachment. IOP may be measured using an applanation tonometer, portable Tono-Pen®, or Schiotz tonometer. Topical anaesthesia (tetracaine) is necessary.

Useful investigations

See also ➔ Chapter 10.

Laboratory tests

A FBC with differential is usually required for any infective, inflammatory, systemic, or neoplastic pathologies.

The ESR should be taken when symptoms suggest the possibility of temporal arteritis.

Plain films

Occipitomental (15 and 30 degrees) and lateral facial views are commonly required in the preliminary assessment of zygomatic/orbital and some mid-face injuries. They are also of use in the preliminary assessment of the maxillary and ethmoid sinuses.

Soft tissue views may be required to locate a foreign body.

CT/MRI

CT has largely replaced conventional plain film radiography in the evaluation of periorbital trauma and other sinus/orbital pathology (tumours, infections, etc.). CT is particularly useful in the evaluation of orbital fractures, intraocular and orbital foreign bodies, globe rupture, and space-occupying lesions. However, radiolucent foreign bodies such as plastic or wood may be difficult to detect on CT or plain film. Standard CT examination should include both axial and coronal views. Sagittal views are also very useful in the evaluation of orbital floor injuries. With today's modern scanners all these views are now easily obtained. Contrast is not necessary in trauma, but may be for other pathologies, so the patient's U&Es may need to be checked. MRI is useful in the evaluation of suspected tumours or soft tissue abnormalities.

Angiography

This may be required urgently following trauma (especially penetrating injuries). If bleeding is active, selective embolization may be necessary. Angiography is also occasionally undertaken in the assessment of vascular swellings (alternatively, CTA or MRA may be performed).

Ultrasound

This has a limited role, but can be of use in identifying some ocular pathologies or foreign bodies.

⊙ Orbital fractures (isolated)

Orbital fractures can affect any of the orbital walls or orbital margin. These may occur in isolation or be part of a larger fracture complex, with involvement of the surrounding bones (e.g. NOE, zygomatic, anterior cranial fossa). *The term 'blowout' fracture refers specifically to an isolated injury to one or more orbital walls (commonly the floor or medial wall) but with the surrounding orbital rims intact.* The orbital floor and medial orbital wall are particularly delicate and are easily damaged, resulting in these fractures. There are two proposed mechanisms. A direct blow to the globe (e.g. squash ball to the eye) can result in the transfer of energy directly to the orbital floor or medial wall. In these cases the globe can also be seriously injured. Alternatively, a blow to the prominence of the cheek, can deform the bone such that it 'buckles', resulting in fracture propagation within the orbit. This type of fracture may be associated with concurrent facial fractures to the zygoma or mid face.

Clinical features

- Swelling/bruising/tenderness (not specific)
- Diplopia (usually on looking up) (Figure 9.2)
- Enophthalmos/vertical ocular dystopia
- Proptosis may occur if there is a lot of swelling or surgical emphysema
- Numbness of the cheek
- Globe injury.

Investigations

- Occipitomental and lateral facial views (for associated cheek or mid-facial injury) may suggest a 'hanging drop' sign. This may represent the herniation of orbital contents into the maxillary sinus. However, it may not be easily seen and not all 'hanging drops' are herniated contents. Nevertheless, it is an important sign and merits further investigation. A fluid level in the sinus suggests there is a fracture somewhere.
- Coronal/axial CT of orbits.
- Orthoptic assessment—Hess chart, measurement of globe projection and fields of binocular vision (to assess restriction of ocular movement). Swelling may preclude immediate assessment.

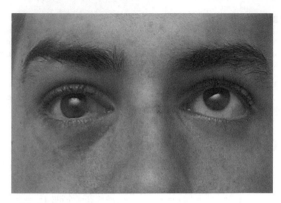

Figure 9.2 Restriction of upward gaze.

Reproduced from *Atlas of Operative Maxillofacial Trauma Surgery: Primary Repair of Facial Injuries*, 'Orbital Fractures', 2014, Figure 9.7a, eds M. Perry and S. Holmes, Copyright © 2014, Springer-Verlag London. With permission of Springer Nature.

Management

In all cases it is important to *advise the patient not to blow their nose*. This is because if they do, pressurized air can pass through the nose and antrum (sinus) into the orbit via the fracture. This potentially could introduce bacteria and result in orbital cellulitis. See Figure 9.3.

Many hospitals advise prophylactic antibiotics specifically. Initial measures include:

- Tell patient not to blow their nose for 3 weeks.
- If they have to sneeze, do so with mouth open.
- Consider antibiotics (co-amoxiclav 375 mg three times daily for 5 days).
- Tell the patient to return if they have increasing swelling, pain, or change in visual acuity.
- Chloramphenicol ointment may be applied to any conjunctival injury.
- Refer to maxillofacial surgery, or specialty that repairs facial fractures.
- If there are ocular symptoms, refer also to ophthalmology.

Never allow a patient with a suspected blowout fracture to go home if you have been unable to assess the eye. Inability to open the eyelids is not an acceptable reason. If you cannot assess the eye, discuss with ophthalmology.

Surgical repair of a blowout fracture is not necessary in every case and is not urgent, *except in children where it can be a surgical emergency*. The eye takes priority. Where an injury to the globe or associated nerves is suspected, an ophthalmic opinion should be sought.

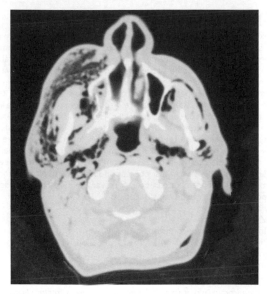

Figure 9.3 Surgical emphysema.

Indications for repair of a blowout fracture include:
- Significant diplopia
- A retraction sign
- Dystopia (displacement of globe)
- Enophthalmos
- A 'large' blowout on CT—said to predispose to the late development of enophthalmos.

The aim of repair is to release entrapped soft tissues and restore orbital geometry and volume. This should release any restrictions on eye movement and restore globe position. Timing of surgery is controversial and dependent on multiple factors. If the tissues are very swollen or there are minimal signs it is common practice to delay surgery for up to 10–14 days post-injury. This allows any swelling to settle and gives an idea of any disability.

In children, the orbits are shallow and there is a greater chance of muscle entrapment and ischaemic incarceration of the orbital soft tissues or muscles. Inappropriate pain, blepharospasm, or vomiting may suggest this. Immediate surgical intervention is indicated.

⊙Zygomatic (malar) fractures

Cheek fractures are common injuries and comprise a spectrum from relatively simple fractures resulting in minimal cosmetic problems, to complex patterns causing gross disfigurement and considerable functional disability. The terminology can also be a little confusing as they often go by a variety of names (zygoma, malar, zygomaticomaxillary, tripod—to name a few!).

The typical fracture pattern is that of a tetrapod. The 'feet' or 'pods' relate to the four main sites of fracture displacement, which can be identified either clinically or radiographically. The arch fractures separately from the remaining sites, which are joined together by a continuous ring of interlinking fractures. Together this allows separation of the entire cheek from the rest of the facial skeleton. Although commonly seen 'en bloc', as the energy transfer increases from mild to moderate to severe, fracture complexity increases correspondingly, with progression to comminution. Management can therefore vary widely. From a practical viewpoint fractures can be considered as:

- Isolated:
  - Zygomatic arch
  - Infraorbital rim (uncommon)
- Minimally displaced
- Significantly displaced
- Comminuted
- Fractures with associated mid-facial or complex orbital floor/wall injury.

All zygomaticomaxillary fractures, by definition, have a fracture line running through the orbit. Patients should therefore be assessed for ocular injury, diplopia, and entrapment. The eye takes priority. Associated ocular problems include:

- Globe/muscle injury
- RBH
- Superior orbital fissure syndrome
- Orbital apex syndrome.

Clinical features

These vary depending on the force of impact and degree of displacement of the cheek. They include:

- Signs of injury:
  - Pain
  - Swelling/bruising
  - Subconjunctival haemorrhage
  - Surgical emphysema
- Signs of orbital involvement:
  - Double vision/limitation of eye movement
  - Enophthalmos
  - Proptosis (exophthalmos)
- Signs of fracture displacement:
  - Flattening of the malar prominence (often masked by swelling immediately after injury)
  - Palpable infraorbital step
  - Antimongoloid slant
  - Hypoglobus (vertical ocular dystopia)
  - Altered sensation of cheek/upper lip

- Restricted jaw movements
- Malocclusion (premature contact of the molar teeth on the side of injury).

A well-defined 'black eye' or a subconjunctival haematoma with no posterior limit, are reliable signs of a fracture involving the orbit. Assess these patients carefully.

Investigations

- Visual acuity/orthoptic assessment.
- Occipitomental, lateral face. Look carefully, sometimes the only clue is a fluid level in the antrum.
- CT scan.
- Ultrasound scan and maxillary sinus endoscopy for orbital floor fractures have been reported as useful techniques but usually have no role in an emergency department setting. They are rarely undertaken.

Interpreting occipitomental views

To the inexperienced, interpreting occipitomental images can be tricky. This is probably due to a combination of complex anatomy, superimposition of the skull (notably vascular markings and sutures), and the relatively oddly angled views compared with images taken elsewhere in the body. The best way to learn is to see plenty of examples. A number of useful approaches have been described to help in interpretation. See Figures 9.4 and 9.5.

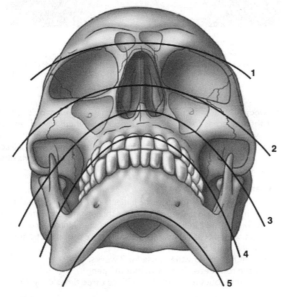

Figure 9.4 Campbell's lines.

Reproduced from *Atlas of Operative Maxillofacial Trauma Surgery: Primary Repair of Facial Injuries*, 'Fractures of the Cheek: Zygomaticomaxillary Complex', 2014, Figure 8.11b, eds M. Perry and S. Holmes, Copyright © 2014, Springer-Verlag London. With permission of Springer Nature.

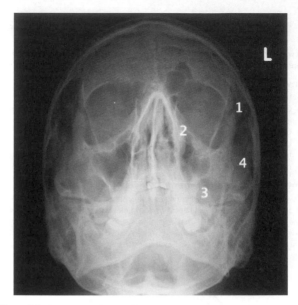

Figure 9.5 Occipitomental view of fractured zygoma.

Reproduced from *Atlas of Operative Maxillofacial Trauma Surgery: Primary Repair of Facial Injuries*, 'Fractures of the Cheek: Zygomaticomaxillary Complex', 2014, Figure 8.13, eds M. Perry and S. Holmes, Copyright © 2014, Springer-Verlag London. With permission of Springer Nature.

Knowledge of a 'tetrapod' fracture configuration enables one to inspect the key areas (or 'pods') on an occipitomental view. These are the sites where displacement is most noticeable. Alternatively the 'baby elephant' interpretation involves checking the sites shown (one infraorbital rim, two frontozygomatic sutures, and three zygomaticomaxillary buttress) and looking for a broken 'trunk'!

Management

In all cases it is important to *advise the patient not to blow their nose*. This is because if they do, pressurized air can pass through the nose and antrum into the orbit via the fracture. This potentially could introduce bacteria and result in orbital cellulitis. Many hospitals advise prophylactic antibiotics specifically. Initial measures include:

- Tell patient not to blow their nose for 3 weeks.
- If they have to sneeze, do so with mouth open.
- Consider antibiotics (co-amoxiclav 375 mg three times daily for 5 days).

- Tell the patient to return if they have increasing swelling, pain, or change in visual acuity.
- Chloramphenicol ointment may be applied to any conjunctival injury.
- Refer to maxillofacial surgery, or specialty that repairs facial fractures
- If there are ocular symptoms, refer also to ophthalmology.

Never allow a patient with a suspected zygomatic fracture to go home if you have been unable to assess the eye. Inability to open the eyelids is not an acceptable reason. If you cannot assess the eye, discuss with ophthalmology.

Surgery is usually carried out either immediately or about 5–6 days following injury. Many fractures are treated by open reduction and internal fixation (ORIF) with titanium miniplates. Surgical access for reduction and fixation is commonly through the mouth to avoid facial scars. Access to the frontozygomatic suture and infraorbital rim may also be necessary to assist reduction and fixation.

① The bulging eye (proptosis/ exophthalmos)

Proptosis, or exophthalmos, is the forward displacement of the eye in the orbit. Since the orbit is essentially a closed cavity, any enlargement of structures located within it will cause this. It can be unilateral or bilateral, acute or longstanding. *When unilateral and non-traumatic, consider un orbital tumour or orbital cellulitis.* Some degree of proptosis, usually minor, is common following trauma to the eye or orbit. Complete or partial dislocation of the globe from the orbit is possible but is very rare. In the vast majority of cases proptosis is not vision threatening despite its obvious cosmetic effects. Nevertheless, many patients complain of symptoms related to a dry eye and if the cornea remains unprotected serious complications can occur.

All cases of proptosis should be investigated for underlying or associated pathology (notably thyroid disease or orbital tumour).

Causes
- Periorbital trauma (from retrobulbar swelling, bleeding, displaced bones/air)
- Graves' ophthalmopathy (hyperthyroidism). This can also cause unilateral proptosis
- Orbital cellulitis
- Dacryoadenitis
- Mucormycosis
- Orbital pseudotumour
- High-altitude cerebral oedema
- Wegener's granulomatosis
- Tumours (leukaemia, lymphoma, meningioma, sarcoma, etc.)
- Haemangioma
- Dermoid cyst
- Carotid-cavernous fistula (look for pulsation)
- High myopia (short-sightedness).

✛ Trauma-related proptosis

Proptosis following trauma occurs in approximately 3% of craniofacial injuries. However, vision-threatening proptosis is a much rarer event. Nevertheless, when it occurs urgent intervention is required if loss of vision is to be prevented. Usually proptosis is apparent by the time the patient arrives in the emergency department, but delayed presentation of up to several days can also occur.

The orbit is essentially a rigid box, except anteriorly. It is therefore at risk of a compartment syndrome following trauma. Bleeding or swelling quickly results in a rapid rise in interstitial pressure, decreased perfusion pressure, and, if untreated, ischaemia and infarction. Re-establishment of perfusion is therefore essential if sight is to be saved. The two most common causes of sight-threatening proptosis following trauma are gross swelling behind the eye (orbital compartment syndrome (OCS)) and bleeding behind the eye (RBH).

⊚ Retrobulbar haemorrhage/orbital compartment syndrome

RBH is usually a clinical diagnosis and needs to be treated as soon as possible. *It is effectively an acute compartment syndrome within the orbit and should be managed with the same degree of urgency as compartment syndromes elsewhere in the body.* Raised intra-orbital pressure is caused by bleeding and oedema. This is contained within the bony orbit, behind the relatively unyielding orbital septum. Bleeding can occur within or outside the muscle 'cone', formed by the recti muscles, intra-conal bleeding being more severe. As the pressure rises, it compresses the ophthalmic and retinal vessels, resulting in retinal and optic ischaemia. In many cases there is no bleeding but oedema. When severe enough, this presents in exactly the same way. This is termed orbital compartment syndrome (OCS).

Clinical features
Consider retrobulbar haemorrhage if there is:
- Severe eye pain
- Acute proptosis
- Visual loss/RAPD
- Severely decreased eye movements in all directions (ophthalmoplegia).

Marked lid oedema may make proptosis difficult to recognize. Inability to open the eyelids with any one of these features is highly suspicious for RBH/OCS. Failure to recognize this may result in blindness. Irreversible damage has been estimated to occur following only 90 minutes of ischaemia. Raised IOP can be assessed with a Tono-Pen®, however many emergency departments will not have this equipment available. Therefore if suspected it is better to err on the side of caution and assume it is present. *Time is of the essence in any patient with deteriorating vision and increasing pain—these are the ones in whom treatment is most likely to be successful.* If you can, perform an immediate lateral canthotomy and cantholysis. If you cannot, get immediate help and learn how to do this. As for a surgical airway, this needs to be done immediately and any delay waiting for a 'specialist' to arrive will worsen the prognosis. Urgent referral to ophthalmology and maxillofacial surgery is also required (depending on local referral pathways). The canthotomy just buys time. Formal decompression may be required, depending on the clinical picture.

Lateral canthotomy/cantholysis

Lateral canthotomy with lateral canthal tendon division can be performed under local anaesthesia in the emergency department. Lignocaine 1% with adrenaline (epinephrine) (1 in 200,000) is injected into the lateral canthal area of the affected eye and the lateral canthus is incised to the orbital rim and the identified canthal tendon cut. The tendon is identified by 'strumming' the tissues, while the eyelid is pulled medially and out. Great care must be taken to avoid damage to the globe. The lower lid attachment is always divided and some authorities recommend division of the upper lid attachment as well. This allows the globe to translate forward, partially relieving the pressure by effectively increasing the retrobulbar volume. The steps for this are:

- Clean the site with sterile saline.
- Inject local anaesthetic into the lateral canthus.
- Crush the lateral canthus with a straight haemostat, advancing the jaws of the clip into the lateral fornix until the rim of the bony orbit is felt.
- Clamp for 30–60 seconds.
- Using straight scissors, make a 1 cm long horizontal incision of the lateral canthal tendon, in the middle of the crush mark.
- Grasp the lower eyelid with toothed forceps, pulling the eyelid away from the face. This pulls the inferior crus (the band of the lateral canthal tendon) tight so it can be easily cut loose from the orbital rim. It will have a 'banjo string' feel against the tip of the scissors.
- Continue to pull the lower eyelid outwards and downwards away from the eye.
- Use blunt-tipped scissors to cut the inferior crus.
- Keep the scissors parallel (flat) to the face with the tips pointed towards the chin. Place the inner blade just anterior to the conjunctiva and the outer blade just deep to the skin.
- The globe should pull freely away. It may also 'pop' forward, relieving the pressure. Cut any residual lateral attachments of the lower eyelid if it does not move freely.
- Do not worry about cutting ½ cm of conjunctiva or skin. The lower eyelid is cut, relieving orbital pressure.
- If the intact cornea is exposed apply ointment or lubricant to prevent corneal desiccation and infection.
- *Do not* apply absorbent gauze dressing to the exposed cornea.

See Figure 9.6.

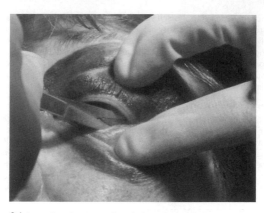

Figure 9.6 Lateral canthotomy and cantholysis.

Reproduced from *Atlas of Operative Maxillofacial Trauma Surgery: Primary Repair of Facial Injuries*, 'Initial Considerations: High- vs. Low-Energy Injuries and the Implications of Coexisting Multiple Injuries', 2014, Figure 1.51d, eds M. Perry and S. Holmes, Copyright © 2014, Springer-Verlag London. With permission of Springer.

Medical decompression

This should be commenced in addition to the canthotomy.

- Mannitol (osmotic diuretic) 20% 2 g/kg IV over 5 minutes.
- Dexamethasone 8 mg IV.
- Acetazolamide (carbonic anhydrase inhibitor, reduces production of aqueous humour), 500 mg IV then 250 mg 6-hourly for 24 hours.

Visual acuity is the key to urgency. If the vision is normal, patients can be investigated urgently to find the precise cause. But if the vision is rapidly deteriorating, or already significantly affected, time is of the essence. Think of the vision as the 'GCS of the eye'.

Assessment of proptosis in the unconscious patient

Comprehensive assessment of proptosis in the emergency department, ICU, or operating theatre is usually not possible in the early stages of management. What is possible is often limited, even more so if the patient is confused, agitated, or unresponsive. Differentiation between RBH and OCS on clinical grounds alone is not always possible since both share similar features.

In awake patients, clinical urgency can be determined by deterioration in visual acuity. However, in the unconscious or agitated patient, this is not possible. Pain and ophthalmoplegia, two further indicators of vision-threatening proptosis, also cannot be determined. It is also worth remembering that a well-made prosthetic eye can fool all but the most astute of clinicians. In unconscious patients, initial assessment of any proptosis is therefore significantly restricted to a relatively crude examination. This includes assessment of the eyelids, pupils, careful palpation of the globes, and, if possible, fundoscopy (or portable slit lamp examination). Each has its limitations. In many patients, the only readily identifiable signs of RBH/OCS will be a 'tense', proptosed globe with an abnormally reacting pupil and swollen disc. The main issue is to maintain a high index of suspicion and to seek advice early.

If the patient requires a CT scan of part of their body and their condition allows, request a CT of the orbits (or head). The additional time required to obtain these scans is now relatively small and you may identify a treatable cause of proptosis.

Remember that proptosis following trauma has several causes:

• Blood (RBH)
• Oedema (OCS)
• Air (surgical emphysema)
• Bone (fractures displaced into the orbit)
• Brain (craniofacial fractures)
• Contrast material (interventional radiology), a rare cause.

:⊕: Orbital cellulitis

This is a severe infection deep to the orbital septum, involving the orbital contents. The commonest source of infection is from infected periorbital sinuses (especially the ethmoid), or from spread of a preseptal cellulitis. The orbital septum is therefore a key anatomical landmark, which acts as a barrier to spread of infection during the initial stages. Tooth abscesses and organisms introduced by trauma are other, less common causes.

Patients with orbital cellulitis are often unwell with a high fever and a painful, swollen eye. There is a quick onset of rapidly worsening symptoms often with a history of sinus disease, periorbital infection, or injury. There is marked proptosis, chemosis, and lid oedema, which is red, hot, and tender to touch. Visual acuity and colour vision are reduced, together with an RAPD, if the optic nerve is involved. Eye movements are reduced and painful. Fundoscopy may show swollen optic nerve head and artery or vein occlusions.

The main differential diagnosis is pre-septal cellulitis, which is less severe and represents an infection anterior to the septum. This generally follows an eyelid infection. *If there is blurred vision, or the conjunctiva is injected, even without other signs of posterior involvement, assume orbital cellulitis until proven otherwise.*

Management

• Patients should be urgently admitted. Refer to ophthalmology.
• FBC, biochemistry, and blood cultures should be performed.
• CT of the orbit and brain is necessary to look for intracranial involvement, pus, and to assess the sinuses.
• Commonly associated pathogens are *Staphylococcus aureus*, *Streptococcus pneumoniae* and *pyogenes*, and (in children) *Hamophilus influenzae*. High-dose, broad-spectrum IV antibiotics that cover both anaerobic and aerobic organisms should be administered after the blood cultures have been taken. Metronidazole and ceftazidime is one such combination.
• Urgent surgical drainage of orbital, sinus, tooth, and brain abscesses is usually required.

The prognosis is good if treated early. Optic neuropathy and vascular occlusions carry poor visual prognosis. Cavernous sinus thrombosis has poor prognosis (see ⟳ Chapter 3).

In children, a rhabdomyosarcoma can mimic orbital cellulitis.

Orbital cellulitis can lead to meningitis, brain abscess, cavernous sinus thrombosis, septic shock, and death. It is vital for it to be diagnosed and managed promptly.

ⓘ Sinusitis

Sinusitis may present in many ways and may be confused with atypical facial pain, dental infections, orbital infections, osteomyelitis, or a tumour. The majority of infections are related to an initial rhinitis (as rhinosinusitis), but some can arise secondarily to dental infections in the upper teeth. Untreated sinusitis can spread to involve all four sinuses (maxillary, ethmoid, frontal, and sphenoid) sometimes referred to as pansinusitis. This is a potentially life- and sight-threatening condition. See Figure 9.7.

Sinusitis often arises following an URTI. Blockage of the draining ostia, paralysis of the cilia, and stagnation of secretions within the sinus predisposes to superadded infection. Any sinus can be affected, but the maxillary and ethmoid sinuses are the more common. Dental infections involving the upper teeth can also cause maxillary sinusitis. The roots of the molar and premolar teeth are sometimes separated from the sinus mucosa only by 'wafer-thin' bone, or dehisced bone. Infection within the pulp chamber can therefore pass through the tip (apex) of the root into the sinus relatively easily. The absence of toothache does not rule out dental causes.

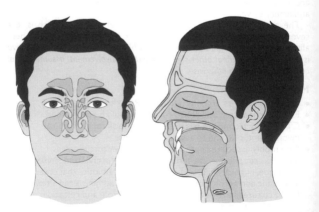

Figure 9.7 The sinuses of the face. kowalska-art/istockphoto.

⊕ Acute maxillary sinusitis

This is commonly caused by upper respiratory commensals (pneumo-cocci, staphylococci, streptococci, and anaerobes), or untreated upper dental infections. There is often some predisposing obstruction to the opening of the middle meatus, preventing the sinus from draining freely. This results in stagnation and then infection.

Clinically there is:

- Systemic upset
- Severe cheek pain, worse on bending
- Swelling over the cheek
- Numbness of the cheek
- Mobile upper teeth, which are tender to percussion (in severe cases).

Patients usually present with unilateral swelling of the face, sometimes referred to as a 'fat face'. Untreated, sinusitis can result in bacteraemia, or even septicaemia. The latter can occasionally lead to septic shock.

Usually the FBC will show an increased WCC. Blood cultures and a raised ESR may indicate the presence of bacteraemia or septicaemia. Radiographically there is radio-opacity of the involved sinus on an occip-itomental view. CT scan is required to assess the extent of infection. Infected large dental cysts should also be considered. If these are not identified a sinus washout will not remove all the pus.

Closure of the eyelids from swelling should be taken seriously—*the eye should be assessed and the patient often needs to be admitted.*

⊘ Chronic maxillary sinusitis

An underlying cause should be considered (dental disease, cystic fibrosis, or Kartagener's syndrome). Symptoms are similar to the acute infection but much less in severity. CT and MRI scans are useful diagnostic tests, although a high percentage of asymptomatic people have 'abnormal' scans. Diagnosis and treatment is therefore on clinical grounds.

⊕ Acute frontal sinusitis

(See ➜ Chapter 3.) This is potentially serious due to the risk of intracra-nial infection. Patients complain of frontal headache, which is tender to percussion. Untreated, the infection can spread intracranially or involve the orbit.

⊕ Acute ethmoid sinusitis

(See ➜ Chapter 7.) This usually occurs in association with other sinus infections. Patients complain of deep-seated pain and throbbing deep to the bridge of the nose. The medial orbital walls are paper thin, so orbital cellulitis can rapidly develop.

Management of sinusitis

Antibiotics and, in some cases, sinus washout with drainage using func-tional endoscopic sinus surgery. Ephedrine nasal drops and menthol inhalations may help reduce congestion and improve sinus drainage. Consider screening for diabetes and other causes of immunosuppres-sion. Symptoms requiring urgent assessment or referral include:

- Pyrexia
- Headache

- Swollen eyelids
- Blurred vision
- Significant malaise.

These patients probably need to be admitted for IV antibiotics and close observation.

① Fungal sinusitis

The most common fungus is *Aspergillus*. *Microsporidia* can also infect the sinuses. This may occur in otherwise healthy individuals. However, look for underlying causes of immunosuppression. The infection is seen as an opacity on X-ray or CT. Surgical debridement may be required.

⑦ Thyroid eye disease

Thyroid eye disease (TED) is frequently termed Graves' ophthalmopathy and is part of an autoimmune process that can affect the orbital and periorbital tissue, the thyroid gland (hyperthyroidism), and rarely pre tibial skin. An antibody-mediated reaction with lymphocytic infiltration of the orbital tissues results in an increase in volume of the orbital contents. This involves both the extraocular muscles and fat. This can cause bilateral or unilateral proptosis. Patients present with irritation around the eye, painful eye movements, a red eye, and, if severe, decreased vision. There is lid retraction, proptosis, chemosis, periorbital oedema, and altered ocular mobility. Initially an acute or subacute stage can make the differential diagnosis of orbital cellulitis difficult. In the latter there is usually a fever. Untreated, TED can cause vision-threatening exposure keratopathy, diplopia, and compressive optic neuropathy. Look for systemic features of hyperthyroidism. TED can also occur in euthyroid state. Investigations include thyroid function tests (thyroid-stimulating hormone, T3, and T4 levels) and thyroid autoantibodies.

Management

Ocular irritation without inflammation can be managed with artificial tear supplements. Mild ocular surface inflammation can be managed with topical steroids. Acute severe TED that can compromise optic nerve function should be referred urgently to ophthalmology urgently for management with IV methylprednisolone. Surgical decompression of the orbits is rarely indicated acutely.

⑦ Diplopia (double vision)

Diplopia occurs when one or both eyes are either moved out of alignment (by displacement of a fracture or by an orbital mass/swelling), or they lose their ability to move precisely together (either because of nerve/muscle weakness, or mechanical restriction). This is called binocular diplopia. Less commonly, diplopia may occur secondary to a problem within just one of the globes. This is called monocular diplopia.

Binocular diplopia is a common complaint following injuries to the orbit/eye, but in most cases it is temporary and secondary to swelling/

bruising around the extraocular eye muscles. Nevertheless, it can also be a symptom of significant orbital or globe injury, and in some cases requires surgical repair (see ➔ 'Orbital fractures (isolated)', pp. 267–9). Diplopia can also occur in other non-traumatic conditions, notably tumours, and therefore needs careful evaluation.

Causes of diplopia

These include ophthalmologic, traumatic, infectious, autoimmune, neurological, and neoplastic causes:

- Alcohol intoxication
- Fractures to the zygoma/orbit/NOE/skull
- CN III, IV, VI injury
- Orbital/extraocular eye muscles, swelling/bruising
- Orbital myositis
- Tumours
- Migraine
- Neurological disease (MS)
- Sinusitis
- Orbital abscess
- Graves' disease
- Strabismus
- Globe disorders.

Investigations

In gross cases, confirmation of diplopia may be possible by clinical examination of eye movements and looking at the corneal light reflex. However, in more subtle cases diplopia may only be apparent at the extremes of eye moments. All cases require an orthoptic assessment.

Diplopia associated with proptosis is worrying and requires an urgent CT (to look for a space-occupying orbital lesion). Other investigations are guided by the history (notably of trauma, or the presence of visual impairment, and/or pain). Progressive, persistent, or significant diplopia requires urgent referral to either ophthalmology or maxillofacial, depending on local protocol.

Management

This is dependent on the underlying cause.

The eye and eyelids

Common presentations

Common presentations for the eye and eyelids:
- Black eye (periorbital haematoma)
- Double vision (see ➲ Chapter 9, pp. 280–1)
- Dry eyes
- Foreign body sensation
- Injuries
- Loss of vision (painful)
- Loss of vision (painless)
- Painful eye
- Proptosis (see ➲ Chapter 9, p. 273)
- Red eye (painful)
- Red eye (painless)
- Swollen (puffy) eyelids.

Common problems and their causes

Black eye (periorbital haematoma)

Common
- Trauma to the eye, nose, or forehead
- Basal skull fracture (especially if bilateral)—racoon eyes
- Recent surgical procedures to the eye or face.

Uncommon
- Pre-septal or orbital cellulitis
- In children—non-accidental injuries.

Rare
- Tumours, e.g. rhabdomyosarcoma, neuroblastoma (in children).

Dry eyes

Common
- Ageing
- Blepharitis
- Meibomian gland dysfunction
- Rheumatoid arthritis
- Sjögren's syndrome
- Drugs, e.g. diuretics, tricyclic antidepressant drugs, antihypertensives, beta-blockers.

Uncommon
- Wegener's granulomatosis
- Systemic lupus erythematosus (SLE)
- Congenital alacrima
- Lacrimal gland ablation
- Sarcoidosis
- Tumours
- Post-radiation fibrosis.

Foreign body sensation

Common
- Grit/dust
- Hairs
- Eyelashes
- Corneal scratch
- Dry eyes.

Uncommon
- Glass
- High-velocity objects
- Corneal ulcer.

Injuries

Common
- Foreign bodies
- Corneal abrasions
- Arc eye.

Uncommon
- Ruptured globe
- Penetrating/perforating
- Eyelid lacerations
- Chemical burns.

Loss of vision (painful)

Common
- Acute angle-closure glaucoma (AACG)
- Uveitis—especially posterior and intermediate uveitis
- Corneal ulcers
- Scleritis—especially posterior scleritis
- Orbital cellulitis
- Herpes zoster ophthalmicus.

Uncommon
- Arteritic anterior ischaemic optic neuropathy—temporal arteritis
- Optic neuritis
- Chemical burns
- Blunt and penetrating ocular trauma
- Retrobulbar haemorrhage
- Endophthalmitis—exogenous and endogenous.

Loss of vision (painless)

Common
- Amaurosis fugax—TIA of the optic nerve
- Retinal artery/vein occlusion
- Retinal detachment
- Vitreous haemorrhage
- Age-related macular degeneration (gradual onset)
- Cataract (gradual onset)
- Non-arteritic ischaemic optic neuropathy
- Advanced glaucoma (gradual onset).

Uncommon
- Neurological diseases—occipital cortex strokes, lesion involving the visual pathways: optic tract, chiasm, lateral geniculate nucleus, cortex.

Painful eye

Common
- All the causes listed under painful loss of vision
- Corneal abrasion
- Foreign bodies
- Conjunctivitis
- Contact lens problems
- Blepharitis
- Dry eyes
- Glaucoma
- Infective keratitis
- Chalazion
- Cluster headache/migraine
- Sinusitis.

Uncommon
- Iritis/uveitis
- Optic neuritis
- Scleritis.

Red eye (painful)

Common
- Acute conjunctivitis—viral, bacterial, allergic
- Keratitis (bacterial/viral), e.g. herpes simplex, herpes zoster
- Keratitis marginal
- Corneal abrasion
- Corneal foreign body
- Subtarsal foreign body
- Arc eye/flash burn
- Contact lens-related problems
- Chronic conjunctivitis—chlamydia, allergic, *Molluscum contagiosum*
- Angle-closure glaucoma.

Uncommon
- Anterior uveitis (iritis)
- Scleritis and episcleritis
- Atypical microbial keratitis, e.g. *Acanthamoeba* keratitis.

Red eye (painless)

Common
- Blepharitis
- Ectropion/entropion
- Trichiasis
- Subconjunctival haemorrhage.

Uncommon
- Pterygium
- Carotico-cavernous fistula.

Swollen (puffy) eyelid(s)

Common
- Blepharitis
- Chalazion
- Allergic reaction
- Stye
- Oversleeping/sleep deprivation
- Normal ageing.

Uncommon
- Cellulitis
- Tumour
- Graves' disease
- Infectious mononucleosis
- Fluid retention—many conditions (including pregnancy)
- Diet—excess salt
- Nephrotic syndrome
- Trichinosis—from eating raw, infected pork
- Superior vena cava obstruction
- Cavernous sinus thrombosis.

Essential questions

Irrespective of the presenting complaint, a detailed history is required.
The two main symptoms to ask about are pain and visual disturbances.
   Ask about the following specific symptoms.

Pain
- Onset and duration
- Gritty/foreign body sensation
- Ache/pain within or around the eye

- Headache and associated symptoms (jaw claudication)
- Photophobia.

Visual disturbance
- Establish the extent of reduced visual acuity, e.g. from blurring to total loss of vision
- Any unusual visual experiences, e.g. floaters, photopsia, shadows/scotoma, distortion
- Any diplopia.

In trauma
- The mechanism of injury—was the injury of low velocity (grinding) or high velocity (hammering, drilling)? Sharp or blunt injury? Size of the offending object.
- Was eye protection used?
- Presence of chemical or organic matter.

Previous ocular history
- Previous ocular surgery (recent and old)
- Pre-existing ocular conditions, e.g. squints, glaucoma
- Any refractive error or amblyopia (lazy eye/poor vision since childhood)
- Does the patient wear contact lens?

General medical history
- Systemic conditions, e.g. hypertension, diabetes
- Drug history including eye drops
- Allergies
- Social history (occupational/travel abroad)
- Family history.

Examination of the eye and eyelids

Corneal abrasions (loss of corneal epithelium) are very painful and can prevent examination. Patients often have intense blepharospasm. If this is present and there is no contraindication, place a few drops of topical anaesthetic (e.g. oxybuprocaine). Rapid pain relief is almost diagnostic. This can then be followed by a drop of 2% fluorescein. All but the smallest of abrasions can be seen as a green patch on the corneal surface. Be careful when looking—a total corneal epithelial defect (due to chemical injury) can be missed easily as the whole cornea is then stained.

Visual acuity
Options include a Snellen chart, Sheridan–Gardner chart (designed for children, disabled people, those with learning difficulties, or patients who do not speak your language) or a Kay picture chart for children who cannot read. Use a pinhole if spectacles are not available.

The vision is recorded as a fraction. The numerator (upper number) is usually 6 (i.e. the test is usually performed at 6 m). The denominator (lower number) corresponds to the line on the chart the patient could read. Start at the top of the chart, where the letters are biggest and work your way down the chart to the smallest size, testing one eye first and then the other. If the patient only manages to read the top line (60 line), the vision is recorded as 6/60. This means that the patient was tested at 6 m yet could only read the line a normal person should have managed to read at 60 m.

If the patient fails to read the top line, try to ascertain if they can count fingers at 1 m (counting finger vision). Failing that, ascertain if the patient can see movements of hand in front of the eye (hand movement vision). Failing that, test the vision with a light source (light perception or no light perception vision). *Test each eye separately.*

If the Snellen chart is not available, a mini Snellen chart can be used with the patient wearing their reading glasses.

Colour vision

Test with Ishihara colour plates. Test each eye separately. Colour vision defects are common in men and affect one in eight males (most commonly confusing reds and greens). Loss of colour perception can be a manifestation of optic nerve pathology, e.g. optic nerve compression after trauma and optic neuritis.

Visual fields

Test each eye separately. Test each quadrant (four quadrants) in turn with your fingers or a hatpin.

Pupils

Assessment of these is vital in assessing optic nerve and retinal function. Ask the patient to look in the distance. Use a bright torch. Assessment includes both the afferent (sensory) and efferent (motor) visual pathways. Normally the pupils of both eyes should respond identically to a light stimulus, regardless of which eye is being stimulated. Light entering one eye produces a constriction of the pupil of that eye (direct response), as well as a constriction of the pupil of the unstimulated eye (consensual response).

Afferent pupillary defect (APD)

This is recorded if a bright light in one eye fails to constrict either pupil (i.e. no stimulus is reaching the midbrain). If one of the pupils constricts, then it is likely that either a pupillary defect (sphincter muscle tear or topical dilating drops), or efferent pathway defect is responsible for the abnormality.

Relative afferent pupillary defect (RAPD)

An important test of the afferent pathway is the 'swinging light test' or RAPD test. In the swinging flashlight test, a light is alternately shone into the left and right eyes with delay of 1 second. Normally there should be equal constriction of both pupils, regardless of which eye the light is shone into. This indicates an intact direct and consensual pupillary light reflex. When the test is performed in an eye with an APD, light shone into the affected eye will result in only mild constriction of both pupils. This is due to a decreased response to light from the afferent defect. Light shone into the unaffected eye will cause a normal constriction of both pupils. *Thus, light shone in the affected eye will produce less pupillary constriction than light shone in the unaffected eye.* This test is undertaken because an APD may be subtle and the pupil may react sluggishly.

Eye movements

Ask the patient to look straight and then follow a target to the eight positions of gaze. Report if the patient sees double vision at any stage.

Observe for any restricted range of eye movement.

Eyelids

The eyelids should be examined with good illumination. Look first at (1) the relative height of the two eyelids and (2) the surface and edge of the eyelids (skin and lashes). The relative heights are best observed casually, rather than under a bright light. If the difference between each palpebral fissure is >2 mm in height, there may be pathology. However, many patients may have a 1 mm difference. When a difference is observed, try to determine which eyelid is abnormal: the upper or lower. If the upper eyelid exposes the white sclera above the limbus in the 12 o'clock position, it is abnormally high (lid retraction). If the upper eyelid covers the pupil, it is abnormally low (ptosis). Extra skin from the upper lid may be seen sagging over the lid margin. This can partially block vision. If it does not, it is a cosmetic issue only.

If a superficial conjunctival foreign body is suspected, the upper eyelid may need eversion. *Never evert the upper eye lid if a penetrating injury or corneal thinning (from ulceration) is suspected.*

- Instil a drop of local anaesthetic and fluorescein dye.
- Ask the patient to look down.
- With one hand, hold the eyelashes of the upper eyelid between thumb and index finger.
- With the other hand, place a cotton bud (or paper clip or other small blunt object) along the lid, midway from its margin.
- Evert the eyelid over the cotton bud.
- If a foreign body is seen, gently remove it with a moistened cotton bud.
- On completion, ask the patient to look up and the eyelid will return to its normal position.

Look at the lower lid. Sometimes the edge can be turned inwards (entropion) or outwards (ectropion). When the lid is turned inwards, the lashes can rub directly on the cornea. When turned outwards, the cornea can become exposed and dry.

Following injury, the eyelids should both be examined for lacerations (noting position, length, and depth). If a wound is present, care must be taken to look for underlying globe damage and retained foreign body. Consider also the possibility of penetrating orbital and brain injuries. When opening a swollen eyelid, *do not press on the eye*, as this can cause or exacerbate globe injury. The direction of applied force should be up and down towards the orbital rims. Remember that medial canthal injuries can involve the lacrimal drainage system.

Slit-lamp examination

Slit-lamps provide a superior, magnified, and three-dimensional view of ocular contents. Use of these requires training.

- Examine systematically from anterior to posterior.
- Eyelids: lid margins for lacerations.
- Conjunctiva: subconjunctival haemorrhage/follicles. If blood is reported in the tear film after trauma in the absence of a lid laceration, then at least a conjunctival laceration must have occurred to account for the blood. Consider globe damage.
- Cornea: clarity, arcus senilis, foreign bodies, keratic precipitates, prolapsed tissues, e.g. iris or uveal tissues which normally appears dark in colour.
- Intraocular pressure (IOP): this is approximately between 10 and 20 mmHg. If you cannot measure this, assess the IOP using your fingers to see if the globe is hard. This can help diagnose acute glaucoma. Ask the patient to close the eye and look down. Using your two index fingers, press through the upper eyelid to feel the consistency of the eyeball. Compare it with your own eye. *In postoperative patients or if globe rupture/penetrating injury is suspected, the IOP should not be assessed this way, as pressure on the eyeball can open up the wound or further expulse the ocular contents.*
- Anterior chamber: this should be deep and clear. Blood and inflammatory debris can settle and form a fluid level called hyphaema and hypopyon, respectively.
- Iris: should be round and reactive to light. Any irregularity in shape is abnormal. Look for defects in in the iris periphery (called a dialysis). This indicates significant trauma with avulsion of the iris root from the ciliary body.
- Lens: this should be clear. Any opacity in the lens is known as a cataract.

See Figure 10.1.

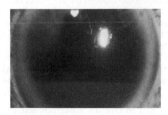

Figure 10.1 Hyphaema. Note some blood is in suspension and obscuring the view of iris and pupil. (See also Plate 1.)

Fundoscopy

Look for the red reflex and examine the optic disc and retina. A poor red reflex indicates opacity in the media (cataract, vitreous haemorrhage). Visualize the disc (if you do not see the disc, follow the branching of the vessels towards the disc). Once on the disc, assess its margin (distinct or blurred), rim colour (pale or hyperaemic), cup (full or empty), and blood vessels (congested, pulsating, or attenuated).

Papilloedema is suspected if the margin is blurred, colour hyperaemic, cup is full, and vessels congested. The rest of the fundus is examined by rotating the ophthalmoscope to view different quadrants and macula.

Paediatric examination

Assessing a child in distress can be difficult. Obtain a detailed history from an adult witness if possible. If this is not available, always suspect an injury being the cause of a red or painful eye.

Assess the visual acuity—fixing and following objects of interest, reaching out for objects of interest or the Sheridan-Gardner test, depending on the age and verbal ability of the child. Test each eye in turn if possible. Note the following:

- General observation, e.g. periorbital redness or bruising.
- Test pupil responses.
- Test for red reflexes.
- If globe injury is suspected, do not try to pry the eyelids open as this can exacerbate a perforating eye injury.
- If periorbital bruising is present, especially if associated with injuries in other part of the body, suspect non-accidental injury.
- If the eyelid is red, tender, and swollen, especially if the child is febrile, suspect periorbital cellulitis.
- If a purulent discharge is present in the eye(s) in a baby in the first month of life, suspect ophthalmia neonatorum as a cause for the red eye(s). This should be investigated for gonorrhoea or chlamydia.
- If a white pupil or leucocoria is present (absent red reflex), congenital cataract and retinal abnormalities (retinoblastoma, Coat's disease, toxoplasma) must be ruled out.
- A white blowout fracture should be suspected if there are signs of a sunken globe, minimal periorbital haemorrhage, or restricted eye movements (especially if associated with severe pain on eye movements). The child is often distressed and vomiting.
- If an eyelid laceration is present, always consider the possibility of a penetrating injury no matter how small the size of the laceration, e.g. a toddler falling on a pencil and penetrating the orbit.

Ocular assessment in the unconscious patient

Visual acuity testing and colour perception are reliable tests in the early recognition and documentation of loss of vision. However, they require a patient who is fully awake and cooperative. Unfortunately, visual assessment in the unconscious patient is extremely difficult. It is in these patients that early and possibly treatable threats to sight may be easily overlooked. Initial clinical assessment therefore usually relies on the assessment of pupillary size, reaction to light and careful assessment of globe tension by palpation, if there is proptosis. The presence of a RAPD is regarded as a sensitive clinical indication of visual impairment. Initial fundoscopy is difficult to perform without dilating the pupil, (which would be contraindicated in an unconscious head-injured patient), but should be attempted anyway. Fundoscopy can also appear misleadingly normal, as the optic nerve takes time to atrophy. However it may be possible to detect intraocular haemorrhage, retinal oedema/detachment, and avulsion or swelling of the optic disc. If fundoscopy is not possible, the red reflex should at least be checked and compared between each eye.

Never press on the globe if a rupture or perforation is suspected.

Useful investigations

Laboratory tests
- ESR/CRP in inflammatory conditions, notably suspected temporal arteritis.
- Eye swabs are required in suspected chlamydial or unusual infections.

Plain films
Plain orbital X-rays may reveal fractures and retained foreign bodies but CT scan is the investigation of choice if the history suggests a likely presence.

CT/MRI scanning
CT scan is the investigation of choice for complex trauma and foreign body detection and localization. MRI is useful in the assessment of the globe, optic nerve, and in the assessment of orbital swellings/masses.

Ultrasound
This can often detect an intraocular foreign body (IOFB), haemorrhage, retinal detachment, and define globe integrity. Ultrasound B-scan may be required to show scleral thickening in posterior scleritis.

Portable tonometry
Portable tonometry can be used to measure the IOP in suspected glaucoma and following trauma. Handheld IOP-measuring devices are now available and reported to be reliable.

Schirmer's test
This measures the amount of moisture bathing the eye. This test is useful for determining the severity of conditions resulting in dry eyes.

Tear breakup time test
This measures the time it takes for tears to break up in the eye. The tear breakup time can be determined after placing a drop of fluorescein in the cul-de-sac.

Visual-evoked potential
This tests the integrity of the visual pathway. It can be useful in assessing the pathway in unconscious patients and in the confirmation of demyelination conditions. However, it is not widely available.

☺ Ocular/eyelid injuries

These can be broadly divided into:
- Lid trauma
- Perforating/penetrating (sharp) trauma
- Blunt trauma—closed globe injury or ruptured globe.

☺ Open globe injury

This refers to a full-thickness wound in the corneoscleral wall of the eye. This may be caused by blunt trauma (globe rupture) or by a sharp object (laceration or penetrating/perforating injury, with or without a retained IOFB).

☺ Closed globe injury

This does not have a full-thickness wound in the eye-wall and includes lamellar lacerations, superficial foreign bodies, and contusion of the globe. *Generally speaking, initial poor visual acuity, presence of an RAPD, and posterior involvement of the eye, carry a bad prognosis.* This holds true for both closed and open globe injuries.

Vision-threatening globe injuries may not always be obvious and a high index of suspicion is required. Lid laceration, subconjunctival haemorrhage, bruising, and oedema are all commonly associated and should lead to suspicion.

> *Vision-threatening injuries*
> - Penetrating globe injuries
> - Blunt injury
> - Ruptured globe
> - Loss of eyelids
> - Retrobulbar haemorrhage/orbital compartment syndrome
> - Traumatic optic neuropathy
> - Chemical injuries.

☠ Penetrating/perforating globe injuries

With penetrating trauma, the globe is disrupted by a full-thickness entry wound. This may be associated with prolapse of the ocular contents. In perforating trauma, the globe is disrupted by a through and through injury, with both an entrance and exit wound. This is a severe injury. These injuries are usually caused by a sharp object causing full-thickness penetration into the cornea or sclera. There may also be a retained IOFB. *Blood-stained tears may indicate the possibility of an open globe injury.* The eye can look collapsed—uveal tissue, retina, and the vitreous gel may be seen prolapsing. A hyphaema and vitreous haemorrhage are usually present and the lens may be damaged and cataractous. The IOP is low and aqueous fluid may be seen leaking from the wound if fluorescein drops are instilled.

Examination

- Visual loss depends on size, location, and extent of injury.
- Lid lacerations, bruising, and subconjunctival haemorrhage.
- Direct ophthalmoscopy: look for loss of red reflex (cataract or vitreous haemorrhage), check pupil reactivity.
- Cornea and sclera: a wound may be seen and the eye may look collapsed, uveal tissues (iris) and vitreous may be seen prolapsing.
- Examine anterior chamber: look for hyphaema, cataract, irregular or distorted pupil, collapsed or flat anterior chamber.
- IOP may be low and the eye may feel soft.
- Instil a drop of fluorescein and look for leaking fluid (Siedel sign).
- Examine the retina if possible, looking for IOFB, vitreous haemorrhage, retina injury.

See Figure 10.2.

These injuries can be deceptive. In cases of small high-velocity objects (such as metal and glass chips) the eye may appear intact and a small entry wound overlooked. The history is therefore important. Care must be taken not to apply pressure to the eye as this can further expulse the ocular contents. The possibility of associated brain injury should also be borne in mind. If intraocular blood or lid oedema prevent examination, ultrasound or CT scan can detect IOFB, retinal detachment, and globe integrity.

Management

- Analgesia and antiemetics as required.
- A hard plastic shield should be taped over the eye to protect it.
- Check tetanus status.
- NBM (in case surgery is needed under general anaesthesia).
- Refer urgently for surgical repair (undertaken as soon as possible).
- The use of oral ciprofloxacin is thought to reduce the risk of endophthalmitis.
- Prognosis depends on visual acuity at presentation, size, and location of defects (large/posterior defects carry poor prognosis). Corneal scarring, glaucoma, cataract, and retinal detachment are the main complications leading to poor vision.

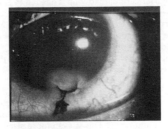

Figure 10.2 Penetrating eye injury. Note jagged corneal laceration with shreds of iris prolapsing. (See also Plate 2.)

☉ Blunt injuries

Blunt trauma can result in intraocular damage with an intact eyeball, or cause a ruptured globe. This is a similar type of injury as seen when a tomato is dropped from a height—the impact may only cause bruising of the fruit or cause rupture of its skin. Anteroposterior compression of the eye during trauma expands the globe at the equator. This is the mechanism of tearing of structures within the eye. The force of trauma may not appear to be severe but an object small enough to fit within the bony orbital rim will transmit all its energy to the eyeball.

In blunt trauma, visual acuity is usually reduced without an APD. The patient may report floaters and that the vision has improved since the incident. This is because any intraocular blood has settled at the bottom of the eye with the patient in an upright posture.

Examination

- Look for associated lid laceration, bruising and subconjunctival haemorrhage.
- Look for iris sphincter muscle tears, iris dialysis, hyphaema, and a displaced or subluxated lens.
- Check IOP. This can be high if blood blocks the trabecular meshwork in the drainage angle.
- Look for posterior segment complications of trauma—vitreous haemorrhage, choroidal ruptures, retinal commotio, and retinal tears leading to a retinal detachment.
- If the view of the fundus is poor, an ultrasound scan can detect globe rupture, retinal tears, and detachment.

If the eye appears soft or collapsed in the setting of blunt trauma, a globe rupture must be excluded. With closed globe injuries, the eyelid injuries and subconjunctival haemorrhage can be similar to those of open globe injuries. However, the globe shape looks normal.

Management

- If a rupture is suspected, or vision is affected, refer urgently.
- Control inflammation, pain, and IOP—steroid drops, cycloplegic, and antihypertensive drops need to be initiated.
- With minor injuries careful follow-up is needed to assess for late complications—retinal detachment, glaucoma, cataract, and retinal membrane formation.
- Prognosis is generally good and depends on whether any of the above-listed complications arise.
- Choroidal rupture and retinal detachment involving the macula carry the worst prognosis.

☉ Ruptured globe

Ruptured globe is defined as the loss of integrity of the eyeball following blunt trauma (Figure 10.3). The bony orbit offers protection to the eye but is deficient anteriorly. This is even more significant in individuals with prominent eyes, as they are more susceptible to blunt trauma. Interpersonal violence and falls are the commonest causes of globe rupture. There is a history of significant blunt ocular trauma, usually with

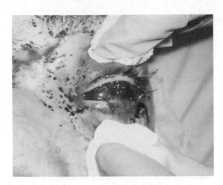

Figure 10.3 Ruptured globe.

Reproduced from *Atlas of Operative Maxillofacial Trauma Surgery: Primary Repair of Facial Injuries*, 'Initial Considerations: High- vs. Low-Energy Injuries and the Implications of Coexisting Multiple Injuries', 2014, Figure 1.49a, eds M. Perry and S. Holmes, Copyright © 2014, Springer-Verlag London. With permission of Springer.

an object small enough to fit within the bony orbital rim, e.g. knuckles, squash ball, or the edge of an object. Previous ocular surgical history is important as any scar is a potential site of rupture. Patients present with *severe pain and sudden loss of vision*. Visual acuity is usually down to perception of light with APD. An associated lid laceration and bruising may be seen. A subconjunctival haemorrhage is invariably present. Uveal tissue, retina, and the vitreous gel may be prolapsing out of the eye. The eye is collapsed, and if the rupture is posterior, the anterior chamber looks very deep. The lens may be displaced and a hyphaema is usually present. The IOP is very low and eye movements are reduced.

If severe lid bruising and oedema are present, it will be difficult to examine the eye. *Care must be taken not to press on the eye in an attempt to open the lids, as this will further expulse ocular contents*. If severe lid oedema prevents examination and a rupture is suspected, then an ultrasound or CT scan can detect globe integrity.

Management
- Analgesia and antiemetics should be given as required. Globe injuries can be painful and vomiting is common (uncontrolled vomiting can further expulse ocular contents).
- A hard plastic shield should be taped over the eye to stop eye-rubbing, especially in children.
- Check tetanus status.
- Refer urgently. Primary surgical repair should be arranged as soon as possible.
- Oral ciprofloxacin may be used to prevent endophthalmitis.
- Prognosis is generally poor, depending on the site and extent of rupture (posterior rupture and large defects carry the worst prognosis).

☼ Traumatic optic neuropathy

Traumatic optic neuropathy (TON) occurs in approximately 0.5–5 % of closed head injuries. These can sometimes be relatively trivial in nature. Visual loss is permanent in approximately half. Injuring forces transferred to the optic canal results in damage to the optic nerve. Stretching, contusion, or shearing forces can injure the nerve as it passes through the relatively thick bony canal into the orbit. Deceleration injuries and blunt trauma to the face and head are the common causes of TON. Motor vehicle collisions, falls, and assault account for the majority of cases. Displaced fractures around the orbital apex together with bleeding and oedema compress the nerve.

Diagnosis
- The diagnosis of TON is a clinical one.
- Loss of consciousness is commonly associated.
- Visual loss is usually sudden and profound although it can be moderate and delayed.
- There is decreased visual acuity and a relative APD.
- When the eye appears normal but there is reduced vision and an APD, injury to the nerve near the optic canal should be suspected.
- Optic nerve avulsion, or nerve compression resulting in nerve head swelling or central artery and vein occlusion are readily recognizable on fundoscopy.

Management
TON needs immediate referral. Treatment has long been controversial and may be medical or surgical:
- Medical treatment aims to reduce oedema and inflammation however the role of high dose steroids is controversial with a growing consensus against this.
- Surgical decompression is even more controversial. It may be indicated for optic nerve haematoma or if a bony fragment is seen (on CT) to be impinging on the optic nerve.

☼ Corneal abrasion

This is an area where part of the corneal epithelium is deficient. The patient complains of pain, watering, and has a foreign body sensation. They have difficulty keeping the eye open. Usually there is a history of trauma or contact lens wear. The eyelids may be in spasm and the conjunctiva is injected. With topical anaesthesia, the vision is normal. The area of abrasion stains with fluorescein.

Management
- Chloramphenicol drops or ointment should be prescribed four times daily for 5 days.
- Ensure that there is no opacity of the cornea (which indicates a secondary infection of the underlying stroma) and that there are no foreign bodies.
- Although an eye pad is not essential, it helps keep the eye closed and patients tend to feel more comfortable. It can be kept on for 1 day.

- Repeated blinking and rubbing the eyes prevents epithelial healing.
- No contact lens should be worn for 2 weeks and after the patient has seen his/her own optician.
- If the patient is very distressed, cycloplegic drops and oral analgesia will provide some relief until abrasion heals.

Abrasions usually heal rapidly and the patient should be a lot more comfortable in 2 days. Refer only if a secondary corneal ulcer or a recurrent erosion syndrome develops. Long-term use of lubricating eye ointments, bandage contact lens, and occasionally surface treatment by needle puncture or laser may then be required.

☼ Arc eye

This is a specific condition caused by ultraviolet injury from welding, tanning lamps, and high-altitude snow (sometimes seen in inexperienced skiers who don't wear sunglasses). Ultraviolet light causes oedema and sloughing of the corneal epithelium leading to punctate erosions or abrasions. Patients complain of pain, tearing, blepharospasm, photophobia, and blurred vision several hours after exposure. Treatment is similar to an abrasion.

Tense 'proptosis' in the elderly
Care is required when assessing the eyes in the elderly. AACG can be precipitated by dim light, and some drugs. In some patients the dilated pupil may precipitate ocular problems. This should be considered in any elderly patient who develops a painful, tense, 'red eye', even after an injury. It may be misinterpreted as proptosis.

---

① Eyelid lacerations

These require careful assessment and often referral to an appropriate specialty (ophthalmology, oculoplastics, plastics, maxillofacial), depending on local protocols. The main concerns here are:
- The possibility of an associated, yet hidden globe injury
- Loss of function of the eyelids following treatment
- Injuries to the lacrimal drainage system.

Assess the eye carefully. A normal appearance does not rule out a serious injury. The mechanism of injury may provide clues to possible globe problems. Small lid lacerations may conceal a large retained foreign body. *Always consider retained foreign bodies* and image accordingly. Damage to the canalicular system can occur with injuries to the medial aspect of the lid margins. Suspected canalicular injuries should be referred. Conjunctival, corneal, and scleral lacerations, hyphaema, lens dislocation, and globe rupture must all be excluded. Upper lid injuries may affect the levator muscle and its function should be noted. Penetrating globe, orbital, and cranial injuries must be excluded in all penetrating lid lacerations.

☼ Lacerations and loss of eyelid integrity

Inability to effectively close the eyelids quickly results in drying of the cornea, ulceration, and potentially loss of sight. Even relatively minor eyelid lacerations may predispose to this and may be easily overlooked. Avulsion of the eyelids is a rare but devastating injury and extremely difficult to reconstruct.

Examination

- Visual acuity, visual fields, ocular movements, the pupil, and the fundus should all be examined
- The position, length, and depth of the wound(s) should be documented.
- Medially sited eyelid injuries can damage the lacrimal drainage system and require special attention.
- Upper lid injuries may affect the levator muscle and its function should be noted.
- Neurological examination is required if penetrating brain injury is suspected. Even small lid lacerations may be the entry wound for a significant penetrating injury.

Plain orbital films may reveal fractures and retained foreign bodies, but CT scan is the investigation of choice.

Management

- Any associated injury must be treated accordingly.
- Refer urgently.
- Check tetanus status.
- Eyelid remnants should be pulled over to provide corneal cover.
- Apply plenty of chloramphenicol or artificial tears.
- Covered with a wet gauze swab.

① Lid lacerations not involving the lid margin

Eyelids have an excellent blood supply and delayed primary closure is not necessary. Simple lacerations can be explored and cleaned under local anaesthesia and closed in layers as with any laceration. Eyelid function (protecting the globe) is the primary consideration. Begin with irrigation, antisepsis (non-irritant to the globe), and a check for retained foreign bodies. Superficial lacerations of the eyelid, not involving the eyelid margin, may be closed with running or interrupted 6-0 suture (Prolene®, Ethilon®, Vicryl®, etc.).

Consider a penetrating eye injury if there is:

- Loss of vision
- Blood in the anterior chamber (hyphaema)
- Obvious corneal or scleral lacerations
- Dark uveal tissue presenting on the surface of the eye (indicating an open globe)
- Pupil distortion
- Proptosis.

Deep lacerations should include the orbicular muscle and skin in the repair. Care must be taken to ensure suture ends do not rub the cornea and cause abrasions. Many shallow cuts can be apposed without sutures; they scab over and heal extremely well. If skin is missing, seek advice on possible reconstruction. Antibiotic ointments may be prescribed. Skin sutures can be removed in 5 days.

Complex lacerations (including any involving the lid margin, lateral and medial canthal regions, medial third of the lids, and levator muscle) must be referred for repair. These lacerations can disrupt the lacrimal drainage system and functional integrity of the lid. As the lid is very vascular, even necrotic-looking tissue can survive and thus no tissue should be excised.

① Lid lacerations involving the lid margin

These usually require referral to a specialist. Primary closure is often possible if there is <25% tissue loss. Irregular edges may be excised (minimally) by creating a pentagonal wedge, removing as little tissue as possible. A 4-0 silk or nylon traction suture is placed in the eyelid margin 2 mm from the wound edges and 2 mm deep and is tied in a slipknot. Symmetric suture placement is critical to obtain good alignment. Approximately 2 or 3 absorbable Vicryl® 5-0 or 6-0 sutures are placed internally to approximate the tarsal plate. The skin and conjunctiva should not be included in this internal closure. Ensure that the wound edges are everted. Skin can be closed with 6-0 nylon/Prolene®/Vicryl® sutures. Skin sutures are removed in 5–7 days.

If there is tissue loss >25% this will require a flap or graft and is best managed by a specialist. In the upper eyelid, if orbital fat is seen, or if ptosis is noted, damage to the orbital septum and levator aponeurosis should be suspected.

If an eyelid is avulsed, the missing tissue can be sometimes reattached if soaked in diluted antibiotic solution, wrapped in moistened sterile gauze, and preserved in ice. Refer urgently. If necrosis is present, minimal debridement should be undertaken to prevent further tissue loss.

Timing of repair of lid lacerations depends on the general condition of the patient and the presence of other injuries. Repair can be safely deferred up to 48 hours (so long as the eye is protected), if other injuries take precedence. However, if unprotected, the cornea can dry very quickly. Under these circumstances, until the defect is repaired, eyelid remnants should be pulled over the globe and supported to provide corneal cover. If a delay in repair is expected, the wound should be cleaned and irrigated with saline. Superficial foreign bodies should be removed. Copious amounts of saline irrigation under light pressure (using a 20 mL syringe and 18-gauge cannula) can be used to wash out foreign bodies and reduce microbial load. IV antibiotic cover (e.g. co-amoxiclav 500 mg three times daily) is needed for all bite injuries and contaminated wounds.

:☠: Chemical injuries

Chemicals that have a pH different to that of the eye (pH = 7.4) can cause a burn. Domestic and industrial accidents are the commonest causes of chemical burns to the eye. Alkalis cause more damage than acids, as they dissolve lipid membranes and penetrate deeper. Loss of vision results from severe dry eyes and scarring. Complications include cataract formation, glaucoma, and uveitis. Patients present with severe pain, blepharospasm, watering, and variable reduction in vision.

Management

- If the chemical is a dry powder, quickly brush as much of this off as possible. Once you start irrigating any residual powder will dissolve producing more active agent.
- Irrigate with copious amounts of saline (litres) as soon as possible. This must continue until the pH is normal before anything else is done (it is not unusual to use over 5 L).
- It is important to irrigate the fornices as residual chemicals tend to settle here.
- Try to obtain the pH of the chemical and establish the baseline pH of both eyes.
- Apply local anaesthetic drops if necessary.
- Note vision, epithelial defects, corneal clarity, cataract, and residual particulate matter.
- Immediate referral to ophthalmology is then made, once the pH has come back to normal.
- Further management with involves antibiotics, steroids, potassium ascorbate, cycloplegia, and vitamin C.
- Patients usually require admission especially if both eyes are involved and vision is impaired.

The prognosis can be extremely poor. This depends on the pH of the chemical and the extent damage. Hence first-aid treatment received on site and in casualty is vitally important.

① The red eye

This usually refers to injection and prominence of the superficial blood vessels of the conjunctiva or sclera. This is different from the subconjunctival haemorrhage seen in trauma. There are many causes.

Examination

Causes of red eye (painful and painless)
- Acute glaucoma
- Injury
- Keratitis
- Iritis/uveitis
- Scleritis
- Episcleritis
- Conjunctivitis

- Blepharitis
- Inflamed pterygium
- Inflamed pinguecula
- Dry eye syndrome
- Airborne contaminants or irritants
- Drug use (cannabis).

If an obvious cause is absent carefully examine the following.
- Visual acuity: any reduction indicates serious ocular disease, notably keratitis, iridocyclitis, and glaucoma.
- Eyelids: blepharitis, entropion, ectropion, trichiasis.
- Conjunctiva: conjunctivitis, subconjunctival haemorrhage.
- Ciliary flush: this is a ring of redness spreading out from around the cornea of the eye. Seen in corneal inflammation, iridocyclitis, or acute glaucoma.
- Sclera: episcleritis (usually sectoral and relatively painless), scleritis (usually painful and tender).
- Cornea: look for corneal foreign body, contact lens, and corneal opacities. Stain with fluorescein and look for corneal staining (abrasion, ulcer, punctate staining). Corneal opacities are the fourth leading cause of blindness.
- Anterior chamber: look for cells, hyphaema, hypopyon, and depth of anterior chamber. A shallow chamber may indicate a predisposition to narrow-angle glaucoma. Any 'red eye' with a shallow anterior chamber suggests acute glaucoma.
- Pupil: in iridocyclitis, the involved pupil will be smaller than the uninvolved one, due to spasm of the sphincter muscle of the iris. With AACG, the pupil is generally fixed in mid-position, oval, and responds sluggishly to light, if at all.
- IOP should be measured. This is mostly normal or low in iritis. It is elevated only in herpetic uveitis (which is not common). In traumatic perforating ocular injuries, the IOP is usually low.

⊙ Glaucoma

Glaucoma is a common condition with an estimated prevalence in the over 40s of 1%. It is usually asymptomatic. It comprises a group of eye diseases in which there is damage to the optic nerve head and visual field loss, usually associated with abnormally elevated IOP (although a significant number of patients can have normal eye pressures). If left untreated this will ultimately lead to loss of vision.

IOP is normally maintained by a balance between formation of aqueous within the eye and its subsequent drainage via a trabecular network of tissues at the 'drainage angle'. Increase in IOP usually occurs as a result of obstruction to the outflow of the aqueous. Obstruction can occur if the periphery of the iris becomes displaced forwards so that it covers the drainage angle of the anterior chamber. This results in angle closure and affects patients whose angle is very narrow. This will result in 'closed'-angle glaucoma. In open-angle glaucoma, pathological changes occur within the microstructure of the drainage system and so obstruct the outflow of aqueous. In these cases the angle is not closed but remains 'open'.

ⓘ Acute angle-closure glaucoma

AACG occurs when sudden closure of the drainage angle leads to a rapid rise in the IOP. Patients with narrow drainage angles are predisposed to this when the pupil dilates. This bunches up the peripheral iris over the angle and blocks it. The increasing size of the lens in the ageing eye also pushes the iris forward, which further narrows the angle. Hence the condition mainly affects the elderly. Long-sighted patients are also at risk, as they have smaller eyes and therefore narrower angles.

Diagnosis

Patients present with a short history of increasing eye pain. This becomes very severe. They also complain of nausea, vomiting, reduced vision, and haloes seen around lights. Some patients may be mistakenly diagnosed as having an abdomen problem, due to severe nausea and vomiting. The cornea becomes cloudy and the pupil unreactive and mid-dilated. The globe becomes hard to palpation. Both eyes have shallow anterior chambers. There may have been previous milder attacks during the night when the pupil naturally dilates. These may have resolved spontaneously.

Management

• Refer immediately to ophthalmology, as the pressure in the eye must be reduced urgently.
• IV acetazolamide 500 mg stat, topical apraclonidine 1% three times daily, timolol 0.25% twice daily may also be given to reduce the pressure (if there are no systemic contraindications).
• Dexamethasone 0.1% four times daily is used to control inflammation.
• Pilocarpine 1% is given to the opposite eye to prevent acute closure.
• Laser peripheral iridotomies may be performed to prevent an attack of angle closure.
• In resistant cases, administration of IV mannitol or oral glycerine can reduce the IOP by drawing fluid out of the eye. Caution must be observed in patients with heart failure.
• If the pressures are controlled quickly, the prognosis is good.

ⓘ Open-angle glaucoma

Open-angle glaucoma is the commonest form of glaucoma. It is an insidious, slowly progressive disease, which occurs bilaterally and with no symptoms until considerable visual impairment has occurred. Early diagnosis is therefore imperative and may be achieved by regular screening of the over 50s or those with a known family history.

Treatment can be both medical and surgical, the medical treatments aim to increase the outflow and/or suppress the secretion of aqueous. Surgical treatment aims to create an alternative outflow for the aqueous or partially destroy ciliary body to reduce inflow.

① Secondary glaucoma

In secondary glaucoma, the raised IOP is secondary to a local cause such as iritis, injury, rubeosis (iris neovascularization due to diabetes or central retinal vein occlusion), and inappropriate use of steroid eye-drops. Treatment involves controlling the underlying factors and then medical or surgical treatment of glaucoma, as appropriate. Secondary glaucomas generally have a poorer prognosis.

① Congenital glaucoma

Congenital glaucoma may present at birth or in the ensuing months and years. The condition is caused by the abnormal development of the drainage angle, which results in raised IOP. This in turn causes the immature eye to enlarge. This is referred to as buphthalmos, which literally means 'ox eye'. Treatment is almost invariably surgical. Urgent ophthalmic referral is required.

:⚙: Keratitis

This is a condition in which the *cornea becomes inflamed*. It is usually painful and often associated with blurred vision. The patient may also describe feelings of itchiness each time they blink. Two types are generally described:

- Superficial keratitis. This involves the superficial epithelium of the cornea. After healing, there is usually no scarring.
- Deep keratitis. This involves the deeper layers of the cornea and therefore heals with scarring. This can permanently impair vision if it is on visual axis. Treatment involves topical corticosteroid eyedrops.

Keratitis has multiple causes.

:⚙: Viral keratitis

Herpes simplex keratitis (dendritic keratitis) is a viral infection of the cornea with herpes simplex virus. It frequently leaves a 'dendritic ulcer'. Herpes zoster keratitis is another cause.

:⚙: Bacterial keratitis

Bacterial infection of the cornea can follow from an injury or from wearing contact lenses. Common organisms are *Staphylococcus aureus* and *Pseudomonas aeruginosa*, respectively.

:⚙: Amoebic keratitis

This is a protozoal infection of the cornea. It is a rare but severe complication of contact lens wear caused by washing and storing lenses in water or swimming and bathing with contact lenses in the eye. The infection is extremely difficult to diagnose and treat. Therefore the disease is usually diagnosed late and runs a long course with severe inflammation.

:⚙: Onchocercal keratitis

This follows infection of a blackfly bite. This is also known as 'river blindness'.

⚙ Fungal keratitis
Although not common, this can occur in injuries involving organic material.

⚙ Exposure keratitis
This is due to dryness of the cornea caused by incomplete or inadequate eye-lid closure.

⚙ Photokeratitis
Keratitis due to intense ultraviolet radiation exposure (e.g. snow blindness or arc eye.)

⚙ Ulcerative keratitis
This can be due to infective or inflammatory causes.

① Contact lens acute red eye (CLARE)
In CLARE, an infective cause must be ruled out first.

① Severe allergic response
This may lead to corneal inflammation and ulceration.

Management
This depends on the cause of the keratitis:
- Infectious keratitis can progress rapidly, and generally requires urgent antibacterial, antifungal, or antiviral therapy. Aciclovir is the mainstay of treatment for herpes simplex virus.
- Contact lens wearing should be prohibited.
- Steroids should not be used for infective keratitis.

Important warning symptoms
- Reduced visual acuity often indicates serious ocular disease. If blurriness improves with blinking, it suggests ocular surface discharge. Coloured halos occur with corneal oedema, and are a warning that acute glaucoma may be present.
- Severe pain suggests serious disease such as keratitis, corneal ulceration, iridocyclitis, or acute glaucoma.
- Photophobia is often seen in iritis and injury to the cornea, but may also occur in acute glaucoma.

⚙ Iritis/uveitis

This is inflammation of the uveal tract of the eye (the pigmented layer—the iris, ciliary body, and choroid). If only the iris is involved, it is called iritis or anterior uveitis. Uveitis can be associated with systemic inflammatory diseases, such as sarcoidosis, SLE, and various arthritides.

Patients usually have a dull ache over the eye and may have blurred vision and floaters. Photophobia can be severe. Conjunctival injection, either ciliary (around the cornea) or generalized is often present. On slit-lamp examination, inflammatory cells can be seen in the anterior chamber, which can stick to the corneal endothelium (keratic precipitates) or form a hypopyon. The pupils may be irregular and immobile if the iris adheres to the lens (due to posterior synechiae). Vitritis and yellow retinal infiltrates may be present on fundoscopy in posterior uveitis.

Refer as soon as possible to ophthalmology. Investigation is not required initially if the patient is otherwise well. Steroids (topical, local injections, and systemically, depending on severity) and cycloplegics must be started under ophthalmology supervision. Generally the prognosis is very good but uveitis can be chronic and recurrent.

Scleritis and episcleritis

This is an inflammation of the scleral or episcleral layer of the eye. It may be associated with systemic and connective tissue diseases, such as rheumatoid arthritis and SLE. Onset is generally over a few days. Usually there is unilateral aching in the eye associated with sectoral (localized) injection of the eye. Scleritis is much more severe and can cause reduced vision, chemosis, proptosis, and pain on eye movement. Episcleritis should not affect any eye functions. Exudative retinal detachment, disc oedema, and vascular occlusions can occur with scleritis. Secondary uveitis and keratitis may occur. Ultrasound B-scan may be required to show scleral thickening in posterior scleritis.

Episcleritis is generally self-limiting over a period of around 4 weeks and can be managed conservatively if mild. Episcleritis and mild scleritis respond well to NSAIDs (e.g. ibuprofen 400 mg three times daily for 4 weeks). Moderate to severe scleritis usually requires systemic and topical steroids under ophthalmology supervision. The prognosis is very good for episcleritis and depends on system associations for scleritis.

Refer as soon as possible for scleritis. Although this is not required for episcleritis, refer in severe or non-resolving cases and when diagnosis is in doubt. Local irritation from lashes and foreign bodies need to be excluded if there is sectoral injection of the eye with a gritty sensation.

Foreign bodies

Surface foreign bodies occur on the cornea, conjunctiva, or under the lids (Figure 10.4). Slow velocity (grinding, welding, and wind-borne) foreign bodies do not have the force to penetrate the eye and only embed themselves superficially in the epithelium. There is a foreign body sensation or grittiness in the eye, watering, and variable photophobia. A clear history of a foreign body may not always be present or it may precede symptoms by hours. On examination the vision is normal, unless the foreign body is on the visual axis. The eye is injected and may be in spasm until anaesthetic drops are instilled.

Foreign bodies in and around the eye can be divided into:
• Subtarsal foreign bodies
• Corneal foreign bodies
• Intraorbital foreign bodies
• Intraocular foreign bodies.

Management
- Instil local anaesthetic drops.
- Everting the lids is essential.
- Foreign bodies can sometimes be seen more readily if fluorescein drops are instilled.
- Surface foreign bodies should be directly visible and do not require radiological investigation.
- A moistened cotton bud is effective for removing most conjunctival and subtarsal foreign bodies. However, a green needle used with a slit-lamp is often needed for corneal foreign bodies.
- Prescribe chloramphenicol ointment four times a day for 5 days and padding for the first day.
- Referral is not required unless a rust ring remains on the cornea or an infected corneal ulcer has developed under the foreign body.

IOFBs that have penetrated the eye as a result of high-velocity injuries are discussed under penetrating injuries. IOFBs usually occur due to high-velocity injury like gunshot injury or industrial accidents. CT scan is the investigation of choice for foreign body detection and localization. Referral to ophthalmologist is necessary.

① Rust rings
These can develop within hours from the iron in a metallic foreign body. Removal may be deferred for a day or so, to allow the ring to become more superficial. Antibiotic ointment may help to prevent infection. Rings persisting for >72 hours should be removed or referred. See Figure 10.5.

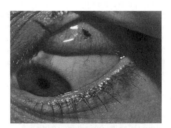

Figure 10.4 Eversion of upper lids showing foreign body. (See also Plate 3.)

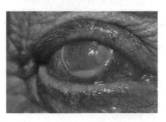

Figure 10.5 Corneal ulcer with hypopyon. (See also Plate 4.)

⑦ Contact lens-related problems

Contact lenses are widely used by many patients but are not looked after, replaced, and cleaned properly. This can lead to sight-threatening complications. Contact lenses can be hard, gas permeable, or soft. The latter can be flexed between fingers and generally speaking are more comfortable than the others. Many soft lenses are disposable and are therefore thrown away after each use. Hence they are less likely to get infected or build-up lipoprotein deposits that can reduce oxygen permeability, comfort, and clarity. Extended-wear lenses (worn for weeks) and lenses designed for yearly disposal are more likely to cause problems.

Over-wear is by far the commonest cause of problems. This leads to hypoxia and damage to the epithelium of the cornea. Epithelial microcyst formation, abrasions, blood vessel growth, and increased risk of microbial keratitis can occur.

Key questions

- What type of lens is worn?
- How old is the lens?
- How old is the lens case and solutions? (Look at how clean/dirty the case is.)
- What cleaning regimen is used?
- Does the patient ever clean the lens in water, or swim with the lenses in?
- How many hours and continuous days are lenses worn?
- Pre-existing eye diseases. Dry eyes, blepharitis, and corneal scarring increase infection risk.

☼ Abrasions

These are usually caused by over-wear and hypoxic damage to the epithelium, which swells and easily sloughs off when the lens is removed.

⑦ Contact lens intolerance

The patient complains of increased discomfort and redness leading to reduced wear time. The commonest reason is dry eyes. Artificial tear drops (preservative free) may alleviate the problem. Other reasons for intolerance are build-up of deposits on lens, lens solution allergy, and giant papillary conjunctivitis (large papillae are seen under the upper lids). This is an allergic response to lens deposits or mechanical irritation.

① Lost contact lens

Everting the eyelids will usually reveal any lost lens.

☼ Infections

Conjunctivitis and microbial keratitis need to be referred promptly as serious complications can arise.

Management

- General advice on contact lens care, cleaning, and avoiding over-wear must be emphasized.
- Dry eyes can be managed with artificial tears suitable for the type of lens being worn.

- Patients must be told to stop lens wear when the eyes are inflamed.
- Abrasions can be treated chloramphenicol four times daily for 5 days.
- No lens should be worn for at least 2 weeks after the eye has settled and after the patient has seen their optician for a check-up to assess suitability to continue wear.
- All infections should be referred to an ophthalmologist.

☉ Loss of vision

Loss of vision can have many causes, some obvious, others less so. It can occur instantly or over a brief period of time. Although all require urgent referral to an ophthalmologist, some conditions are treatable and therefore need rapid diagnosis. The key elements in the history are:
- Speed of onset of symptoms.
- Whether it is binocular or monocular.
- Whether it is associated with pain or headache.
- Associated systemic risk factors (hypertension, diabetes, hypercholesterolaemia).
- Ocular history.
- Whether the patient is on anticoagulants.

To aid in diagnosis, loss of vision can be classified into painful and painless.

Painful loss of vision
- AACG
- Arteritic anterior ischaemic optic neuropathy—temporal arteritis
- Optic neuritis
- Chemical burns
- Corneal ulcers
- Blunt and penetrating ocular trauma
- Uveitis—especially posterior and intermediate uveitis
- Scleritis—especially posterior scleritis
- Orbital cellulitis
- Herpes zoster ophthalmicus
- Retrobulbar haemorrhage
- Endophthalmitis—exogenous and endogenous.

In painful loss of vision, acute angle-closure glaucoma must be ruled out.
- Examine the cornea to rule out corneal pathology, e.g. corneal ulcers. Consider chemical keratitis and blunt/penetrating injury.
- Exclude uveitis.
- Consider arteritic anterior ischaemic optic neuropathy secondary to *temporal arteritis or giant cell arteritis in anyone over 50*—ask about headaches, jaw claudication, malaise, weight loss, and appetite loss. Palpate for tenderness and non-pulsating superficial temporal arteries. Examine pupils for relative afferent pupil defect and look for signs of swollen optic disc. Urgently check the ESR and CRP, which are usually raised in this condition.
- Optic neuritis is commonly associated with demyelinating disease (MS). It is usually associated with unilateral loss of vision deteriorating over a few days, reduced colour and light perception, pain on eye

movements, and is typically seen in young (20–50 years old) females. Examine for reduced visual acuity, red colour desaturation, RAPD, central field defects, and a swollen optic disc.

- If the patient has undergone recent eye surgery (e.g. cataract surgery, trabeculectomy, vitrectomy, penetrating trauma), or received a recent injury consider exogenous endophthalmitis as a diagnosis. In addition to pain and reduced vision, the eye is red, there is fibrin in the anterior chamber, a hypopyon, and loss of red reflex (red reflex may be present early)—urgent referral to ophthalmologists is mandatory.

Painless loss of vision

Sudden onset
- Amaurosis fugax—TIA involving the optic nerve
- Retinal artery occlusion—central or branch
- Retinal vein occlusion—central or branch
- Non-arteritic anterior ischaemic optic neuropathy
- Retinal detachment
- Vitreous haemorrhage
- Neurological diseases—occipital cortex strokes, lesions involving the visual pathways.

Gradual onset
- Age-related macular degeneration—loss of central vision
- Cataract
- Advanced glaucoma.

:Ö: Retinal detachment

Retinal detachment is the separation of the retina from the underlying retinal pigmented epithelium as a result of fluid gathering between the two layers. The majority of cases follow vitreous degeneration and its shrinkage, resulting in vitreous separation from the retina (posterior vitreous detachment). If there are abnormal adhesions between the two, the retina can tear as the vitreous shrinks, allowing fluid to gather beneath it. This is the commonest form of retinal detachment. Less commonly, ocular vascular abnormalities, cancers, or fibrosis in the vitreous (advanced diabetic retinopathy) can cause detachment. Trauma, short-sightedness (myopia) and family history are risk factors.

The main clinical features are:
- Flashing lights (like lightning).
- Floaters (dots, lines, spider's web or flies floating in front of vision) occur because the collapsed strands of vitreous gel are moving around within the eye and cast a shadow on the retina.
- Shadowing (dark curtain covering a part of vision).

There is usually a short history of hours to days. There may be reduced vision if the macula is involved. Examine the visual acuity, visual fields, and pupils (an APD may be detected if a significant portion of the retina is detached). Fundoscopy reveals an elevated retina with or without folds.

If the patient presents at the retinal-tear stage, laser or cryotherapy can be utilized to 'weld' the retina down around the tear to stop fluid leaking underneath it. Surgery is often required to flatten the retina if a significant detachment has occurred. The prognosis depends on the cause and extent of detachment. If the macula is unaffected, prognosis for vision is good.

Most patients with flashes and floaters only have a vitreous detachment. It is, however, difficult to predict which ones go on to develop retinal detachment from the history alone. Therefore all need urgent ophthalmology review.

☼ Optic neuritis

Optic neuritis is an inflammatory optic neuropathy. It is commonly associated with demyelinating disease (MS). However viral infections, compressive lesions, or systemic diseases such as sarcoidosis need to be borne in mind. Usually there is unilateral loss of vision deteriorating over a few days, reduced colour and light perception, typically in the young (20–50 years old) patients. Periocular pain, especially on eye movement, is often present. Examine for reduced visual acuity, red colour desaturation, RAPD, and central or para-central field defects. Swelling of the optic nerve and other focal neurological defects (e.g. weakness) may be present. During the acute attack, vision deteriorates for 1 week and then gradually resolves over the ensuing 3 months to near normal. Investigations should be directed towards this diagnosis if systemic or other neurological associations are present, or if the clinical picture is atypical.

In an acute attack of demyelinating optic neuritis, a course of IV steroids followed by oral steroid has been shown to speed recovery and reduce recurrence in the short term. However, the long-term prognosis is not altered. With other causes, the systemic associations dictate prognosis. Prognosis is best for post-viral optic neuritis. Refer as soon as possible to a neuro-ophthalmologist or neurologist.

☼ Retinal artery occlusion

An occlusion of the central retinal artery or any of its branches can result from an embolus or thrombosis. Less common causes are temporal arteritis and collagen vascular diseases. There is sudden unilateral painless loss of vision, which may be severe and total (central retinal artery occlusion, CRAO) or partial with sectoral field defect (branch retinal artery occlusion, BRAO). The patient may have a history of ischaemic heart disease, diabetes, stroke, amaurosis fugax (sudden loss of vision which resolved within 24 hours), and smoking. The following features are noticed on examination:

• CRAO: visual acuity is at best counting fingers or light perception. There is RAPD, narrow arteries, and a white oedematous retina with a cherry-red spot at the macula. If the patient has a cilioretinal artery (separate artery to the macula from the choroidal circulation, found in 20% of the population), central vision is spared in CRAO. The patient may have 6/6 vision with restricted fields.

• BRAO: vision is variably reduced (depending on how much the macula is affected). The pupils usually react normally and there is sectoral whitening of retina and arterial attenuation.

Refer immediately to ophthalmology. *Get an ESR and CRP urgently to exclude temporal arteritis*. A full cardiovascular work-up can be done, routinely including fasting glucose, cholesterol, triglyceride, ECG, and carotid Dopplers.

The aim of management is to try and dislodge the embolus by reducing the eye pressure within 24 hours of occlusion. The simplest method is ocular massage but IV acetazolamide 500 mg stat or paracentesis (fluid drainage from the anterior chamber) is more effective, although the latter can cause severe complications. The above measures generally have a poor success rate. Usually the occlusion is not reversible and the visual loss is permanent.

Temporal arteritis must be excluded in all patients >50 years.

:Ö: Retinal vein occlusion

Occlusion may involve the central retinal vein or any of its branches. The retinal vein and artery share a common sheath. The artery can therefore compress the vein as they cross, leading to stasis and occlusion. The condition generally affects the elderly.

Patients present with unilateral, painless loss of vision developing over a few hours. There may be a history of hypertension, diabetes, glaucoma, hormone replacement treatment, or hypercoagulable state. The vision is variably reduced and there may be an RAPD, visual field defect, and a raised IOP. On fundoscopy, a swollen disc, congested and dilated veins, retinal haemorrhages, and cotton-wool spots are seen in the area supplied by the occluded vein. FBC and coagulation profile should be investigated. A fluorescein angiogram may be performed later.

No treatment is shown to reverse acute vein occlusion. Control of vascular risk factors, hypertension, IOP, and hypercoagulability states aim to protect the second eye. Patients require long-term ophthalmic follow-up to screen for treatable complications (such as neovascularization, macular oedema, and glaucoma). The prognosis depends on the degree and extent of ischaemic damage and ensuing complications. Poor initial vision and an RAPD carry the worst prognosis. Up to 5% of patients can have the second eye affected.

Vein occlusion should be suspected in asymmetrical diabetic retinopathy.

:Ö: Vitreous haemorrhage

Sudden bleeding into the vitreous can occur for many reasons:
- Diabetes
- Retinal tear ± detachment
- Posterior vitreous detachment
- Retinal vein occlusion
- Trauma
- Subarachnoid haemorrhage (Terson's syndrome).

Patients present with sudden painless loss of vision. There is loss of the red reflex (without the presence of cataract), and fundoscopy is unable to view the retina. Ultrasonography can confirm the diagnosis

Any unexplained vitreous haemorrhage is due to retinal tear(s) until proven otherwise.

☼ Amaurosis fugax

Amaurosis fugax is painless and transient monocular visual loss. It can be considered as a type of TIA, during which an embolus obstructs the lumen of the retinal or ophthalmic artery, causing a decrease in blood flow to the retina. The most common source of these emboli is from an atherosclerotic carotid artery. Other pathophysiological mechanisms exist.

Patients present with monocular visual loss that usually lasts for seconds to minutes. The fundus usually appears normal. Check for atrial fibrillation, carotid bruit, and examine for neurological defect elsewhere. FBC, fasting lipids, and blood sugar to rule out diabetes. Other investigations include carotid Dopplers, echocardiography as an outpatient. Commence aspirin if no contraindications and refer to ophthalmology or a TIA clinic.

① Eyelid problems

The main function of the eyelids is to regularly spread the tears and other secretions across the surface of the eye to keep it moist. This keeps the eyes from drying out. The blink reflex protects the eye from foreign bodies. Any disorder of the eyelids affecting these functions can result in irritating symptoms and the risk of corneal injury.

Common eyelid disorders

- Stye (hordeolum) is an infection of the glands by *Staphylococcus aureus*. The main symptoms are pain, redness of the eyelid margin, and swelling. Styes usually disappear within a week without treatment or with warm water compresses.
- Chalazion is caused by the obstruction of the oil glands. They can be mistaken as styes but they are less painful and it tends to be chronic.
- Blepharitis is a common infective condition that causes inflammation of the eyelids. Treatment includes maintaining good hygiene and warm compresses on the affected eyelid to remove crusts. Antibiotics may be prescribed.
- Ectropion is the turning outwards of the lower lid from globe. It usually results from ageing, but sometimes can be a complication of surgery, injury, or disease. Entropion is where the lid turns inwards.
- Eyelid oedema can occur during an allergic reaction to food, drugs, plants, or secondary to infections.
- Eyelid tumours (e.g. basal cell carcinoma).
- Blepharospasm (eyelid twitching) is involuntary spasm of the eyelids.
- Ptosis is when the upper eyelid droops as a result of weakness of the levator muscle or dysfunction of the nerves to it. It can be part of the normal ageing process or secondary to pathology elsewhere (diabetes, stroke, Horner's syndrome, myasthenia gravis).

⑦ Watery eyes

The lacrimal apparatus

The lacrimal drainage system consists of the puncta, canaliculi, lacrimal sac and nasolacrimal duct. Tears are produced by the lacrimal gland and swept over the eye surface with each blink. Tears drain via the lower canaliculus predominantly (70%) and upper canaliculus (30%) by the lacrimal pump mechanism (the action of the eyelids contracting and pumping the tears into the lacrimal sac).

It is important to differentiate between hypersecretion and epiphora as both can present with watery eye.

Acute
- Microbial keratitis
- Corneal foreign body
- Corneal abrasion
- Allergic reaction
- Acute dacryocystitis.

Chronic
- Nasolacrimal obstruction—congenital or acquired
- Mucocoele
- Ectropion
- Punctal stenosis
- Functional, e.g. lacrimal pump failure, lower lid laxity
- Entropion or trichiasis
- Dry eyes.

⑦ Epiphora

Reduced tear drainage from lacrimal system obstruction at any point from the punctum, canaliculus, sac, and nasolacrimal duct. Nasolacrimal duct obstruction is the commonest.

⑦ Hypersecretion

Excess production of tears in response to stimulation from corneal irritation (e.g. corneal foreign body), dry eye, or conjunctival irritation (e.g. blepharitis, conjunctivitis).

⑦ Functional epiphora

Epiphora in the presence of patent nasolacrimal drainage pathway without hypersecretion. This can be due to eyelid malposition, e.g. lower lid ectropion (lid turned out), lacrimal pump failure, (facial palsy) punctual, canalicular, and nasolacrimal duct stenosis (without complete obstruction).

⑦ **Mucocoele**

This is a dilated lacrimal sac filled with mucous. It can present as a lump around the medial canthus and is often confused with a skin cyst (dermoid, sebaceous). Patients also complain of epiphora. If these get large they can cause considerable distortion of the local anatomy, with canthal drifting. This can then appear like a tumour. Mucocoeles can also become infected (dacryocystitis). *Consider this in any patient presenting with an abscess along the side of their nose.*

History taking in epiphora
- Is stickiness/watering constant or intermittent? Is it worse outdoors?
- Any inflammation or lump at the medial canthus?
- History of nasal disease, sinusitis, polyps, or nasal trauma.
- Any photophobia, red eye?
- Previous conjunctivitis, eye drops and drugs.

Examination
Look specifically for periocular and medial canthus pathology notably eyelid malposition and a mucocoele.
- Fluorescein dye retention test. A drop of fluorescein 2% will rapidly disappear from the conjunctiva if the system is patent. The dye will be retained if blocked.
- Slit lamp examination to exclude corneal causes, blepharitis, punctual stenosis, tear meniscus.
- Probe and syringe/irrigate the lacrimal system (use topical anaesthesia).
- Special clinical tests—Jones' tests used to confirm and localize functional epiphora are performed by ophthalmologists.

Aetiology of the watery eye

Management
Epiphora secondary to blockage of the nasolacrimal duct and functional epiphora need a non-urgent referral to ophthalmology for surgical management. In cases of entropion (turning in of eyelid) steri-strips can be used temporarily to prevent the eyelid rolling in and causing damage to the cornea with the lashes. Trichiatic lashes (misdirected) can cause corneal abrasion and can be removed.

⑦ **Acute dacryocystitis**

This is an acute infection of the lacrimal sac. There is usually a pre-existing swelling close to the medial canthus. Patients present with pain, erythema, a watery eye, and oedema.

Management—oral or IV antibiotics depending on the severity. *It is important to remember that acute dacryocystitis can cause orbital cellulitis and requires urgent ophthalmology assessment if not responding to oral antibiotics.*

The upper jaw and midface

Common presentations

Some common problems in the upper jaw/midface:
- Infections
- Injuries
- Numbness
- Pain
- Paralysis
- Swellings/lump.

Although the term 'midface' refers to those structures situated between the skull base and the occlusal plane, for the purposes of this chapter, the nose and naso-orbitoethmoid (NOE) region, and the cheeks and orbits are excluded as they are covered elsewhere (see ➲ Chapters 7 and 9, respectively). Inevitably, however, there is some overlap between injuries and pathologies in all these regions, including the teeth.

Common problems and their causes

Infections

Common
- Odontogenic (dental) infections
- Parotitis
- Sinusitis.

Uncommon
- Osteomyelitis.

Injuries

Common
- Dentoalveolar
- Soft tissue bruising/lacerations.

Uncommon
- Le Fort fractures
- Craniofacial/panfacial fractures.

Numbness

Common
- Idiopathic
- Iatrogenic (following dental treatment)
- Post-trigeminal neuralgia
- Viral trigeminal neuropathy.

Uncommon
- Demyelinating diseases
- Tumours (sinus, intracranial, skull base, nerve sheath)
- Sinus pathology (including large odontogenic cysts)
- AVM
- Hypothyroidism
- Peripheral neuropathy.

Pain

Common
- Atypical facial pain
- Trauma
- Infected tooth/dental cyst/sinusitis/parotitis
- Trigeminal neuralgia.

Uncommon
- Atypical odontalgia
- Tumours—sinus/parotid/nose
- Herpes zoster
- Maxillary osteomyelitis
- Bisphosphonate-related osteonecrosis of the jaw (BRONJ).

Paralysis

Common
- Cerebrovascular accidents
- Bell's palsy
- Trauma
- Iatrogenic (following surgery)
- Temporal bone fracture.

Uncommon
- Cerebral tumours
- Acute/chronic otitis media, other middle ear disease
- Ramsay Hunt syndrome
- Congenital or birth injury
- Neoplastic (middle ear/acoustic neuroma/parotid malignancy)
- Parotid disease (tumours/infiltrative disease)
- Sarcoidosis
- MS
- Guillain–Barré syndrome.

Swellings/lump

Common
- Odontogenic (dental) cysts/tumours
- Parotid tumour
- Post traumatic.

Uncommon
- Osteomyelitis
- BRONJ
- Fibrous dysplasia
- Extramedullary haematopoiesis
- Paget's disease
- Metastases/myeloma/lymphoma.

Useful questions and what to look for

Infections

Ask about
- Onset and duration
- Recent injuries, dental infections or treatment
- Pain, erythema, and swelling
- Changes in bite
- Systemic symptoms
- Medical history/medications taken.

Look for
- Site and extension
- Skin erythema and swelling
- Systemic involvement (pyrexia, sweating, lethargy)
- Numbness of the cheek
- Intraoral/dental examination.

Injuries

Ask about
- Mechanism of injury
- Loss of consciousness
- Any other injuries
- Lost/loose teeth
- Change in bite
- Numbness of the cheek or change in vision/diplopia
- Alcohol or medications taken.

Look for
- Assess GCS/C-spine
- CSF leaks
- Assess visual acuity/eye movements
- Lacerations or foreign bodies
- Assess bones of orbit, maxilla, forehead, and mandible
- Intercanthal distance >40 mm
- Numbness of cheek.

Numbness

Ask about
- Onset/duration
- Recent injury/dental treatment
- Pain/swelling
- Define site
- Other neurological symptoms.

Look for
- Cranial nerve deficits
- Facial asymmetry/swellings
- Intraoral masses/upper dental pathology
- Peripheral neuropathy.

Pain

Ask about
- Onset/duration/type of pain
- Recent injury/dental treatment
- Swelling/deformity
- Define site
- Other neurological symptoms
- Any other symptoms.

Look for
- Cranial nerve deficits
- Intraoral masses/upper dental pathology
- Infections/tumours/exposed bone (intraorally).

Paralysis

Ask about
- Onset/duration
- Previous episodes
- Recent treatments
- Painful vs painless
- Otalgia/discharge/aural fullness/loss of hearing/dizziness
- Other neurological symptoms.

Look for
- Cranial nerve deficits
- Peripheral neurological deficits
- Parotid lumps/swelling
- Examine the ear (including vesicle formation)
- Determine extent of weakness.

Swellings/lump

Ask about
- Onset/duration/progression
- Single episode or recurrent
- Recent dental infections or treatments
- Painful/painless
- Change in bite/nasal obstruction/discharge
- Systemic symptoms.

Look for
- Assess lump/swelling
- Relevant cranial nerve deficit
- Intraoral masses/upper dental pathology
- Infections/tumours/exposed bone (intraorally)
- Systemic involvement (pyrexia/malaise).

Examination of the upper jaw (and midface)

Applied anatomy

Although the term 'midface' refers to those structures situated between the skull base and the occlusal plane, for the purposes of this chapter, the nose, NOE, cheeks, and orbits are excluded. Inevitably, however, there is some overlap between injuries and pathologies in all these regions, including the teeth.

Unlike the mandible (the lower jaw), the upper jaw is not a single bone, but a complex structure composed of a number of different bones:
- maxillae
- palatine bones
- the pterygoid plates of the sphenoid.

It supports the upper teeth. The remainder of the midface is made up of:
- inferior conchae
- ethmoid vomer
- lacrimal bones
- zygomatic processes of the temporal bones
- zygomas
- nasal bones.

The two maxillary bones are joined in the midline. They support the teeth and along with the palatine bones separate the mouth from the nose. Not surprisingly therefore, pathology in one region can cause symptoms in the other. The maxillary bones also make up part of the lateral wall of the nasal cavity, contain the maxillary sinus (antrum), and make up part of the infraorbital rim and orbital floor. *High-energy fractures can therefore propagate between these different sites. Tumours and infections in any one of these cavities can also extend into another.*

The overall arrangement of all these bones, together with the presence of the sinuses, essentially converts the midface into a series of vertical bony struts, known as 'buttresses'. These pass upwards from the teeth and attach to the skull base. Three pairs of buttresses act as 'pillars', supporting the load of any vertically applied force (i.e. during biting). These are:

- Anterior—which form the piriform fossa lateral to the nose, passing into the frontonasal process.
- Middle—which is formed by the buttress of the zygoma passing between the maxilla inferiorly and the frontal bone above.
- Posterior—which is made up by the pterygoid plates attaching the maxilla to the base of skull.

Between these buttresses lie the sinuses, eyes, and part of the upper respiratory tract. They are joined together by wafer-thin bone, to which the soft tissues of the face are attached. Consequently, the face has evolved into a structure that is very good at resisting vertically directed forces (i.e. chewing). However, there are very few strong horizontally directed buttresses and the face is therefore not as good at resisting horizontally directed forces (i.e. a significant vector in most trauma). It has been argued that the function of the sinuses is to effectively convert the face into a 'crumple zone', thereby absorbing kinetic energy and protecting the brain from injury (much like the chassis of a car protects the driver by crumpling). Physiologically, Wolff's law would have also contributed to their development. This arrangement defines the three-dimensional shape of the face.

Because the mid-facial skeleton sits on the inclined skull base (at 45 degrees to the horizontal plane), severe injuries can result in the bones collapsing along this plane, in a downwards and backwards direction. Clinically this results in an elongated face and a deranged bite where the back teeth meet prematurely (anterior open bite). In severe cases, there may be significant swelling, severe bleeding, and airway compromise (particularly in the supine patient).

Embedded in the lower part of the maxilla are the roots of the upper teeth. Not surprising therefore, disease in one can affect the other (notably dental infections and sinusitis).

Examination

Examination of the upper jaw is really just one aspect of the examination of the face. *It also includes examination of the oral cavity* (see ➔ Chapter 13). The entire face should be inspected from the front and the side of the patient. It should also be viewed from above, looking down over the brow. *If there is any orbital involvement, early assessment of the eye is essential—its management initially takes priority.*

Swellings should be examined both externally and intraorally. Cysts related to the teeth are a common cause of swelling in the upper jaw. Be careful during your palpation, some cysts are covered only by a thin layer of bone and may deceptively feel like soft tissue cysts, rather than cysts arising within the bone. Always request imaging (usually an OPT). Even if a cyst is palpable externally, it may also be expanding internally. It may therefore be palpable within the mouth, either in the upper sulcus (between the soft tissues of the cheeks and teeth) or expanding into the palate (within the oral cavity). The teeth themselves will need to be assessed and this aspect of the examination is described in ➋ Chapter 13). Some cysts/tumours may also bulge into the nasal cavity, which itself may also require careful examination (see ➋ Chapter 7).

Examination following injury

Specifically following injury, the 'level' of any midface fracture (usually classified using the 'Le Fort' classification) can in theory be determined by detailed clinical examination. However, in practice, 'pure' fractures are uncommon. Other fractures of the facial skeleton are often present. The clinical picture can therefore be a little uncertain. This is not a major concern nowadays, since such high-energy injuries usually require CT evaluation, which will ultimately define the fracture pattern. Nevertheless, a thorough examination is still required, not so much to decide which level the fracture is, but to assess for associated problems. For the inexperienced, a simplified 'check list' can be useful. This list is applicable to all injuries to the midface, not just the upper jaw.

Abnormal mobility of the midface can be detected by grasping the anterior maxillary bone and gently rocking the upper jaw. At the same time the other hand palpates the sites commonly known to fracture (nasal bridge, inferior orbital margins, or frontozygomatic sutures). Care is required if the neck has not been 'cleared,' and if concerns exist about the neck this part of the examination is best deferred. Alternatively, the head must be fully supported:

• If the teeth and palate move but the nasal bones are stable, a Le Fort I fracture is present (or it is a denture!).
• If the teeth, palate, and nasal bones move but the lateral orbital rims are stable, it is a Le Fort II fracture.
• If the whole midface feels unstable, it is probably a Le Fort III or some other complex fracture pattern.

Split palate

This is an important part of the examination following an injury to the upper jaw, yet something that can easily be overlooked. Midline or segmental splits of the palate occur following high-energy impacts and are often associated with widespread fractures of the midface. They rarely occur in isolation. If the palatal fragments are separated laterally they can sometimes act as a wedge, displacing the zygomatic buttresses laterally as well. If this is not recognized during repair, the bones may be plated in the wrong position. Clues to a split palate include *palatal bruising in the region of the greater palatine vessels (Guerin's sign), palatal mobility, or the patient having difficulty getting their teeth together normally.*

Clinical examination of the midface following injuries
• General features:
  • ATLS®/ABCs, notably progressive facial swelling, active bleeding, and cervical spine injuries
• Neurosurgical:
  • GCS
  • CSF rhinorrhoea/otorrhoea (cranial fossa fractures).
  • Complications of CSF leaks (meningitis or aerocoele)

- Ophthalmic:
  - Visual acuity, signs of globe injury, pupil reaction to light
  - Enophthalmos/ocular dystopia
  - Diplopia
- Maxillofacial:
  - Abnormal mobility of the midface
  - Posterior oropharyngeal collapse
  - Anterior open bite
  - Apparent trismus—premature contacts in the molar region
  - Lengthening of the midface
  - Is the palate split?
  - 'Dishfaced' deformity
  - Crepitus.

Investigations

Laboratory tests

A FBC with differential is usually required for any infective, inflammatory, systemic, or neoplastic pathologies.

Plain films

Occipitomental (OM) views may provide some useful information in the assessment of swellings and injuries. Similarly an OPT often includes much of the upper jaw and is a useful 'first-line' investigation. These will identify most cysts and bony tumours in the upper jaw.

Patients with suspected midface fractures and those with large cysts should ideally undergo CT scanning. A CXR and soft tissue views of the neck may be required if teeth are missing and cannot be accounted for. Specialized periapical and upper occlusal views are useful in the assessment of dentoalveolar fractures.

CT/MRI

Although CT is undoubtedly more accurate in defining facial fractures, its true value in the early stages of assessment is in determining the presence of 'deep' or occult injuries (those that may not be apparent on clinical examination):

- Cervical spine injuries
- Skull base fractures/intracranial air (CSF leaks)
- Skull base fractures around vascular foramina (notably carotid tears)
- Globe rupture/vitreous haemorrhage
- Orbital apex fractures/optic nerve compression.

Patients may be neurologically impaired, very swollen, or already intubated and clinical examination can therefore be difficult and unreliable. CT helps overcome some of these limitations. Disimpaction and manipulation of midface fractures can also potentially manipulate deep, mobile fragments around the skull base and optic nerve. Only with CT will these fractures be confirmed (or excluded) and the risks of manipulation recognized.

CT is also essential in the assessment of suspected cyst, tumours, and some spreading infections. Some cysts can be surprisingly larger than expected on clinical examination, and present with relatively few symptoms.

MRI may also be of value in the assessment of the associated soft tissues. It is commonly used in the assessment of patients presenting with facial pain and palsy. Although uncommon, skull base tumours and demyelinating conditions can present with either of these symptoms and must be therefore excluded before the patient is diagnosed with 'atypical' facial pain/Bell's palsy.

Ultrasound

This may help in the assessment of the associated soft tissues, but it provides less information than a MRI or CT. However, it will distinguish an abscess from a tumour in most cases.

ⓘ Fractures to the upper jaw and midface

Fractures of the midface tend to result from high-energy impacts and can therefore be both life-threatening as well as disfiguring. But not all do. Patients may also walk into an emergency department with these injuries even if they are significant.

Upper jaw and midface fractures overlap somewhat and may also include dentoalveolar fractures. Conventionally fractures to the upper jaw and midface are referred to as Le Fort fractures, although in reality injuries are often more widespread. With higher-energy impacts there may also be fractures of the nose, NOE region, and zygoma. Fractures may also extend upwards, into the anterior cranial fossa. From a practical point of view injuries in this site can be considered as:
• Dentoalveolar fractures
• Le Fort fractures
• Extended fractures.

ⓘ Dentoalveolar fractures

These can occur in both the upper and lower jaw. Injuries to the teeth themselves are discussed in ➲ Chapter 13. Dentoalveolar fractures are defined as fractures to the teeth and their supporting bone ('alveolar bone') (see Figure 11.1).

The involved teeth may also have fractures of the crown or root, or may be loosened or avulsed. Clinical signs include intraoral bleeding, tooth malposition or mobility, a change in the patients bite and pain. *Dentoalveolar fractures should be regarded as open fractures. Any missing teeth should be accounted for.* Consider the possibility of an associated fracture to the supporting jaw. Management includes appropriate imaging (OM/OPT/CT as indicated), antibiotics, tetanus prophylaxis (when necessary), and reduction and support of the fractures. Refer urgently to the patient's own dentist, dental school, or maxillofacial department (depending on local circumstances).

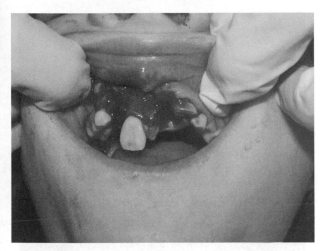

Figure 11.1 Significant dentoalveolar trauma with loss of teeth, gingival tears, and damage to the supporting bones.

Splinting the teeth is usually the treatment of choice, although very occasionally large dentoalveolar fractures may be plated. Many types of splint are available. Since the bone is fractured splinting may be required for around 4–6 weeks. During this time the patient should eat soft foods, avoid biting on the splinted teeth, and keep the mouth as clean as possible.

Consider antibiotics and tetanus prophylaxis in patients with accompanying significant soft tissue injuries. Mucosal tears should be repaired to cover any exposed bone.

① Le Fort fractures
The levels described in this classification refer to the level of the fracture in relation to the skull base (see Figure 11.2). Often these fractures occur in various combinations.

Le Fort I ('low level')
The fracture is orientated horizontally at a level just above the nasal floor, passing around from the piriform aperture, above the alveolar (tooth supporting) bone, to below the zygomatic buttress. It passes along the lower third of the nasal septum and lateral walls of the nose to join the lateral aspects of the fracture across the lower third of the pterygoid plates. This is essentially the tooth baring part of the midface (think of a denture).

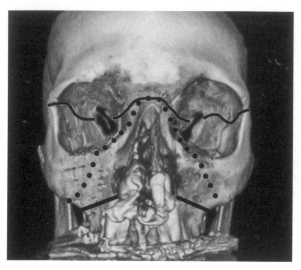

Figure 11.2 Le Fort fracture patterns.

Le Fort II ('pyramidal')

Starting at the nasal bones, this fracture crosses the frontal processes of the maxillae into the medial orbital walls. It passes through the lacrimal bones and crosses the inferior orbital margin near to the infraorbital foramen. It then continues downwards and backwards through the lateral wall of the antrum below the zygomaticomaxillary suture. Posteriorly the fracture passes midway through the pterygoid plates. It also passes through the nasal septum and may involve the cribriform plate of the anterior cranial fossa.

Le Fort III ('high transverse' or 'craniofacial dysjunction')

Starting at the nasal bones, this fracture passes from the frontonasal suture backwards through the ethmoid bone (and cribriform plate). It passes laterally through the orbit below the level of the optic foramen to reach the posterior aspect of the inferior orbital fissure. From here the fracture passes laterally through the lateral wall of the orbit and frontozygomatic process. Posteriorly it crosses the pterygomaxillary fissure and the base of the pterygoids. This separates the entire facial skeleton from the skull base.

Both Le Fort II and III fractures involve the orbit (with risk to the eyes) and potentially involve the anterior cranial fossa (with associated head injury/ CSF leakage)

Clinical features

Consider multiple facial/midface injuries in anyone with gross swelling. Clinical features may be the result of the impact itself, or as a consequence of the effects of this force on disruption and displacement of the midfacial skeleton. Although this list is long it would be a very unlucky patient indeed if they had all these findings. Nevertheless many of them may be present:

- General features:
  - Airway compromise (uncommon).
  - Haemorrhage—associated with mucosal tears in the nasopharynx or facial wounds/lacerations. Rarely torrential, although may require nasal packing or immediate manual reduction of the fracture to stem the flow. If the patient is shocked, always consider another cause.
- Neurosurgical related:
  - CSF rhinorrhoea (anterior cranial fossa #).
  - CSF otorrhoea (middle cranial fossa #).
  - 'Tramlining' may be seen when blood mixes with CSF and leaks from the nose or ear. Along the periphery of this flow the blood clots while the CSF washes it away centrally forming two parallel lines: hence 'tramlining'.
  - Complications of CSF leaks (meningitis, aerocoele or fistula formation with significant CSF loss)
- Facial swelling—this can rapidly progress with high-energy impacts. Consider early intubation.
- Abnormal mobility of the midface—checked by holding the anterior maxillary alveolus and gently attempting to mobilize the maxilla. *Do not attempt this if the patient has been bleeding significantly from the face—it may restart.*
- Eye/orbit related:
  - Bilateral periorbital ecchymoses ('panda faces' or 'racoon eyes'). These are often associated with a significant degree of facial swelling. Seen in any fracture that passes into the orbit.
  - Bilateral subconjunctival ecchymoses (bright red). This is bleeding within the conjunctiva adjacent to an orbital fracture.
  - Enophthalmos—this may initially be masked by oedema.
  - Diplopia—this has many causes and may be difficult to assess at an early stage, unless it is obvious.
  - Traumatic mydriasis (dilated pupil)—spasm of dilator pupillae secondary to a direct blow.
- Features related to the displacement of the midface skeleton:
  - Obstructed airway—this results from a combination of soft palate displacement, swelling, and bleeding.
  - Anterior open bite (see Figure 11.3 for lateral open bite).
  - Apparent restricted mouth opening caused by premature contact in the molar region which results in gagging of the occlusion.
  - Lengthening of the face (long face).
  - 'Dishfaced' deformity—comminution of the bones may result in collapse of the central part of the face, rather than displacement of the whole face.

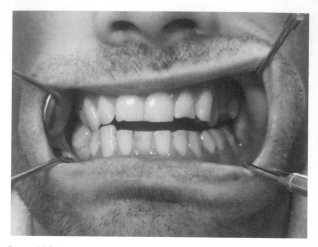

Figure 11.3 Lateral open bite in a midface fracture. Note that the upper dental midline does not correspond with the lower, or the nose.

- Pain and crepitus.
- Upper buccal sulcus/palatal bruising.
- Numbness—commonly in the distribution of the infraorbital nerve.

Investigations
- CXR—remember the possibility of inhaled foreign bodies (e.g. from dental trauma).
- Plain films of the face. *Plain films of the face have no role in the resuscitation room and add little diagnostic information in obvious fractures where CT is clearly indicated.* However, they may be undertaken in the 'walking wounded' as a preliminary view, if fractures are not obvious. One or two OM projections (15 and 30 degrees) together with a good clinical examination should be able to exclude most fractures. A true lateral projection may also show displacement of the maxilla. It is also useful for assessment of the frontal sinuses (fluid levels, posterior wall fractures) and visualizing the pterygoid plates. Specialist periapical and upper occlusal views are useful in the assessment of dentoalveolar fractures. OPT is very useful if a mandibular fracture is suspected. It may also show low-level Le Fort I fractures, dentoalveolar fractures, and dental injuries.
- CT scan. This is now the investigation of choice in obvious midface fractures. MRI may be of value in the assessment of soft tissue injuries, particularly to the brain, cervical spine, and orbit, but is rarely undertaken urgently.

Management

High-energy injuries should be initially assessed using ATLS® principles (see ➲ Chapter 2). *Midface injuries not associated with airway obstruction or major bleeding, should be only treated after the patient has been stabilized and life-threatening injuries managed.* Consider first:

- Airway with cervical spine protection
- Breathing
- Circulation
- Head injuries
- Ocular injuries.

Beware the patient who keeps trying to sit up—they may be trying to clear their airway.

First aid measures

- Le Fort fractures can present with significant epistaxis. As a first-aid measure, nasal packs may tamponade the flow. Posterior nasal packing is discussed in detail in ➲ Chapter 7. Custom-made devices (or if necessary urinary catheters) may be inserted and the balloons inflated to sit in the nasopharynx. This facilitates nasal packing with ribbon gauze.
- Replace lost fluids—patients with midface fractures should have IV access and appropriate fluid resuscitation.
- Dentoalveolar fractures should be reduced and temporarily stabilized. If teeth have been avulsed or subluxed they should ideally be re-implanted or repositioned as soon as possible and then splinted.
- Lacerations should be inspected for contamination and foreign bodies (see ➲ Chapter 2). If the patient obviously needs to go to theatre then formal wound closure can be delayed. A few tacking sutures and a simple dressing should be placed.
- Prevent infection—Le Fort fractures are almost always open (compound) injuries via the sinuses or facial wounds. Antibiotics should be commenced. Many regimens exist and include Augmentin®, or benzylpenicillin + metronidazole. Consider tetanus prophylaxis.
- Analgesia—although often prescribed facial fractures are often not as painful as one may think. Avoid opiates until the patient is cleared of a head injury
- Advise the patient not to blow their nose. They are at risk of both surgical emphysema and tension pneumocephalus.

Definitive management

Not all patients require immediate admission, depending on the severity of their injury. Some minimally displaced upper jaw/midface fractures are managed non-surgically, especially in children, the elderly, or those patients without any teeth. The remainder usually require reduction and repair, or intermaxillary fixation.

⊕ Infections

Infections confined exclusively to the upper jaw tend to be dental in origin and are described in ➲ Chapter 13. Initially contained within the supporting bone, these usually present as toothache. If left untreated an infection may either spread into the surrounding soft tissue facial spaces, or it may spontaneously discharge into the mouth through a sinus, with minimal symptoms.

Fascial spaces related to the upper jaw and midface

These are potential spaces between fibrous tissue planes and the adjacent muscles, which can become distended with serous fluid, pus, blood, or (rarely) tumour. These planes open up relatively easily and bacteria can therefore spread quickly along them by breaking down the friable connective tissue within. Many spaces are interconnected. They include.

Buccal space

This is the most commonly affected space and often presents to casualty as a 'fat face'. *Infections can spread into it from both the mandibular and maxillary teeth.* It is bounded by the buccinator and the masseter muscle medially. Laterally is the deep fascia from the parotid capsule and the overlying platysma. The inferior boundary is the insertion of the deep fascia into the mandible, and its superior boundary the zygomatic process of the maxilla. It contains the buccal fat pad. Posteriorly it is continuous with the pterygoid space.

Masticator space

This is bounded laterally by the temporalis fascia, zygomatic arch, and masseter muscle and medially by the medial and lateral pterygoid muscles. The temporalis muscle and mandibular ramus further divide the space into superficial and deep compartments. The superficial compartment contains the submasseteric space below and the superficial temporal space above. The deep compartment contains the superficial pterygoid space (or pterygomandibular space) below and the deep temporal space above. The superficial pterygoid space communicates with the deep pterygoid space. The superficial and deep temporal spaces together are also known as the infratemporal fossa space.

Parotid space

This contains the parotid gland, the parotid lymph nodes, the facial nerve, the external carotid artery, and retromandibular vein. It is formed by the splitting of the deep cervical fascia, to enclose the parotid gland. The fascial covering is generally thin, but thickens to form the stylomandibular ligament.

Upper lip

Infection here can result in severe swelling of the upper lip, usually deep to orbicularis oris, draining into the mouth. It is usually secondary to periapical infections of the upper incisor teeth.

Canine fossa

This is bounded by the muscles of facial expression around the orbicularis oris (levator labii superioris, levator anguli oris, zygomaticus minor and major) and the overlying skin. Infections usually originate from the upper canine or first premolar teeth. Depending on the length of their roots and their inclination, infections can spread either between these muscles, or it can track to the buccal sulcus within the mouth. Non-dental causes of swelling include skin infections. If bilateral consider an allergic reaction. Also consider sinusitis and nasolacrimal dacryocystitis—infection of the tear drainage pathway.

Potentially infection can spread superiorly and then, via the ophthalmic veins, intracranially (see ➔ 'Cavernous sinus thrombosis', pp. 92–3). This is rare.

ⓘ Facial space infection

This is usually due to a localized or spreading bacterial infection in one of the fascial spaces. Most often the underlying cause is a dental infection. However, be thorough and exclude all other possible causes. *Although initially mild, if left untreated, these can rapidly progress and in some cases become life-threatening.*

Spread of infection depends on the local anatomy, in which tooth the infection originates in, and in which jaw. Virulence of the organism and host resistance are also important factors. The face has a very rich blood supply which helps in its resistance to infection. However, the rich venous drainage of the face also communicates with the cavernous sinus, potentially draining infections intracranially. These veins are often valve-less, allowing infection to pass in a retrograde direction. The communications are mostly around the orbit, the most important being between the angular veins on the face and ophthalmic veins. These then pass through the orbit into the cavernous sinus. *Infected emboli can therefore result in cavernous sinus thrombosis and intracranial abscesses.*

Clinical features

Symptoms and signs depend on the severity of the infection. This is determined by the health of the patient, the virulence of the micro-organism, antibiotic sensitivity and the fascial space or spaces involved. Patients usually present with a localized, or more commonly a diffuse swelling on the face. There may be cervical lymphadenopathy. If advanced they are often unwell, feverish, with signs of systemic inflammatory response syndrome.

Investigations

- Usually the FBC will show an increased WCC.
- Blood cultures and a raised ESR may indicate bacteraemia or septicaemia.
- If the patient is very ill and dehydrated, the haematocrit will be raised and the urea and creatinine will be elevated.
- Never forget to take a random serum glucose sample—the patient may be an undiagnosed diabetic.
- Depending on the extent of infection and the suspected source imaging will be required (OPT/OM/CT). US will often determine if a swelling is oedematous only, or contains pus.

Management

Not all fascial space infections require admission. If minor they can be prescribed antibiotics and referred to their own dentist for assessment of the teeth. Treatment depends on the extent of the infection, its location, the patient's general health, and the response to previous treatments. Presentation varies from the ambulant patient with mild cellulitis to the severely ill, toxic, and bed-bound individual requiring urgent admission and drainage of infection. Keep the following principles in mind:

- If in doubt, refer or admit.
- Screen for diabetes (random blood sugar) and immunosuppression (WCC).
- Never underestimate a fascial space infection. In fact, never call it a 'dental abscess' as this terminology will put you, the anaesthetist, and theatre staff in the wrong state of mind and a lower gear of alertness. It is a 'fascial or cervical space infection'.
- Do not underestimate the rapidity with which these infections can spread. If you suspect the airway may potentially be threatened, do not 'wait and see' by treating with antibiotics. Electively secure the airway with endotracheal intubation and drain the abscess.
- Never treat a fascial space infection of an identifiable cause with antibiotics alone, try to remove the cause.
- If a collection has formed, it will never resolve with antibiotics alone, but requires incision and drainage. The space containing it must be incised and drained, with appropriate drains left *in situ*.

ⓘ Osteomyelitis of the upper jaw

Osteomyelitis of the jaws is uncommon and most commonly associated with odontogenic infection (infections of the teeth). It can occur following extractions, trauma, or irradiation to the mandible. It can also occur in patients taking bisphosphonates (BRONJ). Infection is more common in the lower jaw, as the upper jaw has a relatively better blood supply. Before the antibiotic era, however, it was frequently fatal. Acute osteomyelitis is less common than chronic osteomyelitis, with patients rarely presenting with obvious suppuration. A small amount of pus exuding from around a tooth is more likely to be a periodontal abscess, but *if multiple adjacent teeth are involved, mobile, and the overlying soft tissue are inflamed, there is probably acute osteomyelitis.*

Clinical features

These depend upon the type and extent of infection and may include:

- Pain—in acute osteomyelitis, this can be severe, throbbing and deep seated. Chronic infection has a less intense but still deep seated and unremitting character.
- Swelling, erythema, and tenderness. Initially soft, swelling is secondary to inflammation and oedema. This may later progress to a firm subperiosteal abscess.
- Trismus.
- Dysphagia.
- Cervical lymphadenopathy.
- Halitosis.
- Pyrexia, anorexia, and malaise.

- Friable granulation tissue, exposed necrotic bone, and sequestrum formation are all common in chronic infection. *It is important to make sure these features are not those of a malignancy.*

Usually there is an obvious cause such as a decayed tooth. This may be tender and mobile. Most patients are either malnourished or immune deficient to some extent. This condition is therefore commonly seen in smokers, diabetics, and alcoholics as well as other well-known at-risk groups.

The infection is usually a polymicrobial in nature. It is caused by a mixture of streptococci and anaerobic bacteria, which pass into the bones from the infected tooth. Haematogenous spread is rare. Osteomyelitis may also arise in an infected fracture. This tends to be chronic. Smokers are at particularly high risk of this. *Actinomycosis* is an unusual but specific infection, also known to occur. This results in recurrent and chronic jaw abscesses. These can discharge large amounts of pus, which often contains characteristically appearing bright yellow granules (referred to as 'sulphur granules'). *Consider actinomycosis in any patient with chronic bone abscesses and discharging sinuses.*

Management

Acute osteomyelitis needs urgent referral for admission, IV antibiotics, and drainage of pus. Chronic osteomyelitis may be managed as an outpatient with appropriate long-term antibiotics. If so, close follow-up is required. The decision to admit for IV antibiotics depends on a number of factors including the severity of symptoms, signs of systemic involvement (which are usually rare), extent of the infection (patients require CT) and patient compliance. Any associated contributing factors should also be identified and treated if possible. Surgical debridement may be required.

ⓘ Parotid sialadenitis

Mumps is the commonest cause of parotid swelling, even unilaterally. It has a peak incidence in childhood but can occur in adults. In teenagers, coxsackieviruses and echoviruses can also cause acute parotid sialadenitis. Clinically there is pyrexia and malaise. Pain is the most striking symptom. There is diffuse swelling of the gland and often trismus. Treatment is supportive.

'Ascending' infection, i.e. bacteria in saliva passing back along the ducts into the gland, can involve the parotid (and submandibular) glands. In such cases, predisposing conditions are often associated, e.g. dehydration, diabetes, or immunosuppression. Fibrosis following radiotherapy or pre-existing obstruction from a calculus or stricture may also predispose to infection.

Clinical features include:
- Fever
- Pain
- Erythema
- Tender swelling
- Discharge of pus from the duct.

If the infection is not treated early, this may develop into chronic or recurrent infection. Progressive destruction occurs that aggravates the situation resulting in a non-functional gland.

Management

In the absence of an obvious abscess, management initially consists of IV antibiotics, rehydration, analgesia, and correction of any systemic conditions (e.g. diabetes). If an obstruction is found (e.g. stone), this needs to be removed to enable drainage. Gland massage, especially after meals, and 'lemon drops' to stimulate salivary flow, help to maintain a flushing effect and prevent stagnation of saliva. Abscesses need to be incised and drained on an urgent basis. Ultrasound may help distinguish an abscess from swelling. If infection persists or continues to recur, excision of the gland may be necessary. This is best done when there is no active infection.

ⓘ Facial pain

See also ⮑ Chapter 3.

Anatomy and physiology of orofacial pain

The upper cervical nerves carrying pain impulses from the back of the head and the neck converge with trigeminal sensory neurons in the dorsal horn—the 'trigeminocervical complex'. This convergence is the basis for referred pain from the neck to the face and head. Facial sensation is principally from the trigeminal nerve, although there is some contribution from the facial and vagus nerves. The posterior aspect of the tongue, tonsils, tympanic cavity, and the pharynx are innervated by the glossopharyngeal nerve. The cornea and dental pulp are predominately innervated by pain fibres. There is a large representation of the orofacial region in the cerebral somatosensory system, accounting for the exquisite sensibility of the orofacial tissues.

Types of pain

- Somatic pain is pain arising from structures which one is generally aware of (skin, oral mucosa, joints, etc.). This pain often subsides following healing. It is usually described as sharp or sore.
- Neuropathic pain is due to injury to the nociceptive (pain) pathway and may persist long after healing has taken place. It is often described as burning, shooting, or like an electric shock. Injury may occur peripherally or centrally, anywhere along the neural pathway. This can occur for example, following herpes zoster infection—'post-herpetic neuralgia'.
- Deafferentation. This refers to partial or total loss of sensation in a localized area following loss or interruption of sensory fibres. Instead of a decrease in pain sensation in the affected area, spontaneous pain may develop. This is referred to as 'dysaesthesia'. It is occasionally seen following inferior alveolar or lingual nerve injury (e.g. after wisdom tooth removal).
- Allodynia is pain caused by stimuli that would normally not produce pain, e.g. bedclothes producing a burning sensation or shaving causing severe facial pain.

① Orofacial pain syndromes

Trigeminal neuralgia and atypical facial pain are among the most challeng-ing pain conditions in the orofacial area. It is not always easy to distinguish between these and other possible diagnoses, although it is important to do so as treatments and prognoses differ. *All forms of idiopathic facial pain syndromes should be regarded as a 'diagnosis of exclusion'*, that is, all other causes of facial pain should be considered and if necessary, investigated for. Every now and then patients with odd symptoms turn out to have significant underlying disease, notably tumours.

Idiopathic facial pain

This makes up a significant proportion of outpatient attendances. Four symptom complexes are commonly seen:

- Facial arthromyalgia (FAM or TMJ dysfunction syndrome) (see ➔ Chapter 12)
- Atypical facial pain
- Atypical odontalgia
- Oral dysaesthesia (burning mouth) (see ➔ Chapter 13).

It has been suggested that these symptoms may form part of a whole-body pain syndrome, involving the neck, back, abdomen, and skin. Adverse life events and impaired coping ability are well-known associa-tions. The precise aetiology of idiopathic facial pain is still unknown. It has been suggested that stress-induced neuropeptide inflammation within the tissues (e.g. TMJ) causes pain and local production of free radicals. Eicosanoids have been suggested as responsible for unexplained pain in non-joint areas including the teeth.

① Atypical odontalgia

This is a severe throbbing pain in the tooth and jaw without significant pathology. Often described as severe continual throbbing pain, it may vary from mild to intense pain, especially with hot or cold stimuli. It may be widespread or well localized, frequently precipitated by a dental pro-cedure and may move from tooth to tooth. It may last a few minutes to several hours. This is often a symptom of hypochondriacal psychosis or depression and there is often excessive concern with oral hygiene. Treatment involves counselling, avoidance of unnecessary pulp extirpa-tions and extractions, antidepressants, and phenothiazines.

① Herpes zoster (shingles)

This is an acute herpetic infection in any dermatome, commonly the fifth (V) cranial nerve. It commonly involves the side of the face or forehead, presenting with burning or a tingling pain in the skin with skin eruptions. These are confined to the distribution of a nerve. *If near the orbit, involve-ment of the eye is possible and requires urgent referral to ophthalmology.* Post-herpetic neuralgia is chronic pain with skin changes following acute herpes zoster. There may be burning or tearing sensations, or itching and crawling dysaesthesias in skin. In the acute phase, stellate ganglion blocks using local anaesthetic such as bupivacaine, may help for severe pain. Transcutaneous nerve stimulation, capsaicin cream, and tricyclic antidepressants are also useful.

① Trigeminal neuralgia ('tic douloureux')

Trigeminal neuralgia is most commonly a disorder seen in middle-aged and elderly patients. It is more common in women with a peak incidence between 50 and 60 years of age. *In young patients it may be an early feature of MS, HIV disease, or as a consequence of a lesion irritating the trigeminal nerve.* Patients complain of a sharp, intense, lancing/'electric-type' pain induced by a specific trigger point that radiates across the distribution of a branch of the trigeminal nerve. The pain is almost always unilateral, with over 30–40% of patients showing a distribution affecting both the maxillary and mandibular divisions. In approximately 20% of patients, the pain is confined to the mandibular division, and the ophthalmic division in 3%. Episodes may last up to several hours. The aetiology of trigeminal neuralgia is presumed to be multifactorial, with local nerve microcompression within the skull base and possible demyelination.

Management

- Always consider skull base pathology and intracranial disease/demyelination. Imaging may be required.
- The mainstay of treatment remains medical, typically with anticonvulsant agents. Usually, trigeminal neuralgia responds well to carbamazepine and/or amitriptyline, and a muscle relaxant such as baclofen. Carbamazepine remains the drug of choice with an initial regime of 100 mg three times daily being gradually increased to a maximum of 1200 mg daily titrated against effect. About 20% of patients may develop side effects such as tremor, dizziness, double vision, and vomiting, which will obviously limit its use. They should have regular monitoring of FBC, electrolytes, and LFTs. Approximately 20% can develop folic acid deficiency with megaloblastic anaemia, and hyponatraemia in the elderly. Withdraw therapy slowly.
- Alternative agents include phenytoin, sodium valproate, lamotrigine, and baclofen.
- Local surgical procedures may be considered in trigeminal neuralgia not responsive to medical management. This can include cryotherapy to the nerve, alcohol/glycerol injections.
- Neurosurgical decompression in severe cases following imaging confirming there is nerve compression.
- Gamma Knife® (stereotactic radiosurgery). High-resolution imaging provides excellent definition and allows a focus beam of ionizing radiation to irradiate the proximal trigeminal nerve at its entry into the pons. Results are very promising (see http://www.gammaknife.org.uk).

① Atypical facial pain

Atypical facial pain has many distinguishing features that make it a clinical entity in its own right and not just a 'catch all' diagnosis for seemingly unexplained facial pains. It is, however, *essentially a diagnosis of exclusion that should only be made after all other possible organic causes have been excluded*. These patients therefore often undergo extensive investigation.

Clinical features

Patients often have a 'flat affect' and the more they are questioned about the pain the more vague their answers become. The pain is typically described as being a deep, dull ache, sometimes fluctuating, sometimes continuous, with intermittent severe episodes that the patient can find no causative factor for. Often the pain has been present for several years and analgesics rarely affect its nature. It is most commonly bilateral, but ill defined, and its distribution cannot be explained on an anatomical basis. The patient may say they are kept from sleeping by the pain but usually look well rested. When they do admit to sleeping, the pain does not wake them. A proportion of these patients may show symptoms of depressive illness or anxiety states, and patients often complain of other symptoms such as back and neck pain and irritable bowel syndrome. The patient's mood often does not correlate to the description of their symptoms and they may show exaggerated responses to examination and report stressful life events.

Management

Often the ill-defined nature of the patient's pain results in unnecessary dental work being carried out. In light of the association of atypical facial pain with the neuroses (particularly depression), and the belief that it essentially has a psychogenic basis, emphasis has been placed on the use of antidepressant agents as the main treatment option.

- Dothiepin, a tricyclic antidepressant, has been shown to be effective in reducing the painful symptoms (as it has in TMJ dysfunction).
- Selective serotonin re-uptake inhibitors (SSRIs).

ⓘ Facial numbness

Facial numbness is a problem that presents from time to time. In most cases either the cause is benign or cannot be found. Many cases spontaneously resolve without a firm diagnosis ever being made—idiopathic facial numbness. *Nevertheless, numbness, especially if it corresponds to the distribution of a nerve, should be taken seriously.* It can occasionally be the first symptom of a serious problem.

Causes

- Idiopathic
- Migraine
- Following dental treatment (nerve injury)
- Post-trigeminal neuralgia
- Viral trigeminal neuropathy. Temporary dysfunction of the nerve following a viral infection
- Demyelinating diseases (notably MS)
- Tumours (sinus, intracranial, skull base, nerve sheath)
- Sinus pathology (including large odontogenic cysts) affecting the infraorbital nerve
- AVM
- Hypothyroidism
- Peripheral neuropathy (common causes are vitamin deficiency, diabetes, excessive alcohol intake, and lead poisoning, but there are many other causes).

Investigations
These are tailored towards the suspected cause, but include the following:
• FBC and ESR/CRP
• Electrolytes (notably calcium, potassium, and sodium)
• LFTs
• Thyroid function tests
• Measurement of vitamin levels
• Heavy metal or toxicology screening
• Imaging may include MRI or CT. MRI is useful for demyelinating and other intracranial disease, CT in the assessment of the sinuses, but it is often best to discuss these with a radiologist.

Management
This is directed to the underlying cause (if one is found). Sometimes reassurance and review is all that is required.

⊙ Facial palsy

Assessment of a patient with facial palsy requires careful examination of the ear—see ➜ Chapter 6 for details.
The cranial nerve VII (facial nerve) supplies:
• Motor fibres to the muscles of facial expression, post belly of digastric, and a branch to the stapedius muscle in the middle ear.
• Taste sensation from the anterior two-thirds of the tongue via the chorda tympani.
• Secretomotor fibres to the submandibular, sublingual salivary glands, and to the lacrimal glands.

Extracranial course of the facial nerve

The facial nerve exits the stylomastoid foramen, just in front of the mastoid process and passes almost immediately into the parotid gland. Here it lies in a fibrous plane separating the deep and superficial lobes of the gland. The nerve then divides into two major divisions: an upper 'temporofacial' and lower 'cervicofacial' branch. These then divide further into its five terminal branches:
• Temporal
• Zygomatic
• Buccal
• Marginal mandibular
• Cervical branch.

Sometimes the marginal mandibular branch divides immediately into two, making six main branches of note. Frequent interconnections exits between these branches—the 'pes anserinus'.

Causes of facial palsy

• Cerebrovascular accidents
• Cerebral tumours
• Bell's palsy
• Acute/chronic otitis media/other middle ear diseases

- Ramsay Hunt syndrome (herpes zoster infection of the geniculate ganglion)
- Trauma
- Surgical (iatrogenic—possibly intentional)
- Temporal bone fracture (see ➲ Chapter 6)
- Birth injury
- Neoplastic—malignant disease of the middle ear and acoustic neuroma
- Parotid tumours and infiltrative disease (TB)
- Sarcoidosis—Heerfordt's syndrome is sarcoidosis resulting in parotid enlargement, fever, anterior uveitis, and facial nerve palsy
- MS
- Guillain–Barré syndrome (acute idiopathic polyneuritis). Facial palsy does not occur in isolation. An ascending peripheral neuropathy is usually associated. It is believed to occur following a recent viral infection. Potentially a serious condition.

Clinical features

Varying degrees of weakness of the muscles of the face may be seen:
- Upper motor neuron lesions will cause a unilateral facial palsy with sparing of the muscles of the upper face. The upper face receives innervation bilaterally from both motor cortices. All muscles may move normally during emotional responses.
- Lower motor neuron lesions will show a unilateral paralysis of all the muscles, both voluntarily and to emotional stimulus.

This can result in the following:
- Facial asymmetry is exaggerated when attempting to show the teeth, whistle, or close the eyes tightly (the eyes roll upwards—Bell's phenomenon).
- Food collects in the vestibule because of buccinator paralysis.
- Loss of the nasolabial fold as the commissure of the mouth droops.
- Epiphora—tears overflow to the cheek.
- Reduced lacrimation (lesions above the geniculate ganglion).
- Hyperacusis: loss of stapedius reflex (lesions above nerve to stapedius).
- There may also be loss of taste and reduced salivation.

ⓘ Herpes zoster infection (Ramsey Hunt syndrome)

This is a viral infection, usually chickenpox, affecting the geniculate ganglion. In addition to facial weakness, vesicles are visible on the ear canal, pharynx, and face. Management requires the use of systemic antiviral agents (aciclovir). Some specialists also advise steroids.

ⓘ Bell's palsy

Idiopathic facial palsy (Bell's palsy) should be a 'diagnosis of exclusion'. All other causes must be eliminated clinically or following investigations (notably parotid tumours and acoustic neuroma). There is unilateral facial paralysis, sometimes associated with loss of taste and hearing, or occasionally hyperacusis. It is often preceded by mastoid discomfort. High-dose IV steroids may be of use, although this is controversial, and if the diagnosis is wrong (e.g. it is herpes zoster instead) this may lead to rapid spread and deterioration in the patient. Bell's palsy can be easily confused with Ramsey Hunt syndrome (in which the use of steroids is controversial). To differentiate between the two, consider the history and carefully examine for vesicles in the external meatus. The prognosis for Bell's palsy is generally good.

Management of facial palsy
This is dependent on the cause.

Non-infective lumps and swellings

① Parotid obstruction

Obstruction of any part of the duct system of the gland may result in a build-up of salivary secretions and swelling. The classic history is of unilateral swelling on the side of the face, associated with meal times. Patient may also report that the swelling settles a few hours after the end of eating. Parotid calculi are not as common as submandibular and are usually not visible on plain films. Sialography is often required to locate them. Stones may be removed endoscopically. With recurrent bouts of obstruction, infection may eventually supersede due to stagnation of secretions.

① Parotid tumours

70–80% of all salivary gland tumours arise in the parotid. Of these, approximately 80% are pleomorphic adenomas and 10–15% are malignant. Classification of salivary gland tumours is complex. This includes (not an exhaustive list):
- Benign epithelial tumours (pleomorphic and monomorphic adenoma, myoepithelioma, and Warthin's tumour)
- Malignant epithelial tumours (acinic cell, mucoepidermoid, and adenoidcystic carcinoma, salivary duct carcinoma)
- Soft tissue tumours (lymphangioma, haemangioma, and lymphomas)
- Metastatic tumours (skin cancers metastasizing to parotid nodes).

A lump associated with facial nerve weakness suggests infiltrative pathology (i.e. tumour). Patients may present with the following clinical features:
- Swelling
- Pain
- Facial weakness
- Skin changes
- Poor hearing or earache.

Most parotid tumours present as a painless, localized swelling, which have been present for several years. *Pain in the gland suggests infection or malignancy.* Other features suggestive of malignancy include facial nerve weakness, tethering of the lump, and rapid growth. Investigations include CT or MRI scan. FNAC is often undertaken but its value is debatable. Parotid lumps need urgent referral to a head and neck specialty (e.g. maxillofacial/ENT). Imaging is usually required (CT/MRI or ultrasound). Management is usually surgical removal.

Not all swellings of the parotid gland are due to salivary tumours. Tumours can also arise from associated blood vessels, nerves, fat, and lymphatic tissue. 'Tumour-like' conditions presenting as swellings include sarcoid, toxoplasmosis, and sialosis. The latter is painless swelling, which may be associated with alcoholic cirrhosis, diabetes, acromegaly, or bulimia. *Heerfordt's syndrome* is sarcoidosis resulting in parotid enlargement, fever, anterior uveitis, and facial nerve palsy.

ⓘ Odontogenic cysts and tumours

As a group these form the commonest cause of non-infective swelling in the upper and lower jaws. The vast majority which present are benign. The term 'odontogenic' refers to structures arising from the tissues that make up the teeth. Classification of odontogenic cysts and tumours is very complex. Some pathologists specialize in just these and other oral pathology. Odontogenic cysts and tumours can be considered as follows:

Benign odontogenic tumours
- Ameloblastoma
- Squamous odontogenic tumour
- Calcifying epithelial odontogenic tumour (Pindborg tumour)
- Ameloblastic fibroma
- Calcifying odontogenic cyst
- Odontoma
- Odontogenic fibroma
- Myxoma (odontogenic myxoma, myxofibroma)
- Cementoblastoma.

Malignant odontogenic tumours
- Malignant ameloblastoma
- Primary intraosseous carcinoma
- Malignant variants of other odontogenic epithelial tumours
- Malignant changes in odontogenic cysts
- Odontogenic sarcomas
- Odontogenic carcinosarcomas.

Non-neoplastic bone lesions
- Fibrous dysplasia of the jaws
- Cemento-osseous dysplasia
- Periapical cemental dysplasia (periapical fibrous dysplasia)
- Cherubism (familial multilocular cystic disease of the jaws)
- Central giant cell granuloma
- Aneurysmal bone cyst
- Solitary bone cyst
- Traumatic bone cyst of jaw
- Simple bone cyst of jaw
- Haemorrhagic bone cyst.

This is not an exhaustive list.

⑦ Odontogenic cysts

Many types of cyst can occur in the jaws and the classification of these is also very complicated. The vast majority of these present as a well-defined, corticated, radiolucency in the bone, often incidental. A few

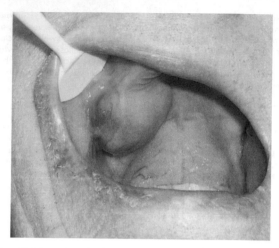

Figure 11.4 Large dentoalveolar cyst in the right maxilla. The overlying bone was eggshell thin.

have characteristic calcification that enables diagnosis. Many can be diagnosed with reasonable certainty from the X-ray (see Figure 11.4). Some require biopsy. All should be referred, but not necessarily on an urgent basis (if small and asymptomatic). The more common ones encountered include:

- Dentigerous cyst
- Odontogenic keratocyst (may be considered as an intraoral basal cell carcinoma)
- Periapical cyst
- Residual cyst of the jaw
- Traumatic bone cyst of jaw
- Stafne cyst.

Other causes of a 'cyst' in the jaws include:

- Ameloblastoma
- Metastases, including lymphoma
- Squamous cell carcinoma invading the bone
- Multiple myeloma
- Periapical abscess
- Giant cell granuloma
- Aneurysmal bone cyst.

Again, this list is not exhaustive but demonstrates the difficulty in triaging and diagnosis of cysts and growths of the jaws.

⑦ Extramedullary haematopoiesis

This should be considered in the differential diagnosis of any diffuse jaw swelling in patients with chronic anaemia. It is the production of blood in sites other than the long bones, pelvis, spine, and sternum. This occurs as a response to increased production of erythropoietin in chronically anaemic patients (such as those with chronic haemolytic anaemia). There is usually hepatomegaly and splenomegaly. Extramedullary haematopoiesis rarely involves the facial bones but has been reported to involve the mandible, maxilla and orbit. It may be misdiagnosed as sinusitis.

① Myeloma

Myelomatous involvement of the maxilla is very rare, but may present as an expansile jaw lesion. Patients may also present with renal failure, bone pain, fatigue, recurrent infections, and neurological dysfunction. Oral manifestations may be the first sign. Treatment involves mainly irradiation and chemotherapy and the prognosis is generally poor.

⑦ Osteoradionecrosis (ORN)

ORN of the upper jaw is less common than the lower, due to its relatively better blood supply. The clinical spectrum of presentation of ORN is wide. The patient will usually have a non-resolving painful mucosal ulcer with evidence of exposed bone or sequestrum. There may be trismus and this usually appears 3–6 months following radiotherapy. At the other end of the spectrum the patients may present with an orocutaneous fistula, increasingly mobile teeth, or a pathological fracture. Typically radiological appearances will include a moth-eaten appearance to the bone, which is best seen on CT. Management principles are based on controlling any acute superadded infection, strict oral hygiene, analgesia, and nutritional support as well as minimal surgical debridement. In severe cases, resection of the bone involved and reconstruction with a free tissue transfer may be required.

⑦ Bisphosphonate-related osteonecrosis of the jaw (BRONJ)

Bisphosphonates inhibit osteoclastic action and reduce bone loss in patients with multiple myeloma, bony metastasis in breast cancer, Paget's disease of bone, and postmenopausal osteoporosis. However, osteonecrosis can occur as a serious side effect in both jaws. Patients present with pain and swelling affecting the mucosa of the jaw, which may be confused with chronic osteomyelitis, ORN, or even malignancy. CT usually shows regions of mottled bone and sequestrum formation. Treatment usually involves meticulous oral hygiene, antibiotics and gentle debridement. Cessation of the drug, if not contraindicated may help some recovery.

⑦ Paget's disease

Paget's disease is a localized disorder of bone remodelling. Usually the bone is mechanically weaker, larger, less compact, more vascular, and more susceptible to fracture than normal adult lamellar bone. Patients can present with bone pain associated with marked deformity. Clinical examination may reveal excessive warmth, due to hypervascularity and paraesthesia of the infraorbital nerve due to bony compression. These symptoms may be confused with chronic infection or a tumour.

⑦ Fibrous dysplasia

This is a disorder of bone growth where normal bone is replaced with immature fibrous bone. It can occur in any part of the skeleton but the skull and face are commonly involved. Patients present with a smooth hard swelling and deformity usually in childhood or early adulthood. During rapid growth this may become painful. Two types of fibrous dysplasia are described.

McCune–Albright syndrome, includes endocrine diseases (precocious puberty) and skin pigmentation. Fibrous dysplasia may also be associated with neurofibromatosis. Management include bisphosphonates and surgical contouring of a cosmetic deformity.

The lower jaw and face

Common presentations

Common presentations around the lower jaw and face:
- Bleeding from the lower jaw/teeth (see also ➔ Chapter 13)
- Clicking TMJ(s)
- Deranged (change in) bite (disocclusion)/dislocation
- Fistula/sinus on the skin overlying the mandible
- Infection
- Injuries
- Limitation of opening
- Numbness/altered sensation of the lower lip
- Painful jaw
- Swellings around the lower jaw.

Common problems and their causes

Bleeding from the lower jaw/teeth

(See also ➔ Chapter 13.)

Common
- Trauma
- Infections (notably dental)
- Gingivitis/periodontitis
- Toothbrush injury, incorrect flossing
- Bleeding from extraction socket/surgical site.

Uncommon
- Drug-related; anticoagulants (warfarin, aspirin, etc.)
- Haematological (leukaemia/idiopathic thrombocytopenic purpura)
- Cysts/tumours
- Plus causes of fistula/sinus (see later).

Clicking temporomandibular joint(s)

Common
- 'Disc' problems (temporomandibular joint dysfunction syndrome (TMJDS)/internal derangement).

Uncommon
- Intra-articular loose bodies
- Subluxation.

Deranged (change in) bite (disocclusion)/dislocation

Common
- Fractures (mandible/midface/zygoma)
- TMJ 'disc' problems (TMJDS)
- TMJ effusion/haemarthrosis

- Dentoalveolar trauma
- Dislocation of the TMJ.

Uncommon
- Condylar hyperplasia
- Large dental cysts
- Osteomyelitis
- Tumour involving bone
- Fibrous dysplasia
- Paget's disease
- Following jaw surgery.

Fistula/sinus on the overlying skin

Common
- Infections (dental/skin cysts)
- Injuries (delayed presentation)
- Infected osteosynthesis plate.

Uncommon
- Chronic osteomyelitis
- Foreign body in the skin
- Necrotic lymph node
- Osteoradionecrosis (ORN)/BRONJ
- Underlying tumour
- Congenital/developmental cysts.

Infections

Common
- Dental
- Jaw cysts
- Infected osteosynthesis plate.

Uncommon
- Chronic osteomyelitis/untreated fracture
- Foreign body in the skin
- Actinomycosis
- ORN/BRONJ
- Acute necrotizing ulcerative gingivitis (see ⊙ Chapter 13).

Injuries

Common
- Fractures
- Haematoma/soft tissue injuries
- Effusions of TMJ.

Uncommon
- Gunshot injuries
- Penetrating injuries
- Blast injuries.

Limitation of mouth opening

Common
- TMJDS/internal derangement of TMJ/disc problems
- Injuries (fractured condyle/midface/zygoma/dislocation)
- Following treatment (dental/removal wisdom teeth)
- Infections (dental/tonsils/ear/parotid).

Uncommon
- Arthritis (osteoarthritis/inflammatory)
- Ankylosis
- Tumour/cholesteatoma
- Radiation fibrosis/submucous fibrosis/myositis ossificans.
- Coronoid hyperplasia.

Numbness/altered sensation of the lower lip

Common
- Trauma (displaced fractures)
- Iatrogenic (following dental treatment).

Uncommon
- Dental cysts and infections
- Tumours
- Demyelinating diseases
- Post herpetic
- Osteomyelitis.

Painful jaw

Common
- TMJ 'disc' problems and associated muscles
- Infections (notably dental)
- Injuries
- Trigeminal neuralgia
- Salivary gland disease
- Jaw cysts
- Postoperative pain.

Uncommon
- Tumours
- Sickle cell crisis
- ORN/BRONJ
- Pathological fracture

- Giant cell arteritis
- Post-herpetic neuralgia/shingles
- Referred pain
- TMJ arthropathy.

Swellings around the lower jaw

Common
- Infections (notably dental)
- Injuries/haematoma
- Salivary gland disease (e.g. mumps/tumours)
- Postoperative swelling
- Callus
- Buried teeth
- Mandibular torus/osteoma.

Uncommon
- Cystic/ossifying lesions of the mandible
- Post traumatic swelling
- Tumours
- Haemangioma/lymphangioma
- Paget's/fibrous dysplasia.

Useful questions and what to look for

Bleeding from the lower jaw/teeth
(See also ➲ Chapter 13.)

Ask about
- Preceding events (extractions, surgery, trauma) or spontaneous
- Previous episodes
- History of anticoagulant use
- History of alcohol consumption or liver disease
- Isolated or bleeding from other sites
- Generalized bruising elsewhere on the body.

Look for
- Haemodynamic instability
- Intraoral bleeding/skin bruising/petechiae
- Fractures/tumours
- Mucosal abnormalities
- Swelling/deformity
- Other causes, i.e. post-nasal and tonsillar bleeding, haemoptysis, or haematemesis.

Clicking temporomandibular joint(s)

Ask about
- Previous episodes
- Duration of symptoms
- Associated with other symptoms—i.e. pain
- Timing of symptoms—i.e. is it constant or only when eating
- Unilateral or bilateral joint involvement
- History of change in bite
- Any history of jaw locking
- Any other joints involved
- Any history of trauma.

Look for
- Clicking or crepitus when opening
- Restriction in mouth opening
- Tenderness of muscles of mastication
- Evidence of trauma
- Deviation of jaw to one side on opening.

Deranged (change in) bite (disocclusion)/dislocation

Ask about
- History of trauma
- Sudden or progressive
- Recent or previous jaw surgery
- Any change in the shape of the jaw
- Pain
- How is the bite different? (e.g. premature contact on one side vs teeth meeting at the back and not at the front)
- Can patient bite at all (dislocation).

Look for
- Examine as for trauma
- Examine the teeth for missing/mobile teeth
- Steps in the horizontal level of the teeth
- Uneven contact on biting (at the back or on one side)
- Inspect any dentures to ensure no obvious fractures
- Range of jaw movements.

Fistula/sinus on the overlying skin

Ask about
- Preceding or precipitating event prior to the appearance of fistula/ sinus (e.g. injury, lump, or swelling)
- Previous facial/jaw surgery
- Previous malignancy or radiotherapy
- Medication (bisphosphonates)
- Any discharge present
- Any pain/swelling associated.

Look for
- Sites of fistula/sinus
- Discharging fluid (pus, blood, or saliva)
- Exposed bone or osteosynthesis plate
- Features suggestive of fracture (mobility/dysocclusion)
- Broken down teeth
- Signs of osteomyelitis of the mandible
- Tumours.

Infections

Ask about
- Onset and duration
- Recent injuries, dental infections, or treatment
- Previous episodes
- Pain, erythema, and swelling
- Changes in bite
- Swelling at mealtimes
- Systemic symptoms
- Medical history/medications taken.

Look for
- Site and extension
- Skin erythema and swelling
- Systemic involvement (pyrexia, sweating, lethargy)
- Numbness of the lower lip
- Intraoral/dental examination
- Salivary gland enlargement/discharge of saliva.

Injuries

Ask about
- When it occurred
- Mechanism of injury
- Any loss of consciousness or signs of head injury
- Any cervical spine injury or symptoms
- Progression of symptoms since time of injury
- Any difficulty swallowing
- Any infective symptoms
- Any altered sensation of lower lip
- Any change in bite
- Tetanus status.

Look for
- Other injuries
- Airway risk factors
- Facial asymmetry/swelling over the mandible
- Limitation of mouth opening
- Bruising under the tongue
- Mobility between fracture fragments

- Dental injuries—all lost or fractured teeth must be accounted for
- Change in bite—uneven contacts
- Soft tissue injuries
- Paraesthesia of lower lip
- Bleeding from the external auditory meatus.

Limitation of mouth opening

Ask about
- Onset (sudden or progressive) and duration
- Symptoms one or both sides
- Recent injuries, dental infections or treatments
- Previous episodes
- Pain (localized or diffuse) and swelling
- Change in bite
- Previous clicking.

Look for
- Degree of limitation (minor vs total)
- Swelling
- Tenderness (joint/muscles)
- Numbness of the lower lip
- Intraoral/dental examination (if access allows)
- Range of jaw movements/palpable click
- Systemic involvement (pyrexia, sweating, lethargy).

Numbness/altered sensation of the lower lip

Ask about
- Sudden or gradual onset
- Static or progressive
- History of recent injury or trauma
- Recent dental or maxillofacial treatment
- Other facial areas affected (especially trigeminal nerve)
- Bleeding or increasing mobility of teeth
- Jaw pain
- Any other neurological symptoms.

Look for
- Full cranial nerve examination
- Objective or subjective paraesthesia
- Map out the area involved—is it anatomical?
- Blisters/vesicles at site of numbness
- Signs of fracture along the path of the inferior alveolar nerve
- Jaw swelling/tenderness
- Exposed bone/mucosal ulceration
- Dental examination
- Tumours.

Painful jaw

Ask about

- Sudden or gradual onset
- Nature of the pain—toothache/sharp/burning
- Define site (local vs diffuse, one side or both)
- Known cause, e.g. trauma
- Associated swelling/bleeding/limitation of mouth opening/swallowing difficulty
- Aggravating and relieving factors
- Recent surgery/dental work
- Previous history of problems with the mandible (surgery/cysts/malignancy)
- Consider referred pain (notably myocardial).

Look for

- Dental decay/broken/bleeding/mobile teeth
- Ulceration/mucosal abnormalities
- Signs of injury
- Swellings of the jaw/neck
- Salivary gland swelling/lumps
- Tenderness in the muscles of mastication
- In the absence of clinical signs—consider referred pain or trigeminal neuralgia.

Swellings around the lower jaw

Ask about

- Onset and duration
- How has the swelling progressed?
- Is the swelling painful or painless?
- Preceding or precipitating events (toothache/trauma)
- Symptoms suggestive of infection (limitation in mouth opening/pain/systemic symptoms)
- Any discharge from the swelling/bleeding from teeth
- Any previous episodes.

Look for

- Site of the swelling
- Nature of the swelling, i.e. hard/soft/cystic
- If thought to be infective:
  - Assess swallow and airway
  - Is the tongue raised?
  - Limitation in mouth opening
  - Redness and heat of overlying skin
  - Signs of systemic sepsis
- Tenderness
- Evidence of trauma
- Condition of the overlying skin (injury/punctum/discharge)
- Assess the dentition for broken/loose/bleeding teeth.

Examination of the lower jaw and face

Applied anatomy

The mandible forms the lower third of the facial skeleton and is responsible for the lower transverse facial width. It has a number of powerful muscles inserted along its length. These include the muscles of mastication (temporalis, masseter, medial, and lateral pterygoid), and the suprahyoid muscles (digastric, geniohyoid, and mylohyoid). These muscles can generate considerable biting forces and are an important cause of mandibular fracture displacement. The mandible also receives the insertion of genioglossus (which forms the bulk of the tongue). *Loss of support for this muscle can place the airway at risk.* Morphologically, the mandible can be considered as a U-shaped long bone articulating at each end with the skull at the TMJs. Anatomically it is divided into:

• Symphysis (in the midline)
• Parasymphysis (anterior to the premolar region)
• Body (premolar and molar region)
• Angle (third molar region)
• Ramus (from third molar to condyle)
• Condyle (neck and head).

The vertical ramus supports the condyle (which articulates with the glenoid fossa) and the coronoid process (which receives the insertion of the temporalis muscle). The condylar head is supported on a relatively slender neck—a frequent site of fracture. On the medial side of the ramus, the inferior alveolar (inferior dental—ID) nerve and vessels enter the bone via the mandibular (lingula) foramen, passing forward through the 'ID' canal. These provide sensory innervation and nutrition to the lower teeth. The mental nerve, a terminal branch, exits the mandible through the mental foramen in the premolar region. This provides sensation to the lower lip. *Numbness of the lower lip may therefore signify fracture or pathology anywhere along the course of this nerve.* High-energy blows to the side of the lower jaw can result in significant displacement of fractures involving the ID canal. This may result in stretching (or even avulsion) to the nerve itself, adversely affecting its likelihood of recovery. *Make sure you record any numbness.* This is a common source of litigation following injuries as well as dental treatment/surgery (notably removal of wisdom teeth).

In a healthy adult the lower jaw is around 3–4 cm in height. However, once a tooth (or teeth) has been lost, there is progressive resorption of the bone. This can weaken the bone locally, predisposing the site to fracture.

Age-related changes

In the child, the dentition will be at various stages of development and developing tooth germs are present within the bone. While these lead to a structural weakening of the bone, this is compensated for by increased elasticity and pliability of the young mandible, compared with mature bone. As a result, relatively higher forces are required to fracture the bone in children. In the edentulous elderly jaw, continued resorption of bone leads to a significant reduction in bone height. This feature, together with age-related conditions such as osteoporosis makes the jaw highly vulnerable to fracture. In some patients the bone can literally be pencil thin, especially if they have been without teeth for many decades.

Examination

Always begin by assessing the airway, notably for obvious signs of compromise and by listening for any stridor. High-energy impacts that are sufficient enough to break the bone (particularly those resulting in comminuted or multiple-site fractures), not only put patients at risk from cervical spine injuries, but can also place the airway at risk from bleeding, swelling, and loss of tongue support. If there are airway problems, call for help and try to identify the cause.

In the absence of any urgent airway problems, start by inspecting the patient from in front. Note any lacerations, bruising, abrasions, swellings and haematomas. Look carefully under the chin—impacts here may suggest the possibility of fractures in the condylar region. The classic 'guardsman's' fracture (a midline/parasymphyseal fracture, associated with bilateral fractures of the condyles) usually occurs following a faint or fall onto the chin. Bleeding from the external auditory meatus may be present, usually as a result of tearing of its anterior wall by a condylar fracture. However, it may also be a sign of a fractured skull base—be careful in your assessment.

Ask the patient to open and close their mouth and note for any limitation in mouth opening. Normal opening should be approximately four finger breadths (40 mm). Ask the patient to swallow and stick out their tongue and report if they have any pain or difficulty during this.

Then stand behind the patient and palpate the inferior border of the mandible passing from the chin to the TMJ on each side. Note any swelling, steps, and tenderness. Assess the movement of each condyle by palpating immediately in front of each tragus and then by placing a gloved finger in each auditory meatus. Ask the patient to open and close while palpating here. Gently stress the joints by pushing backward on the point of the chin with the teeth slightly apart. Then ask the patient to attempt to open their mouth against resistance by placing your hand under the lower border of their mandible. These two manoeuvres help identify fractures of the condyles. Note any areas of paraesthesia, or anaesthesia. If appropriate, assess for a displaced fracture the zygomatic arch—this may impinge on the coronoid process limiting mouth opening.

Following injury, if a fracture is thought *not* to be present, 'springing' the mandible by gently compressing the angles, should be possible without causing pain. Similarly, asking the patient to open their mouth, with increasing force against resistance at the symphysis, should also be pain free. A clinically intact jaw should be able to resist both these deformational forces without discomfort and therefore avoid unnecessary imaging.

It is also important to carefully examine inside the patients mouth (see ➔ Chapter 13). Intraoral examination requires a good light and a tongue depressor to retract the cheeks. Look for:
• Asymmetry/swelling
• Bruising/bleeding

- Damaged, loose, missing teeth (see ➋ Chapter 13)
- Occlusal derangement, or steps in the occlusal plane.

Sublingual haematoma (submucosal blood under the tongue) is highly suggestive of a fracture involving the lingual plate of the mandible. If present, the airway should be reviewed regularly in any patient taking antiplatelet agents or anticoagulants (notably aspirin and warfarin), since continued bleeding may put the airway at risk.

Testing any suspected fracture sites can be done by grasping the mandible on each side of the suspected site and gently manipulating it to assess mobility. Check the patient's occlusion and look for loose teeth. A normal bite will have an even and almost simultaneous contact of all the teeth. Derangement can be assessed by asking the patient to slowly bite together. Look for premature contacts and any teeth that do not come into contact. Also look for any obvious bony or soft tissue swellings.

Following injury, any missing teeth must be accounted for. If their whereabouts are unknown, request a chest and soft tissue X-ray of the neck. Similarly, if associated with a lip laceration, a soft tissue radiograph of the lips is essential.

Examination of the lower jaw for non-traumatic problems follows the same sequence. Although fractures are less likely, keep pathological fractures in mind. These can present without an obvious history of trauma.

Approximately half of patients with a mandibular fracture will have multiple fractures present. In about 10%, three or more sites will be involved. Therefore, if you identify one fracture, look for another (cf. pelvic fractures).

Useful investigations

Laboratory investigations

- FBC: this is usually required in all cases of suspected infection and following significant blood loss. A raised WCC is a useful guide to severity of infection.
- Glucose: screen for diabetes (associated with spreading sepsis).
- ESR/CRP: this is also a useful guide to severity of infection.
- Microbiology: for any pus/discharge.

Plain films

Preliminary investigations commonly include an orthopantomograph (OPT), posteroanterior (PA) mandible film, and lateral oblique films.

Indications for performing these images are as follows:

Patients presenting with a history of trauma and clinical suspicion of a fractured mandible

- Two images should be taken at 90 degrees to each other.
- An OPT requires the patient to sit or stand upright. If this is not possible, a lateral oblique film can be taken.
- If a fracture of the condylar neck is suspected, a reverse Townes view can be helpful.
- It is important that all images include the mandible in its entirety.

Pain in the jaw
- If trauma is involved, then an OPT and PA mandible are required.
- If a dentoalveolar infection is suspected, the patient needs an OPT to examine the teeth and bone morphology.
- If the patient has had recent surgery, an OPT is indicated.

Swelling of the jaw
An OPT should be taken to assess the dentition and underlying bone.

Limitation of mouth movement
- If trauma to the TMJ is suspected, an OPT and PA mandible should be used.
- If dislocation is suspected, an OPT must image both the condyle and glenoid fossa.

Altered sensation of the lower lip
OPT.

Fistula/sinus of the skin
OPT is required to image the teeth and underlying bone.

CT/MRI

Not all patients require a CT of their mandible. Indications are generally as follows:
- Imaging complex fractures including the condylar region. With isolated condylar fractures, this may be done as an outpatient.
- Imaging the mandible and soft tissues to identify the source and extent of severe cervicofacial infections (see ➔ Chapter 5).
- Imaging the TMJ for patients with suspected joint arthropathy (usually as an outpatient).
- Imaging bone when osteomyelitis, ORN, or large cystic pathology has been identified on plain films.
- Imaging of suspected tumours (CT or MRI)

Ultrasound

This has a limited role in lower jaw conditions. It is useful in assessing soft tissue swellings surrounding the lower jaw. This would be primarily to differentiate between solid or fluid filled swellings. Ultrasound also has a role in differentiating salivary gland swellings from lymph nodes.

ⓘ Injuries to the lower jaw

The commonest cause of patients presenting with lower jaw symptoms will be from an injury.

Clinical features

Most patients will give a history of blunt injury to the face, the most common mechanism being interpersonal violence. Sports, falls, and accidents are other common causes. Common symptoms include:
- Pain
- Swelling
- Altered bite

- Numbness of the lower lip
- Difficulty in opening and closing of the jaw.

The hallmark of a mandible fracture is a change in the bite (occlusion); however, a normal occlusion does not rule out a mandible fracture.

Other features include:

- Loosened/missing teeth
- Facial deformity
- Mobility across the fracture
- Bleeding from a tear of the overlying gingival tissue
- Sublingual haematoma (Figure 12.1)
- Trismus.

Initial assessment

(See also ➜ Chapter 2.) *Isolated lower jaw trauma can occasionally present as an emergency.*

Airway

Obstruction can be caused by displaced or broken dentures/teeth or severely displaced fractures. The commonest cause is bleeding and/or saliva, especially if the patient is intoxicated or supine. If the patient is supine, quickly decide if he/she can sit up (this is possible in most isolated low-velocity injuries—see ➜ Chapter 4), or if they need full spinal protection. Sitting up will certainly help the airway. Saliva and blood should be cleared by suction. Displaced fractures should be manually reduced if possible and supported. This usually slows the bleeding. Major bleeding is rare, but if ongoing the airway should be protected with a definitive airway.

Bilateral anterior ('bucket handle') or comminuted mandibular fractures can displace allowing the base of the tongue to fall back. *This is*

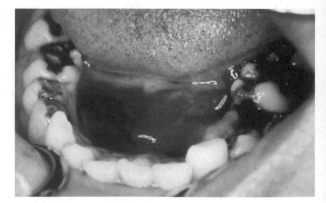

Figure 12.1 Sublingual haematoma.

much more likely when patients are supine with a reduced conscious level. Any obstruction can be initially dealt with by gently pulling the fractured bones forward. This provides only temporary relief and a definitive airway will probably be required. But it may also cause further bleeding.

Bleeding

Bleeding from mandibular fractures although common is not usually life-threatening. If the patient is in shock, look for another cause. *Actively consider facial bleeding, in awake supine patients—they may be swallowing blood.* If bleeding is obvious and significant, it must be controlled during the primary survey. Bleeding from overlying lacerations can be controlled either by pressure or by rapid placement of tacking sutures. These are placed to stem bleeding and are not intended as definitive closure.

① Common fracture patterns

The periosteum is an important structure in maintaining the stability of a mandibular fracture. In young patients it is generally a strong unyielding membrane. Gross displacement of the fractures only occurs after heavy impacts. However, once the periosteum has been torn, displacement of the bones can occur under the influence of the attached muscles. High-energy mandibular fractures therefore tend to be unstable.

Common fracture patterns include those shown in Figure 12.2.

① Angle fractures

Fractures of the angle (wisdom tooth area) can be displaced by the medial pterygoid and masseteric muscles, depending on the fracture orientation (termed 'favourable' or 'unfavourable'). These may pull the posterior fragment lingually, or in an upward direction. This is only important when the periosteum has been torn allowing displacement to occur. See Figures 12.3 and 12.4.

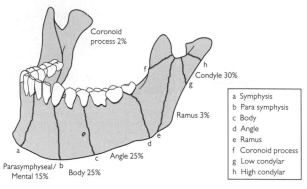

Coronoid process 2%
Condyle 30%
Ramus 3%
Parasymphyseal/ Mental 15%
Body 25%
Angle 25%

a Symphysis
b Para symphysis
c Body
d Angle
e Ramus
f Coronoid process
g Low condylar
h High condylar

Figure 12.2 Common fractures of the lower jaw.

Reproduced with permission from O'Connor I. F. and Urdang M., *Handbook for Surgical Cross-Cover*, Figure 9.7, p. 367, Copyright © 2008 with permission from Oxford University Press.

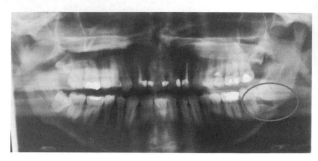

Figure 12.3 OPT showing angle fracture.
Reproduced from *Atlas of Operative Maxillofacial Trauma Surgery: Primary Repair of Facial Injuries*, 'Mandibular Fractures', 2014, Figure 6.32a, eds M. Perry and S. Holmes, Copyright © 2014, Springer-Verlag London. With permission of Springer Nature.

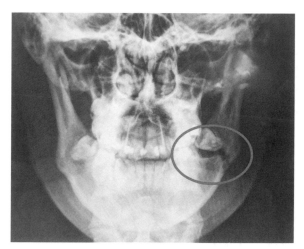

Figure 12.4 PA mandible showing angle fracture.
Reproduced from *Atlas of Operative Maxillofacial Trauma Surgery: Primary Repair of Facial Injuries*, 'Mandibular Fractures', 2014, Figure 6.32b, eds M. Perry and S. Holmes, Copyright © 2014, Springer-Verlag London. With permission of Springer Nature.

ⓘ Fractures at the symphysis and parasymphysis
The mylohyoid muscle passes between the hyoid bone and the inner aspect of the mandible. With midline fractures of the symphysis, the mylohyoid and geniohyoid muscles can act as a stabilizing force. However, oblique fractures will tend to overlap due to the pull of these muscles. With bilateral parasymphyseal fractures (which result from considerable force), the periosteum is often torn and the fragments can displace under the influence of the genioglossus, so-called bucket handle fractures.

ⓘ Condylar fractures
This is a common site of fracture and often occurs in association with fractures elsewhere in the jaw. The classical history is a blow or fall onto the point of the chin, where one or both condyles are fractured, often associated with a symphyseal or parasymphyseal fracture (so-called guardsman's fracture). *Beware the laceration over the chin following a fall—check the condyles carefully. On mouth opening, the jaw deviates towards the site of injury.*

Condylar fractures in adults tend to occur outside the joint space, although the joint can still be damaged with long-term problems. *Effusion or bleeding into the joint space can occur in the absence of a fracture,* the space is distended and the patient complains of an abnormal bite. Intracapsular fractures in children are more common and can result in growth disturbances in the condyle later on. See Figure 12.5.

ⓘ Ramus fractures
These are uncommon and usually follow a direct blow to the side of the face. Check for other fractures (notably the zygomatic arch). Since the ramus is heavily enveloped in muscle the fracture does not displace too much. Treatment is based on the patients bite, not the X-ray appearances.

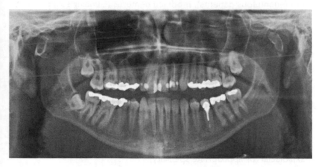

Figure 12.5 OPG showing bilateral fracture dislocations of the condyle.

Reproduced from *Atlas of Operative Maxillofacial Trauma Surgery: Primary Repair of Facial Injuries*, 'Mandibular Fractures', 2014, Figure 6.83, eds M. Perry and S. Holmes, Copyright © 2014, Springer-Verlag London. With permission of Springer Nature.

Management
- ABCs.
- Pain relief is a priority and may be simply achieved by infiltration of local anaesthesia or, if possible, by an inferior dental nerve block.
- Minimize movement across the fracture site. This reduces pain, bleeding, and contamination of the fracture from oral bacteria:
  - A simple method is to apply a soft neck collar but this should only be done after the cervical spine has been formally cleared.
  - If possible, place a bridal wire across the fracture site. This is a loop of wire encircling the teeth either side of the fracture. Care must be taken not to avulse the teeth by over-tightening the wire.
- Any loose dentoalveolar fractures should be splinted.

Non-surgical management
This is possible if the patient is cooperative and has:
- A minimally displaced fracture on imaging
- With no mobility across the fracture line
- No change in occlusion
- No evidence of bleeding or infection.

Treatment involves oral analgesia, antibiotics for 1 week, and a liquid/very soft diet for 4 weeks until a stable callus has formed. Patients still need urgent follow-up but do not need admission.

For painful or more displaced fractures, intermaxillary fixation (IMF) may be applied. The upper and lower teeth are fixed together using wires or elastics. This uses the upper (uninjured) teeth for support and as a guide, to re-establish the bite and immobilize the fracture during healing. Various devices are available to achieve this. Relative contraindications include respiratory disease, the possibility of convulsions, a head injury (GCS score of ≤8), and poor patient cooperation. If the patient has no teeth (edentulous patients), modified dentures (Gunning splints) can be ligated to the jaws to achieve a similar goal. This may be possible in the emergency department, but usually patients need admission or transfer to the appropriate specialty's department for this to be done.

Surgical repair
This is required in displaced or mobile fractures where IMF is not suitable or cannot be undertaken. Surgical exposure of the fracture and anatomical reduction is carried out. The fracture is accurately reduced and fixed using titanium 'mini' plates or screws. This is now the preferred approach to most mandibular fractures, resulting in faster recovery and rehabilitation. However, there is potentially more morbidity, especially injury to the inferior alveolar nerve and tooth roots. The patient still requires a soft diet for the same period of time. Keep the patient fasted and refer to maxillofacial (or appropriate specialty).

⊙ Temporomandibular joint dislocation

TMJ dislocation occurs when the condyle is displaced anteriorly out of its socket, the glenoid fossa, and is prevented from returning to the correct position. It becomes trapped anterior to articular eminence. See Figure 12.6.

Spasm of the powerful masticatory muscles then prevents its relocation. It usually occurs with an audible pop at times of maximal mouth opening, i.e. yawning, or following an injury to the jaw when the mouth is open. Radiographs are not normally required unless there is a history of trauma—to make sure it is not a fracture/dislocation.

The patient will attend with a mouth that is propped open, they cannot close or move the jaw and this will be associated with drooling.

Management

There are many ways to relocate a dislocated jaw. The trick is muscle and patient relaxation (analgesia and sedation). The TMJ is an intrinsically unstable joint and it is the spasm in the powerful masticatory muscles that prevents relocation in many cases. Relocation therefore often requires analgesia and a parenteral short-acting muscle relaxant (e.g. midazolam). Entonox is also a very good drug to use. Local anaesthesia injected directly into the muscles of mastication (both sides) is also very helpful. *Whatever you use, give this plenty of time to take effect.*

The patient is then sat with their back and head resting against a wall. Stand in front and place your thumb(s) inside the patient's mouth, just posterior to the last standing mandibular teeth. Apply downward and

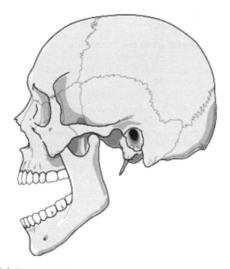

Figure 12.6 TMJ dislocation.

posterior pressure from your thumb(s) and at the same time push up with your fingers on the under surface of the chin. If fully relaxed, the joint(s) should pop back into position and the mouth can fully close.

Be mindful to wrap gauze around your thumbs to avoid trauma when the patient bites down. Once reduced, place a barrel bandage around the patient's head for 30 minutes and monitor closely if parenteral sedative or a muscle relaxant was given.

If this does not work or the jaw immediately dislocates again, refer to maxillofacial for advice.

Patients with dislocation cannot close their wide open mouths. This is a common cause of confusion. If the patient cannot open their mouth or it is only slightly open it is not a dislocation.

ⓘ Infective swellings around the lower jaw and face

General considerations

Acute swellings around the lower jaw are usually due to bacterial infections in the adjacent fascial spaces. These may be localized at first but they can quickly become widespread. *Most often they arise from an underlying dental infection.* However, there are other causes (such as infections of bone cysts, skin lesions, or the salivary glands). Infections localized only to the skin (cellulitis) may also occur. Untreated, some infections can rapidly progress and become life-threatening. Spread of infection depends on the local anatomy, particularly the point of origin of the infection (i.e. which tooth). Virulence of the organism and host resistance are also important factors.

Fascial spaces related to the mandible

The mylohyoid muscle divides the floor of the mouth into two large spaces—the sublingual space above the muscle and the submental and submandibular spaces below it.

Sublingual space

This is a horseshoe-shaped space passing from one side of the floor of the mouth to the other. The superior limit of this space is the tongue and the inferior limit is the mylohyoid. It contains the sublingual glands and the deep lobes of the submandibular glands. It communicates posteriorly with the submandibular spaces. *Swelling here is potentially very serious because of the threat to the airway.* The tissues are delicate and can easily distend, pushing the tongue up and back. Usually infections here are associated with swelling in one or both submandibular spaces. They are almost always due to dental infections. When significant swelling is present, urgent decompression is required.

Submandibular space

This is triangular in shape, bounded above by the mylohyoid muscle (medially) and mandible (laterally), and below by the deep cervical fascia. It contains lymph nodes, the superficial lobe of the submandibular gland, and blood vessels. It communicates with the sublingual space above, the superficial facial space laterally, and the deep pterygoid space and parapharyngeal spaces posteriorly. Surgical access can be made 2–3 cm below the lower border of the mandible. Skin and subcutaneous tissues are incised and sinus forceps are used to penetrate the deep cervical fascia towards the lingual side of the mandible.

Submental space

This is contained by the two anterior bellies of the digastric muscles. Above is the mylohyoid muscle and below is the deep cervical fascia, covered by platysma and skin. It contains submental lymph nodes and communicates with the submandibular space. Surgical access is obtained behind the chin prominence in the neck.

Buccal space

This is a commonly affected space and often presents to casualty as a 'fat face'. Infections can spread into it from both mandibular and maxillary teeth. It is bounded by the buccinator muscle anteromedially, and the masseter muscle posteromedially. Laterally is the deep fascia from the parotid capsule and the overlying platysma. The inferior boundary is the insertion of the deep fascia into the mandible, and its superior boundary the zygomatic arch. Its contents are the buccal fat pad. Posteriorly it is continuous with the pterygoid space. Surgical access is usually obtained from within the mouth. If the abscess points onto the skin, an incision can be made externally, but a scar will result.

Masticator space

This is bounded laterally by the temporalis facia, zygomatic arch, and masseter muscle, and medially by the medial and lateral pterygoid muscles. The temporalis muscle and mandibular ramus further divide this space into superficial and deep compartments. The superficial compartment contains the submasseteric space below and the superficial temporal space above. The deep compartment contains the superficial pterygoid space (or pterygomandibular space) below and the deep temporal space above. The superficial pterygoid space communicates with the deep pterygoid space. The superficial and deep temporal spaces together are also known as the infratemporal fossa space.

☼ Ludwig's angina

This is a rapidly spreading, tense cellulitis of the submandibular, sublingual, and submental spaces bilaterally. When advanced it is an obvious diagnosis, with gross swelling both in the neck and the mouth. Earlier infections still need to be treated seriously and need urgent referral. *Ludwig's angina is a potential airway emergency which if not diagnosed and treated quickly has a mortality rate of around 75% within the first 12–24 hours.* With aggressive surgical intervention, good airway control, and antibiotics this rate has now dropped to 5%.

Usually the cause is a submandibular space infection secondary to an infected wisdom tooth. Other causes include tonsillitis, infected mandibular fractures, and submandibular sialadenitis. From the submandibular space, the infection spreads to the sublingual space around the deep lobe of the submandibular gland. It then passes to the contralateral sublingual space and thence to the other submandibular space. The submental space is also affected by lymphatic spread. Infection can also originate in the sublingual space and spread laterally to both sides. Left untreated, oedema and cellulitis spread backwards in the space between the hypo-glossus and genioglossus to the epiglottis and larynx, resulting eventually in respiratory obstruction.

Clinical features
- Systemic upset.
- Massive firm swelling bilaterally in the neck.
- Swelling in the floor of the mouth, forcing of the tongue up onto the palate.
- A 'hot-potato' voice. This term is used to describe the characteristic pattern of speech, which has been likened to a person speaking with a hot potato in the mouth. It has several causes in addition to Ludwig's angina.
- Difficulty in swallowing and drooling.
- Inability to protrude the tongue.
- Eventually this leads to difficulty breathing.

Management
The first consideration is the airway which can rapidly obstruct. *Difficulty in breathing, swallowing, or talking, and gross swelling are all indications to call for senior help (often anaesthetic) urgently.* Refer to maxillofacial team urgently. Further management includes IV fluids (patients often present after a few days, having not been able to drink), IV antibiotics (e.g. penicillin and metronidazole), together with surgical drainage of the sub-mandibular and sublingual spaces and removal of the underlying cause. If there is respiratory difficulty, give oxygen. These cases are commonly associated with self-neglect (including alcohol and smoking) and immu-nosuppression (e.g. diabetes)

Never underestimate these fascial space infections. They are often referred to as 'dental abscesses' but this terminology will put you, the anaesthetist, and theatre staff, in the wrong state of mind and a lower gear of alertness. Do not underestimate the rapidity with which these infections can come to threaten the airway. If you suspect the airway may potentially be threatened, do not 'wait and see' by treating with antibiotics. Get senior help and consider electively securing the airway with endotracheal intubation before draining the abscess.

Antibiotics alone will not treat these infections. They require incision and drainage.

ⓘ **Acute bacterial submandibular sialadenitis**
The majority of these infections are secondary to a calculus (stone) in the duct. Other causes include surgical scarring or strictures secondary to radiation or other causes of chronic fibrosis. The whole gland swells up and there is malaise, pyrexia, and pain. Submandibular calculi are opaque in 80% of cases, so a radiograph may aid in the diagnosis. Antibiotics are required. If the stone is easily felt in the mouth it can be removed intra-orally. If the infection leads to a collection, then incision and drainage of the submandibular space must be carried out, and the gland removed on an elective basis later. Mumps virus infection involving the submandibular gland is rare but has been reported.

⑦ Chronic submandibular sialadenitis (Kuttner's tumour)

This results from repeated episodes of acute sialadenitis. The structure, parenchyma, and function of the gland are gradually destroyed. The gland ends up feeling very hard to palpation. Treatment is by surgical excision.

① Parotid sialadenitis

Mumps is the commonest cause of parotid swelling, even unilaterally. It has a peak incidence in childhood but can occur in adults. In teenagers, coxsackieviruses and echoviruses can also cause acute sialadenitis. Clinically there is pyrexia and malaise. Pain is the most striking symptom. There is diffuse swelling of the gland over the ramus, which raises the lobe of the ear, and often trismus. Treatment is supportive

'Ascending' infection, i.e. bacteria in saliva passing back along the ducts into the glands, can involve the parotid (and submandibular) glands. In such cases, predisposing conditions are often associated, e.g. dehydration, diabetes, or immunosuppression. Fibrosis following radiotherapy or pre-existing obstruction from a calculus or stricture may also predispose to infection.

Clinical features
- Fever
- Pain
- Erythema
- Tender swelling
- Discharge of pus from the duct.

If the infection is not treated early, this may develop into a chronic or recurrent infection. Progressive destruction of the gland aggravates the situation, resulting in a non-functional gland.

Management

In the absence of an obvious abscess, management initially consists of IV antibiotics, rehydration, analgesia, and correction of any systemic conditions, e.g. diabetes. If an obstruction is found, e.g. stone, this needs to be removed to enable drainage. Gland massage, especially after meals, and 'lemon drops' to stimulate salivary flow, help to maintain a flushing effect and prevent stagnation of saliva. Abscesses need to be incised and drained on an urgent basis. If infection persists or continues to recur, excision of the gland may be necessary. This is best done when there is no active infection.

① Cellulitis

Spreading infection within the skin (cellulitis) is characterized by swelling, warmth, erythema, and pain. The patient may present with minimal signs initially, or they may be unwell with malaise, fatigue, chills, or a fever. Regional lymphadenopathy may also be present. Cellulitis around the lower jaw and face may be a presenting sign of an underlying deeper infection. These include:
- Dental infection (tooth or cyst)
- Skin cyst (e.g. sebaceous) infection
- Infected laceration with or without a retained foreign body

- Infected lymph node (usually cellulitis is in the neck)
- Submandibular infection
- Untreated fracture.

In the absence of these, inflammation is confined initially to the deeper dermis and subcutaneous tissue resulting in an ill-defined red rash. Untreated this can progress to sepsis, abscess formation, or necrotizing fasciitis. The most common infecting organisms in cellulitis are group A *Streptococcus* followed by *Staphylococcus aureus*. These gain access to the dermis through a break in the skin (e.g. during shaving).

Management

Flucloxacillin has become a mainstay of treatment due to its bactericidal effect on both commonly occurring organisms. Benzylpenicillin is particularly affective against streptococci and is also commonly prescribed. In immunocompromised individuals and children, a wider variety of bacteria may be implicated and a broader spectrum of antibiotic cover may be necessary. Oral antibiotics are sufficient for mild disease; more severe cases need admission for IV antibiotics.

Treat cellulitis in the head and neck carefully. This can rapidly deteriorate resulting in abscess formation and necrotizing fasciitis. Always consider an underlying cause (often dental infections) and the possibility of immunocompromise (diabetes and alcohol abuse especially).

① Infected mandibular fracture

Severe infection of a mandibular fracture resulting in osteomyelitis is rare. However, localized infection still happens relatively frequently, particularly when patients have poor oral hygiene, smoke, and present late. Debilitated patients, diabetics, and patients on steroids or chemotherapy are more likely to develop infected fractures because of lowered general resistance. Commonly, these occur at the angle of the mandible, where the patient has retained third molars (wisdom teeth). Comminuted fractures of the mandible may be complicated by the formation of bone sequestra which become a potential source of infection. In some cases the sequestra may extrude spontaneously into the mouth with quite minimal symptoms, but sometimes a localized abscess forms and surgical removal of the dead bone becomes necessary. Infected fractures need urgent referral. Management involves antibiotics and stabilization of the fracture.

① Osteomyelitis

Osteomyelitis of the jaws is uncommon and most commonly associated with odontogenic infection (infections of the teeth). It can occur following extractions, trauma, or irradiation to the mandible. It can also occur in patients taking bisphosphonates (BRONJ). Infection is more common in the lower jaw, as the upper jaw has a relatively better blood supply. Before the antibiotic era, however, it was frequently fatal. Acute osteomyelitis is less common than chronic osteomyelitis, with patients rarely presenting with obvious suppuration. A small amount of pus exuding from around a tooth is more likely to be a periodontal abscess, but *if multiple adjacent teeth are involved, mobile, and the overlying soft tissue are inflamed, there is probably acute osteomyelitis* (see Figure 12.7).

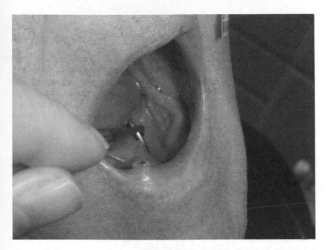

Figure 12.7 Osteomyelitis of the mandible.

Clinical features

These depend upon the type and extent of infection and may include:

- Pain—In acute osteomyelitis, this can be severe, throbbing, and deep seated. Chronic infection has a less intense but still deep-seated and unremitting character.
- Swelling, erythema, and tenderness. Initially soft, the swelling is secondary to inflammation and oedema. This may later progress to a firm subperiosteal abscess.
- Trismus.
- Dysphagia.
- Cervical lymphadenopathy.
- Numbness of the lower lip and jaw.
- Halitosis.
- Pyrexia, anorexia, and malaise.
- Friable granulation tissue, exposed necrotic bone, and sequestrum formation are all common in chronic infection. *It is important to make sure these features are not those of a malignancy.*

Usually there is an obvious cause such as a decayed tooth. This may be tender and mobile. Most patients are either malnourished or immune deficient to some extent. This condition is therefore commonly seen in smokers, diabetics, and alcoholics as well as other well-known at-risk groups.

The infection is usually a polymicrobial in nature. It is caused by a mixture of streptococci and anaerobic bacteria, which pass into the bones from the infected tooth. Haematogenous spread is rare. Osteomyelitis may also arise in an infected fracture. This tends to be chronic. Smokers are at particularly high risk of this. *Actinomycosis* is an unusual but specific infection, also known to occur. This results in recurrent and chronic jaw abscesses. These can discharge large amounts of pus, frequently through multiple skin sinuses, which often contains characteristically appearing bright yellow granules (referred to as 'sulphur granules'). *Consider actinomycosis in any patient with chronic bone abscesses and discharging sinuses.*

Management

Acute osteomyelitis needs urgent referral for admission, IV antibiotics, and drainage of pus. Chronic osteomyelitis may be managed as an outpatient with appropriate long-term antibiotics. If so, close follow-up is required. Any associated contributing factors should also be identified and treated if possible. Surgical debridement may be required.

ⓘ Infected branchial cyst

(See ➔ Chapter 5.) Most branchial cysts present in the neck and are painless, but they may become infected and involve the upper part of the lateral neck/parotid region. These are difficult to treat and recurrence is common. If infected, refer urgently.

ⓘ Infected bone cysts

These can present in a number of ways:
- Chronic jaw pain, with or without swelling
- Chronic swelling, with or without pain
- Acute fascial space infection
- Cellulitis
- Halitosis
- Pathological fracture.

In most cases, the presence of the cyst is not apparent until plain films have been taken, although some cysts may pour pus into the oral cavity on examination, suggesting the presence of a large cavity. Management may be the same as for fascial space infections, depending on the severity of symptoms. Refer urgently if systemic symptoms are present or the cyst is large.

ⓘ Non-infective swellings around the lower jaw and face

ⓘ Osteoradionecrosis

The lower jaw is particularly susceptible to ORN due to its low vascularity and greater bone density. The clinical spectrum of presentation is wide. Patients usually have a non-resolving painful mucosal ulcer with evidence of exposed bone or sequestrum. This is usually in the posterior mandibular region. There may be trismus and this usually appears 3–6 months following radiotherapy. See Figure 12.8.

At the other end of the spectrum, patients may present with an orocutaneous fistula, pathological fracture, and paraesthesia of the inferior alveolar nerve. Typically radiological appearances will include a moth eaten appearance of the bone. Management principles are based on controlling any acute superimposed infection, strict oral hygiene, analgesia, and nutritional support as well as minimal surgical debridement. In severe cases resection of the bone and reconstruction with a free tissue transfer may be required.

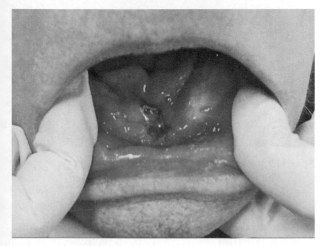

Figure 12.8 ORN of the mandible.

⑦ Bisphosphonate-related osteonecrosis of the jaw (BRONJ)

Bisphosphonates inhibit osteoclastic action and reduce bone loss in patients with multiple myeloma, bony metastasis in breast cancer, Paget's disease of bone, and postmenopausal osteoporosis. However, osteonecrosis can occur as a serious side effect in both jaws. Patients present with pain and swelling affecting the mucosa of the jaw, which may be confused with chronic osteomyelitis, ORN or even malignancy. See Figure 12.9.

CT usually shows regions of mottled bone and sequestrum formation. Treatment usually involves meticulous oral hygiene, antibiotics and gentle debridement. Cessation of the drug, if not contraindicated may help some recovery.

⑦ Paget's disease

Paget's disease is a localized disorder of bone remodelling that typically begins with excessive bone resorption followed by an increase in bone formation. Usually the bone is mechanically weaker, larger, less compact, more vascular, and more susceptible to fracture than normal adult lamellar bone. Although rare for the maxilla to be involved, when it is, patients can present with bone pain associated with marked deformity. Clinical examination may reveal excessive warmth, due to hypervascularity and paraesthesia of the infraorbital nerve due to bony compression. These symptoms may be confused with chronic infection or a tumour.

⑦ Fibrous dysplasia

This is a disorder of bone growth where normal bone is replaced with immature fibrous bone. It can occur in any part of the skeleton but the skull and face are commonly involved. Patients present with a smooth

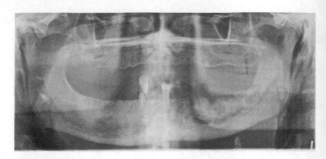

Figure 12.9 BRONJ.

hard swelling and deformity usually in childhood or early adulthood. During rapid growth this may become painful. Two types of Fibrous dysplasia are described.
• Monostotic—involving a single bone, or adjacent bones, such as the upper and lower jaw
• Polyostotic—involving many bones.

The most severe form of polyostotic fibrous dysplasia is known as McCune–Albright syndrome, which includes endocrine diseases (precocious puberty) and skin pigmentation. Fibrous dysplasia may also be associated with neurofibromatosis. The condition is said to burn itself out during puberty but exceptions are well known. Management include bisphosphonates and surgical contouring of and cosmetic deformity.

⑦ Odontogenic myxoma
Odontogenic myxomas are uncommon benign odontogenic tumours arising from embryonic connective tissue associated with tooth formation. It usually occurs in younger patients (10–35 years old). The lower jaw is most commonly involved. Patients generally notice a painless, slow growth in the jaw, sometimes with tooth loosening or displacement. As the tumour expands, it frequently infiltrates adjacent structures and posterior lesions are associated with infiltration of the ramus.

⑦ Mandibular tori
These will rarely present as an emergency. Tori are painless, bilateral bony growths present on the inner aspect of the mandible, usually in the premolar region. In some patients they can grow to the size of a walnut. They have normal overlying mucosa. They are usually an incidental finding in patients with parafunctional habits, but are sometime referred as a 'lump in the jaw' particularly in edentulous patients where they are more noticeable.

⑦ Haemangiomas
Central haemangiomas within the mandible are extremely rare. They arise from a proliferation of vessels within the medullary cavity. They usually present as a painless, firm swelling that can be associated with a subjective sensation of pulsation. They can be locally destructive because of pressure effects and can cause mobility of surrounding teeth.

⑦ Cystic lesions/tumours

(See ➲ Chapter 11.) *The differential diagnosis for any large 'cyst' or cavity in the bone must include AVM. Although rare, these can lead to torrential haemorrhage if breached (i.e. during a dental extraction). Contrast imaging may be required.*

⑦ Temporomandibular joint dysfunction syndrome

This is a controversial topic. TMJDS is a collective term used to describe a number of related conditions affecting the joints, muscles of mastication, and associated structures. These all result in common symptoms such as pain and limited mouth opening. No single condition has been found to cause it. Although up to 70% of the general population may have at least one clinical feature of this disorder, only about 5% will actually seek treatment. Females outnumber males by at least four to one. Patients most commonly present in early adulthood. Temporomandibular dysfunction is not always progressive or destructive. It is a complex disorder involving many interacting factors including stress, anxiety, and depression. Non-surgical treatments, such as counselling, pharmacotherapy, and occlusal splint therapy, continue to be the most effective way of managing >80% of patients.

Three common temporomandibular disorders are myofascial pain and dysfunction, internal derangement, and osteoarthrosis:

• Myofascial pain and dysfunction are by far the commonest. This is primarily a muscular problem resulting from 'parafunctional' habits, such as clenching or bruxism (grinding teeth). Stress, anxiety, and depression are commonly associated.
• Internal derangement describes a disorder in which the articular disc is in an abnormal position, resulting in mechanical interference and restriction of movement. Disc problems can result in both limitation of mouth opening and clicking/crepitus.
• Osteoarthrosis is a localized degenerative disorder that affects mainly the articular cartilage of the joint. Usually in older age groups.

Applied anatomy

The TMJ is a synovial 'ball and socket' type joint. A fibrous sleeve encapsulates the joint. Between the condyle and fossa there is a fibrocartilaginous disc, or 'meniscus'. The muscles of mastication act directly across the TMJ to effect mandibular movements. Of note, the insertion of the lateral pterygoid is into both the condylar neck and the anterior aspect of the disc. Joint movement is complex. On opening the mouth from the closed position, there is initially a hinge-type movement for the first 1 cm. After that a forward translation is added in which the condyle moves forwards and downwards along the slope of the eminence. Very little movement occurs side to side.

Aetiology

Various aetiological factors have been suggested, but in reality it is likely that the condition is multifactorial:

* Parafunction, such as tooth clenching and grinding (often subconsciously or during sleep), or abnormal movements of the jaw (e.g. a swing from left to right, reversed on closing—'chewing the cud'). Such movements often exert unbalanced loads on the joints, resulting in painful muscle spasm.
* Occlusal anomalies are a common feature and there may be a higher frequency of TMJ problems in patients with heavily restored dentitions. However, there are also plenty of patients who have abnormal bites yet do not have any TMJ symptoms.
* Poorly fitting dentures can contribute to TMJ dysfunction. Over closure of the jaws when the back teeth/dentures are severely worn down (loss of posterior support) can put a strain on the joints.
* Trauma either directly from a blow, or indirectly from stretching (e.g. for dental treatment) may cause tears or adhesions around the disc, or a synovitis resulting in pain and altered function.
* Stressful life events and impaired coping mechanisms are more frequent in patients with TMJ dysfunction, compared to non-affected control patients. Anxiety neuroses and affective disorders (particularly depression) are more common. These psychogenic factors are often considered as exacerbating factors, rather than the primary cause of temporomandibular disorders.

Management

This is difficult and controversial. Most patients do not need to be referred and can be treated by their own doctor or dentist. Treatment options include:

* Physiotherapy and jaw exercises.
* Psychosocial and behavioural interventions (such as biofeedback techniques, cognitive behavioural therapy, hypnosis, and relaxation techniques). Reassurance plays an important role in management.
* Occlusal splints (bite plates, bite raising, or intraoral appliances) are made of acrylic and can be hard or soft. They are designed to fit over the upper or the lower teeth. Normally splints are worn during sleep.
* Medications include analgesics, benzodiazepines, and muscle relaxants.
* Botulinum toxin solution (Botox®).
* Occlusal adjustment.
* In selected cases where the joint is damaged, surgery may be indicated (arthrocentesis, arthroscopy, menisectomy, disc repositioning, condylotomy or joint replacement).

⑦ Clicking joints

The commonest cause of a clicking joint is internal derangement. This is managed initially as for TMJDS. Osteochondral loose bodies are uncommon, but should be considered if symptoms are severe or persist. Common clinical features are pain, swelling, joint noise, and sudden onset of impaired joint movements ('locking'). Exclude any history of trauma. In the absence of fractures these patients require outpatient follow-up for imaging (CT/MRI) to confirm the presence of a loose body. This will need to be removed.

⑦ Limitation of mouth opening

Inability to fully open the mouth has many causes, some of which are serious. This may present acutely and is often misdiagnosed as a 'dislocated jaw'. However, in a dislocation the problem is one of closing—the mouth is typically wide open. *'Trismus' is a specific term.* It refers to reduced opening of the jaws caused by spasm of the muscles of mastication. This implies specific pathologies, the commonest being trauma, infection or a tumour.

Normal mouth opening ranges from 35 to 45 mm.

Causes of limitation of mouth opening

These include:

- Trismus (notably trauma, infection, or tumour)
- 'Internal derangement' of the TMJ (meniscus displacement or 'locking')
- Trauma (including an untreated depressed zygomatic arch fracture)
- Infection within and around the joint (notably parotid)
- Osteoarthritis and other types of arthritis (e.g. rheumatoid)
- Ankylosis and osteophyte formation
- Myofascial pain/TMJDS
- Radiation fibrosis
- Submucous fibrosis
- Systemic sclerosis
- Myositis ossificans
- Coronoid hyperplasia
- Psychiatric causes.

Assessment

The history may give some indication of the cause. Differentiate between painless and painful restriction. Plain films, CT, or MRI may be required depending on the suspected cause.

The important thing is not to miss an occult tumour—examine the oropharynx carefully (especially the 'coffin corner'—the deep recess between the side of the tongue and wisdom teeth).

⑦ Closed lock

The TMJ contains an articular disc which overlies the condylar head and prevents direct contact between it and the glenoid fossa. The disc can sometimes displace anterior to the condyle and become trapped between it and articular eminence. If this occurs it can prevent free movement of the condyle during mouth opening. This is usually an acute event but patients may give a history of preceding joint symptoms. This condition may require outpatient referral to maxillofacial if patients have significant pain.

⑦ TMJ ankylosis

True joint ankylosis is unlikely to present acutely. This progressive destructive arthropathy results in loss of joint space and fusion of the condylar articular surface to the glenoid fossa. It usually occurs following untreated fractures of the condyle, or middle ear infections in childhood and is therefore uncommon in the developed world. Imaging of the

TMJ (OPT) will demonstrate gross irregularity of the joint and loss of joint space. In children, severe ankylosis can result in asymmetric facial growth. This requires an outpatient referral.

⑦ Radiotherapy-induced fibrosis

This arises following radiotherapy where the irradiated fields include the TMJ or muscles of mastication. Radiotherapy to the muscles results in atrophy and fibrosis of the muscle fibres. Onset is often gradual, usually noticeable 8–12 weeks after completion of treatment. However, it can continue to develop. Without intervention, mouth opening can be reduced by up to a third after several years. Studies have demonstrated that nearly half of all patients who receive curative intent radiotherapy to the head and neck will experience some limitation of opening.

⑦ Oral submucous fibrosis

Oral submucous fibrosis is a chronic debilitating disease of the oral cavity characterized by inflammation and progressive fibrosis of the submucosal tissues. It causes progressive limitation of opening which if untreated can progress to total inability to open the mouth. The buccal mucosa is the most commonly involved site, but any part of the oral cavity can be involved, including the pharynx. The condition is well recognized for its malignant potential and is particularly associated with areca nut chewing, the main component of betel quid. It is usually associated with a marbled appearance of the buccal mucosa and the presence of taut palpable fibrous bands within it.

⑦ Myositis ossificans

This is heterotopic calcification of muscle. There are two forms:
- Myositis ossificans is when calcification occurs within an injured muscle.
- Myositis ossificans progressiva (also referred to as fibrodysplasia ossificans progressiva) is a condition in which ossification can occur without injury. It is inherited.

Imaging will show hazy densities approximately 1 month after injury, and denser opacities at 2 months. Treatment is usually conservative (NSAIDs and physiotherapy). Surgical removal of the myositis ossificans is rarely required.

⑦ Coronoid hyperplasia

This is a condition of unknown aetiology but is seen in association with submucous fibrosis and TMJ ankylosis. As elongation of the coronoid process occurs, it results in progressive limitation of opening from impingement on the under-surface of the zygoma and its arch. In severe cases, the coronoid can be excised.

Trismus

This is an important sign and should always be taken seriously, especially in infections. Trismus is limitation in mouth opening due to muscle spasm. Most commonly, the spasm is in the masseter muscle, but it can occur in the medial pterygoid or temporalis muscles. It is a marker indicating that any infection is advanced and it is often taken as a sign that the patient needs admission. Untreated infection will rapidly progress, eventually resulting in dysphagia and potential airway problems. *Anaesthetists need to be aware of any trismus if the patient is going to theatre*, as fibreoptic intubation is required.

Trismus can be graded 35–40 mm normal. Mild opening 30–35 mm, moderate 15–30 mm, and severe <15 mm.

Causes of trismus

Most causes can be considered under the headings of *infection, trauma, and tumour*. If you remember these three pathologies you won't overlook serious conditions:

- Muscle spasm (following injury/infection)
- Post-surgical oedema (especially following removal of wisdom teeth)
- Recent dental treatment
- Following an inferior alveolar nerve block (usually from a haematoma in the medial pterygoid)
- Dental infections/pericoronitis/submasseteric abscess
- Peritonsillar abscess
- Cerebrovascular accident/brain injury
- Acute parotitis (e.g. mumps)
- Tetanus
- Malignancy (intraoral and extraoral).

The most common causes will be trauma and abscesses which cause spasm of the medial pterygoid. Following injury there does not have to be a fracture. Occasionally a displaced fracture of the zygomatic arch may impinge on the movement of the coronoid process and prevent normal opening. This is not trismus, but it still requires treatment.

⑦ Oral surgery procedures

Removal of the lower molar teeth may cause trismus as a result of inflammation in the muscles of mastication, direct trauma to the masticatory apparatus, or postoperative infection. Infections require antibiotics. Following this, heat therapy, analgesics, a soft diet, and gentle jaw exercises should eventually resolve the remaining symptoms.

① Inferior alveolar nerve injections

Medial pterygoid haematoma can occur following a dental injection to anaesthetize the inferior alveolar nerve. These patients will present with progressive trismus within a few days of undergoing dental treatment. Be mindful of the possibility of secondary infection. A simple haematoma is managed by prescribing NSAIDs and starting the patient on gentle jaw stretching exercises. If infection is suspected, commence antibiotics and avoid exercises. Refer severe limitation or infections to maxillofacial.

ⓘ Peritonsillar abscesses (quinsy)

(See also ➔ Chapter 8.) These are common infections arising when infection of the tonsil spreads to the surrounding tissue. As the peritonsillar abscess increases in size it is often associated with trismus resulting from spasm of the medial pterygoid muscle. Often they can be drained in the emergency department but if they threaten the airway, general anaesthesia is required.

ⓘ Neurological causes of spasticity of the muscles of mastication

Cerebrovascular accident and traumatic brain injury may result in severe trismus secondary to masseter spasticity. Many patients with severe neurological injury undergo PEG placement secondary to severe masseter spasticity. Botulinum toxin may be effective in reducing this type of trismus.

☼ Tetanus-induced trismus

Tetanus toxin, the product of *Clostridium tetani*, causes muscle rigidity and spasms. This results in trismus, dysphagia, opisthotonos (severe hyperextension and spasticity), and spasms of respiratory and laryngeal muscles. Treatment is with tetanus immunoglobulin, IV antibiotics, and muscle relaxants. Patients may need intubation.

ⓘ Oropharyngeal cancer

(See ➔ Chapter 13.) Oral cancer typically presents as a non-healing ulcer, with raised rolled edges. Although they can occur anywhere in the mouth, the most common locations are the floor of mouth and posterolateral tongue. The patient may have a history of risk factors, including smoking and alcohol. *Any ulcer which is progressively enlarging, and persists >2 weeks, should be referred for urgent biopsy to exclude dysplasia or malignancy.* Management involves further imaging to determine whether there is regional lymph node involvement or distant spread. Following review at a head and neck multidisciplinary team meeting, treatment may be curative or palliative, involving surgery, chemotherapy, and radiotherapy.

Any cancer infiltrating into the muscles of mastication (skin, parotid, sarcoma) can result in trismus.

ⓘ Bleeding from the lower jaw (non-traumatic)

(See also ➔ Chapter 13.) Bleeding from the gums and the mouth in general can be a common symptom. The commonest cause is local inflammation caused by inadequate tooth-brushing—'gingivitis'. However, gingival bleeding may be a marker of an underlying systemic disease and recognition of this fact is important for early diagnosis and management. Certain medical conditions and drugs are known to affect the gingivae. Where oral hygiene is very good consider these other causes. Rare causes include vitamin K deficiency and scurvy.

⑦ Dental causes
Often the cause of bleeding gums is obvious and easily treated. Treatment of infection involves removing the cause—either plaque in the case of gingivitis, or treatment of a dental infection (root canal therapy, extraction). The patient's dentist can treat and advise on oral hygiene/arrange for the patient to see a hygienist.

⑦ Pregnancy
The hormonal changes that are associated with pregnancy will reverse following delivery, but during the pregnancy excellent oral hygiene should be maintained. Local gingival bleeding may also be associated with a pregnancy epulis. This may need to be surgically removed if troublesome, although they usually regress after delivery.

① Drugs
Drug-related gingival bleeding must be managed in close association with the physician who prescribed the medication. Simply stopping any drug thought to be the cause of bleeding may have adverse effects that are potentially far worse for the patient. The degree of urgency in altering a prescription is related to the severity of gingival bleeding as well as the presence of bleeding from other sites (e.g. nasal mucosa and GI tract). In the case of some drugs, immediate reversal is possible (e.g. warfarin), whereas for others it is not.

① Idiopathic thrombocytopenic purpura
This is thought to be an autoimmune disorder and probably the most common cause of thrombocytopenia. Close liaison with a haematologist is essential. Regional local anaesthetic blocks may be contra-indicated if the platelet count is $<30 \times 10^9/L$. The vast majority of cases can be adequately managed by the administration of corticosteroids. If a major surgical procedure is required, platelet transfusions and/or the use of immunoglobulins may be necessary.

① Leukaemia
It is not uncommon for leukaemias, especially the acute types, to present with oral signs and symptoms. These include:
- Bleeding gums—a hyperplastic gingivitis (red, spongy, fragile gums), which bleed spontaneously.
- Infection—the gingivae are highly susceptible to infection. Secondary acute ulcerative gingivitis may be seen.
- Localized masses of leukaemic infiltrates.
- Candida/herpes simplex virus.

① Bleeding dyscrasias
Occasionally persistent bleeding following minor injuries is the presenting sign of an underlying clotting disorder such as haemophilia. Bleeding sockets following dental extractions are rarely life-threatening. However, in the presence of significant co-morbid disease (e.g. in the elderly with poor cardiovascular reserve), a continually bleeding socket may quickly become a problem. You will need to decide whether it is sufficient to simply deal with the local problem, or whether it is necessary to investigate further.

Management of bleeding sockets
Most cases need only simple reassurance and getting the patient to bite firmly on a clean handkerchief or gauze swab placed over the wound for at least 20 minutes. In the vast majority of cases bleeding settles and no further action is required other than care of the airway, if necessary using gentle suction. If bleeding persists, rinse the mouth out to clear any clots and look for the bleeding site. Depending on where the problem is this can be dealt with by further suturing or packing the wound with a haemostatic dressing, such as Surgicel®. Other measures include antifibrinolytic agents, such as tranexamic acid. Patients rarely need to go to theatre. If all else fails, patients need to be admitted for bed rest and investigations for bleeding disorders or liver disease.

⊙ Oropharyngeal cancer

(See ➲ Chapter 13.) Oral cancer is described elsewhere. Ulcers can occasionally bleed. Tumours invading bone can present with bleeding. Bleeding from the throat is a poor prognostic sign, indicating a deeply invasive cancer. These all need urgent referral.

⊙ Cutaneous sinuses and fistulae overlying the lower jaw

A sinus is an abnormal, blind-ending tract, opening onto an epithelial surface. This is not restricted to skin only, but includes any epithelial surface, including mucosa (mouth, pharynx, anus, rectum, vagina, etc.), intestinal epithelium, bronchial epithelium, bladder epithelium, and so on. *A fistula is an abnormal communication between two such epithelial surfaces.* In the lower jaw the two most common causes of these are infection and tumour. Causes include:

• Dental abscesses
• Chronically infected dental root
• Chronic osteomyelitis
• ORN
• BRONJ
• Foreign body in the skin
• Ingrowing hair
• Infected osteosynthesis plate
• Necrotic lymph node
• Underlying tumour
• Furuncles and carbuncles
• Jaw cysts.

See Figures 12.10 and 12.11.
Clinically a sinus on the skin appears as a small opening, sometimes with surrounding induration. There is often a chronic discharge of pus from the sinus. A fistula may occur if the abscess drains both intra-orally and onto the skin. A microbiological swab should be taken from any discharge. If there is no obvious dental or jaw pathology, consider *actinomycosis*. Clinically, this is presents as 'sulphur granules' discharging onto the skin, although they are not always present.

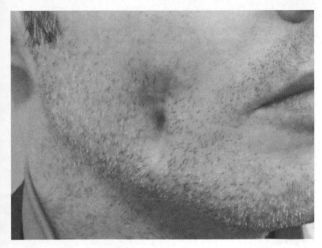

Figure 12.10 Beware discharging sinuses of the lower face—consider dental causes.

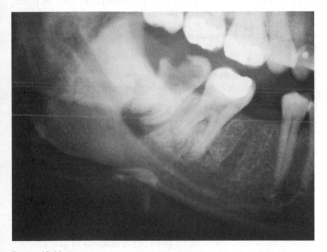

Figure 12.11 The cause of the sinus in Figure 12.10 was an infected tooth.

Management

The treatment of a sinus is primarily the elimination of the underlying condition. A specimen should always be sent for histopathology.

Don't just excise sinuses on the face. They will probably recur. Try to find the underlying cause (often dental). Consider also Actinomyces infection.

Pain in the lower jaw

⑦TMJDS

This is described elsewhere in this chapter (see ➲ 'Temporomandibular joint dysfunction syndrome', pp. 375–6). A common cause of pain.

⑦Toothache

Odontalgia

This is a short-lasting diffuse pain due to exposed dentine that is provoked by local stimuli (hot, cold, touch). The pain can be sharp or dull and is usually mild to moderate in intensity, lasting less than a second to minutes. Treatment is usually with a dressing or restoration and simple analgesics.

Pulpitis

This is a pain due to inflammation of the dental pulp provoked by local stimuli. It can vary from a sharp, poorly localized, dull ache, to throbbing pain which can be severe. Pain can last minutes or hours, with episodes that may continue for several days. Treatment requires removal of the pulp or extraction of the tooth and analgesics (e.g. NSAIDs and paracetamol).

Periapical periodontitis and abscess

These cause severe throbbing pain arising from the periodontal tissues. It is a continuous, well-localized, mild to intense aching.

①Atypical odontalgia

This is a severe throbbing pain in the tooth and jaw without major pathology. Often described as a severe continuous throbbing pain, it may vary from mild to intense pain, especially with hot or cold stimuli. It may be widespread or well localized and may move from tooth to tooth. It may last a few minutes to several hours. This is often a symptom of hypochondriacal psychosis or depression and there is often excessive concern with oral hygiene. Counselling, avoidance of unnecessary dental treatments or extractions, and sometimes antidepressants are required.

⑦Postoperative pain

For these patients prevention is better than cure. NSAIDs are good for relieving bone pain. They may be given perioperatively as 'pre-emptive' analgesia and then continued postoperatively to minimize discomfort. Short-acting opioids, such as IV fentanyl, are commonly used for perioperative analgesia. Many analgesic regimens exist.

ⓘ Dry socket

This is localized inflammation of the cortical bone of a socket following dental extraction, most commonly the lower wisdom teeth. Typically, the patient complains of severe dull throbbing pain, around 4–5 days after surgery and often has a bad taste in the mouth. Pain is often exquisite, with inflammation, exposed bone and halitosis. They are multiple predisposing factors:

- Mandibular extractions
- Difficult extraction
- Pre-existing infection
- Poor blood supply (e.g. Paget's disease, following radiotherapy)
- Smoking—nicotine is a vasoconstrictor
- Systemic disorders (e.g. diabetes)
- Oral contraceptives.

Management

The socket is irrigated with warm saline. It is then dressed with an anti-septic pack, e.g. Alvogyl®. This contains iodoform (antiseptic), eugonal (sedative), and seaweed (for bulk)—this is resorbed as healing occurs. Antibiotics may be necessary.

ⓘ Herpes zoster (shingles)

This is an acute herpetic infection in any dermatome, commonly the fifth (V) cranial nerve. Involvement of the lower jaw is unusual but can occur. It presents with burning and tingling pain in the skin with eruptions on the lower lip. Post-herpetic neuralgia is chronic pain with skin changes following acute herpes zoster. There may be a burning sensation or itching and crawling dysaesthesias in skin. In the acute phase, stellate ganglion blocks using local anaesthetic such as bupivacaine, may help for severe pain. Transcutaneous nerve stimulation (TENS), capsaicin cream, and tricyclic antidepressants are also useful.

ⓘ Trigeminal neuralgia ('tic douloureux')

Trigeminal neuralgia is most commonly a disorder seen in middle-aged and elderly patients. It is more common in women with a peak incidence between 50 and 60 years of age. *In young patients it may be an early feature of MS, HIV disease, or as a consequence of a lesion irritating the trigeminal nerve.* Patients complain of a sharp, intense, lancing/'electric-type' pain induced by a specific trigger point that radiates across the distribution of a branch of the trigeminal nerve. The pain is almost always unilateral, with over 30–40% of patients showing a distribution affecting both the maxillary and mandibular divisions. In approximately 20% of patients, the pain is confined to the mandibular division, and the ophthalmic division in 3%. Episodes may last up to several hours. The aetiology of trigeminal neuralgia is presumed to be multifactorial, with local nerve microcompression within the skull base and possible demyelination.

Management

- Always consider skull base pathology and intracranial disease/ demyelination. Imaging may be required.
- The mainstay of treatment remains medical, typically with anticonvulsant agents. Usually, trigeminal neuralgia responds well to carbamazepine and/or amitriptyline, and a muscle relaxant such as

baclofen. Carbamazepine remains the drug of choice with an initial regime of 100 mg three times daily being gradually increased to a maximum of 1200 mg daily titrated against effect. 20% of patients may develop side effects such as tremor, dizziness, double vision, and vomiting, which will obviously limit its use. They should have regular monitoring of FBC, electrolytes, and LFTs. Approximately 20% can develop folic acid deficiency with megaloblastic anaemia, and hyponatraemia in the elderly. Withdraw therapy slowly.

- Alternative agents include phenytoin, sodium valproate, lamotrigine, and baclofen.
- Local surgical procedures may be considered in trigeminal neuralgia not responsive to medical management. This can include cryotherapy to the nerve, alcohol/glycerol injections.
- Neurosurgical decompression in severe cases following imaging confirming there is nerve compression.
- Gamma Knife® (stereotactic radiosurgery). High-resolution imaging provides excellent definition and allows a focus beam of ionizing radiation to irradiate the proximal trigeminal nerve at its entry into the pons. Results are very promising (see http://www.gammaknife.org.uk).

ⓘ Atypical facial pain

Atypical facial pain has many distinguishing features that make it a clinical entity in its own right and not just a 'catch all' diagnosis for seemingly unexplained facial pains. It is, however, *essentially a diagnosis of exclusion that should only be made after all other possible organic causes have been excluded.* These patients therefore often undergo extensive investigation.

Clinical features

Patients often have a 'flat affect' and the more they are questioned about the pain, the more vague their answers become. The pain is typically described as being a deep, dull ache, sometimes fluctuating, sometimes continuous, with intermittent severe episodes that the patient can find no causative factor for. Often the pain has been present for several years and analgesics rarely affect its nature. It is most commonly bilateral, but ill defined, and its distribution cannot be explained on an anatomical basis. The patient may say they are kept from sleeping by the pain but usually look well rested. When they do admit to sleeping, the pain does not wake them. A proportion of these patients may show symptoms of depressive illness or anxiety states, and patients often complain of other symptoms such as back and neck pain and irritable bowel syndrome. The patient's mood often does not correlate to the description of their symptoms and they may show exaggerated responses to examination and report stressful life events.

Management

Often the ill-defined nature of the patient's pain results in unnecessary dental work being carried out. In light of the association of atypical facial pain with the neuroses (particularly depression), and the belief that it essentially has a psychogenic basis, emphasis has been placed on the use of antidepressant agents as the main treatment option:

- Dothiepin, a tricyclic antidepressant, has been shown to be effective in reducing the painful symptoms (as it has in TMJDS).
- Selective serotonin re-uptake inhibitors (SSRIs).

Salivary gland pathology

Salivary gland pathology can either be obstructive, infective, or neoplastic in origin. Regardless of the origin of the pathology salivary gland disease can present with swelling and pain around the lower jaw. This pain can mimic jaw pain because of the intimate relationship of the major salivary glands to the mandible.

⑦ Cystic lesions of the mandible

(See ➲ Chapter 11.) Cystic jaw lesions comprise an extremely varied group of conditions and to consider each individually is beyond the scope of this book. Slow-growing cysts can present with painless firm swellings of the jaw. But they can present acutely following infection. Oral bacteria gain access to the cavity and a superimposed infection arises. Larger cysts may also present with a pathological fracture. Malignant or invasive lesions can present with paraesthesia of the inferior alveolar nerve. Consequently the most likely presentation of cystic lesions in the emergency department will be pain and swelling.

① Tumours of the mandible

Tumours of the mandible can be:
• Invasive tumours from oral mucosa squamous cell carcinomas
• Primary bone tumours
• Metastatic tumour.

Presentation can be varied. Swelling of the lower jaw and associated cervical lymphadenopathy will usually be present as these tend to be advanced by the time patients seek help. Pain, although not an initial feature, will become more significant as the disease progresses regardless of the type of tumour. Bony involvement may result in paraesthesia of the inferior alveolar nerve or pathological fracture. There is often some degree of trismus. Larger tumours will present with fistulae to the skin, bleeding and occasionally airway compromise. Urgent referral is then required for management of acute symptoms and further investigation (see http://bahno.org.uk/docs/head_and_neck_cancer.pdf).

Referred pain

In the emergency setting always be aware of the common causes of referred pain in the lower jaw. These include:
• Cardiac
• Neoplasms of pharynx, nasopharynx, base of tongue
• Lesions of the ear and Eustachian tube
• Major salivary glands
• Intracranial lesions.

① Giant cell arteritis

Patients can present with lower jaw pain and claudication of the muscles of mastication. This results from involvement of the maxillary artery. Diagnosis is histologically (biopsy of the superficial temporal artery) but this should not delay commencement of treatment with glucocorticoid steroids. Suspect in any elderly patient with a high ESR.

① Pathological fractures of the lower jaw

These are rare, accounting for <2% of all fractures of the mandible. They are defined as fractures that occur in regions where the bone has been weakened by an underlying pathological process. These include:
- Surgical interventions (third molar removal and implant placement)
- Osteomyelitis
- Osteoporosis
- ORN
- BRONJ
- Large cystic lesions
- Benign, malignant, or metastatic tumours.

Treatment of pathological fractures can be challenging and complex. Diagnosis radiologically in the emergency setting then urgent referral is required.

① Acute sickle cell

The most important pathological event of sickle cell anaemia is vascular occlusion resulting in ischaemia. *Pain is typically disproportionately severe.* Other sites may be affected. Patients presenting with a sickle cell crisis need IV fluids, analgesics, and oxygen to prevent further sickling of the cells. Although the pain may be in the mandible, this is a medical emergency, not a maxillofacial one.

① Osteomyelitis

See ➋ 'Infective swellings around the lower jaw and face', pp. 366–72.

⑦ ORN/BRONJ

See ➋ 'Non-infective swellings around the lower jaw and face', pp. 372–5.

① Altered sensation of the lower lip

Patients who present acutely with a non-trauma-associated altered sensation of the lower lip need to be assessed carefully. Many of the serious conditions outlined previously in this chapter can be associated with numbness. These include:
- Tumours
- Cystic lesions
- ORN
- Osteomyelitis
- Pathological fractures
- Paget's disease
- Central haemangiomas/intraosseous AVM
- BRONJ
- Iatrogenic injury.

All patients who present acutely with altered sensation of the lip following jaw surgery should have plain radiography to exclude a pathological fracture. Rarely, the 'numb chin' presentation can be a presentation of a *paraneoplastic neurological disorder* and can be associated with breast, ovarian, and lung cancer.

The mouth, lips, and teeth

Common presentations

Common presentations for the mouth, lips, and teeth:

The lips
- Change in colour/pigmented lesions
- Injuries
- Lumps/swelling
- Pain and numbness
- Ulceration and blistering
- Weakness or paralysis (see also ⟳ 'Facial palsy', pp. 340–2).

The mouth
- Bleeding
- Change in colour/pigmented lesions
- Difficulty swallowing (see ⟳ Chapter 8)
- Halitosis
- Injury
- Lumps (see also ⟳ Chapter 11 and ⟳ Chapter 12)
- Pain and numbness (See also ⟳ 'Toothaches and the wisdom teeth', pp. 429–32)
- Swelling
- Ulceration and blistering.

The tongue
- Bleeding/bruising
- Change in colour/pigmented lesions
- Hairy/coated
- Lumps
- Pain and numbness
- Smooth, sore surface (depapillation)
- Swelling
- Ulceration and blistering
- Weakness/paralysis (see also ⟳ 'Facial palsy', pp. 340–2).

The teeth
- Change in bite (see also ⟳ Chapter 11 and ⟳ Chapter 12)
- Discolouration/staining
- Injury
- Toothache
- Wisdom teeth problems.

The gums
- Bleeding gums
- Change in colour/pigmented lesions
- Lumps and swelling.

The teeth and gums
- Exposed bone
- Bleeding extraction socket
- Painful extraction socket
- Loose teeth
- Miscellaneous—denture/orthodontic appliance (braces)-related problems.

Common problems and their causes

Lips: change in colour/pigmented lesions

Common
- Benign nevus
- Haemangioma
- Actinic keratosis.

Uncommon
- Melanoma
- Perioral freckling (Peutz–Jeghers syndrome)
- Addison's disease
- Cyanosis.

Lips: injuries

Common
- Lacerations
- Bites—animal/self
- Foreign bodies
- Bruising/swelling.

Uncommon
- Projectile/blast injuries
- Fish hook.

Lips: lump/swellings

Common
- Trauma
- Skin abscess
- Dental infection
- Anaphylaxis/allergic reaction
- Mucocoele/polyps/haemangioma.

Uncommon
- Orofacial granulomatosis
- Hereditary angio-oedema
- Dermal fillers and implants
- Salivary gland tumours.

Lips: pain or paraesthesia

Common
- Infection
- Trigeminal neuralgia
- Neurapraxia of nerve (fracture/lower jaw pathology)
- Iatrogenic—dental injection or surgery/lip biting
- Burning mouth syndrome.

Uncommon
- Shingles/viral trigeminal neuropathy (see ➔ Chapter 11)
- Hypocalcaemia
- MS
- Tumours.

Lips: ulceration and blistering

Common
- Primary herpetic stomatitis/'cold sores'
- Angular cheilitis
- Denture-induced trauma.

Uncommon
- Cancer (skin/oral)
- Stevens–Johnson syndrome (SJS)
- Vesiculobullous disorders
- Shingles.

Lips: weakness or paralysis
(See also ➔ 'Facial palsy', pp. 340–2.)

Common
- Stroke
- Bell's palsy.

Uncommon
- Other causes of facial palsy (parotid tumour/middle ear infection)
- Iatrogenic facial nerve injury.

Mouth: bleeding

Common
- Trauma
- Infections
- Gingivitis.

Uncommon
- Oral cancer
- Causes of ulceration and blistering
- Haemoptysis
- Haematemesis
- Anticoagulants
- Haematological disease.

Mouth: change in colour/pigmented lesions

Common
- Normal pigmentation (Fordyce's spots, racial variation)
- Haemangioma/AVM
- Amalgam tattoo
- Oral lichen planus/lichenoid reaction
- Frictional hyperkeratosis
- Candidiasis
- Extrinsic (food stains, e.g. betel).

Uncommon
- Leucoplakia/erythroplakia
- Cancer
- Drugs/heavy metals
- Hyperpigmentation—Addison's disease.

Mouth: difficulty swallowing
(See also ➡ Chapter 8.)

Common
- Infection (odontogenic/HSV/mumps)
- Ludwig's angina
- Trauma/fractures/sublingual haematoma.

Uncommon
- Cerebrovascular accident/TIA
- Causes of swollen tongue/ulceration and blistering
- Neuromuscular disorders
- Eagle syndrome
- Tumours
- Previous surgery.

Mouth: halitosis

Common
- Poor oral hygiene/alcohol/cigarettes/dietary
- Infection (odontogenic, pericoronitis, sinusitis, tonsillitis).

Uncommon
- Bulimia
- Retained foreign body (nose/mouth)
- GORD/tumours in the aerodigestive tract
- Fetor hepaticus, lung abscess, metabolic conditions, and bowel obstruction.

Mouth: injury

Common
- Lacerations/cheek biting
- Denture induced.

Uncommon
- Iatrogenic
- Chemical/thermal/inhalation.

Mouth: lumps
(See also ➔ Chapter 11 and ➔ Chapter 12.)

Common
- Normal lumps (parotid papilla, submandibular duct, taste buds, lingual tonsils)
- Fibroepithelial polyps/haemangioma
- Nicotine stomatitis of the palate
- Torus
- Mucocoele
- Causes of blistering.

Uncommon
- Amyloidosis
- Orofacial granulomatosis
- Crohn's disease
- Flabby ridge/denture fibroma
- Lipoma.

Mouth: pain
(See also ➔ 'Toothaches and the wisdom teeth', pp. 429–32.)

Common
- Infections (dental/mucosal)
- Burning mouth syndrome/atypical odontalgia
- Causes of ulceration and blistering
- Oral lichen planus
- Herpetic gingivostomatitis
- Postoperative.

Uncommon
- Cancer
- Trigeminal neuralgia
- Angina bullosa haemorrhagica
- Osteomyelitis/ORN/BRONJ
- Reflux oesophagitis.

Mouth: swelling

Common
- Infection, abscess, Ludwig's angina
- Sublingual haematoma
- Ranula.

Uncommon
- Anaphylaxis and allergic reaction
- Bone disease (see ➔ Chapter 11 and ➔ Chapter 12)
- Haemangioma/lymphangioma
- Amyloidosis
- Orofacial granulomatosis.

Mouth: ulceration and blistering

Common
- Traumatic
- Primary herpetic stomatitis
- Aphthous ulceration
- Drug-induced (nicorandil/chemotherapy).

Uncommon
- Oral cancer
- ORN/BRONJ/osteomyelitis (see ➔ Chapter 11 and
  ➔ Chapter 12)
- SJS
- Vesiculobullous disorders
- Angina bullosa haemorrhagica
- Necrotizing sialometaplasia (palate)
- Kaposi's sarcoma (palate)
- Syphilitic lesions (palate).

Tongue: bleeding/bruising

Common
- Laceration/tongue biting/sublingual haematoma
- Postsurgical injection/bleeding
- Haemangioma.

Uncommon
- Tongue piercing
- Foreign body
- Erosive lichen planus
- Cancer.

Tongue: change in colour/pigmented lesions

Common
- Oral lichen planus/lichenoid reaction
- Frictional keratosis
- Candida/strawberry tongue
- Poor oral hygiene/smoking
- Antibiotics/mouthwash (chlorhexidine)
- Alcohol/food dyes
- Racial pigmentation.

Uncommon
- Dysplasia/cancer
- Amalgam tattoo
- Erythroplakia
- Haemangioma
- Hairy tongue
- Melanoma.

Tongue: hairy/coated

Common
- Frictional keratosis
- Poor oral hygiene/smoking
- Candida
- Antibiotics/mouthwash (chlorhexidine)
- Alcohol/food dyes.

Uncommon
- Black/brown hairy tongue (lingua villosa)
- Hairy tongue of HIV
- Chronic tooth brushing to clean surface
- Pellagra.

Tongue: lumps

Common
- Fibroepithelial polyps
- Papilloma
- Normal lumps (taste buds, lingual tonsils)
- Ranula/mucocoele
- Chronic biting.

Uncommon
- Tumours (submucosal)
- Amyloidosis/acromegaly
- Orofacial granulomatosis
- Lipoma/myofibroma
- Haemangioma/AVM
- Dermoid/ectopic thyroid.

Tongue: pain or paraesthesia

Common
- Geographical tongue
- Infection (hand, foot, and mouth disease/cold sores)
- Trauma/postoperative
- Causes of ulceration and blistering
- Median rhomboid glossitis
- Lichen planus
- Drugs/mouthwashes
- Atrophic glossitis
- Burning mouth syndrome (glossodynia).

Uncommon
- Cancer
- Trigeminal neuralgia/glossopharyngeal neuralgia
- Reflux oesophagitis
- Behçet's disease
- Vesiculobullous disorders.

Tongue: smooth, sore surface (depapillation)

Common
- Iron/vitamin B12/folate deficiency (atrophic glossitis)
- Trauma/friction
- Geographic tongue.

Uncommon
- Postsurgical resection/reconstruction
- Dry mouth (xerostomia).

Tongue: swelling

Common
- Infection, abscess, Ludwig's angina
- Anaphylaxis and allergic reaction
- Sublingual haematoma/ranula
- Postoperative swelling.

Uncommon
- Tumour (submucosal, leukaemia, and rhabdomyoma)
- Lipoma
- Haemangioma/lymphangioma
- Syndromic macroglossia (acromegaly/Down syndrome/Beckwith–Wiedemann syndrome)
- Orofacial granulomatosis
- Amyloidosis/myxoedema
- Neurofibromatosis
- Pellagra
- Pernicious anaemia.

Tongue: ulceration and blistering

Common
- Frictional from sharp teeth/fillings
- Burns or topical irritants
- Primary herpetic stomatitis
- Aphthous ulceration
- Erosive lichen planus
- Drug-induced (nicorandil/chemotherapy).

Uncommon
- Cancer—squamous cell carcinoma
- Behçet's disease
- Vesiculobullous disorders
- SJS
- Angina bullosa haemorrhagica.

Lips: weakness of paralysis
(See also ➔ 'Facial palsy', pp. 340–2.)

Uncommon
- CVA/bulbar palsy
- Hypoglossal nerve lesions
- Iatrogenic injury
- Tumour.

Teeth: change in bite
(See also ➔ Chapter 11 and ➔ Chapter 12.)

Common
- Jaw/dentoalveolar fracture (see ➔ Chapter 11 and ➔ Chapter 12)
- TMJ effusion
- Recent dental treatment.

Uncommon
- Dislocation/locking TMJ (see ➔ Chapter 12)
- Jaw cysts or odontogenic tumours (see ➔ Chapter 11 and ➔ Chapter 12)
- Over-erupted wisdom tooth.

Teeth: discolouration/staining

Common
- Extrinsic stains (coffee, wine, cigarettes)
- Trauma
- Age related.

Uncommon
- Excessive fluoride exposure during childhood
- Tetracycline
- Dentinogenesis imperfecta.

Teeth: injury

Common
- Crown fractures
- Root fractures
- Dentoalveolar fractures
- Subluxation/avulsion
- Chipped fillings, lost crowns/caps.

Teeth: toothache

Common
- Pulpitis/dental or periodontal abscess
- Dentine hypersensitivity
- Recent treatment.

Uncommon
- Referred—sinusitis
- Pain on biting—cracked tooth
- Teething pain—infants.

Teeth: wisdom teeth problems

Common
- Pericoronitis/dental decay/pulpitis
- Erupting
- Postoperative pain.

Uncommon
- Infected dentigerous cyst.

Gums: bleeding gums

Common
- Poor oral hygiene/periodontal disease
- Trauma—laceration or fracture
- Ill-fitting dentures.

Uncommon
- Pregnancy
- Anticoagulants
- Haematological disorders—leukaemia, haemophilia, thrombocytopenia

- Liver disorders
- Tumours
- Scurvy
- Vitamin K deficiency.

Gums: change in colour/pigmented lesions

Common
- Frictional keratosis
- Oral lichen planus/lichenoid reaction
- Amalgam tattoo
- Racial pigmentation/nevi
- Smoking.

Uncommon
- Cancer
- Anaemia
- Heavy metal poisoning (lead, bismuth, and mercury)
- Addison disease
- Albright syndrome
- Blue nevi
- HIV
- Peutz–Jeghers syndrome.

Gums: lumps and swelling

Common
- Dental/periodontal abscess
- Gingivitis
- Drugs (calcium channel blockers, antiepileptics)
- Pregnancy.

Uncommon
- Pyogenic granuloma
- Unerupted teeth
- Pregnancy
- Cancer
- Leukaemia
- Malnutrition
- Poorly fitting dentures.

Teeth and gums: exposed bone

Common
- Dry socket
- Fracture (see ➲ Chapter 11 and ➲ Chapter 12).

Uncommon
- Osteomyelitis/ORN/BRONJ
- Cancer
- Denture trauma.

Teeth and gums: bleeding extraction socket

Common
- Normal/reactionary haemorrhage—local anaesthetic wearing off
- Iatrogenic—poking the socket/sucking/spitting
- Infection
- Anticoagulants.

Uncommon
- Clotting disorders, liver disease, haematological disease.

Teeth and gums: painful extraction socket

Common
- Normal postoperative pain
- Dry socket
- Abscess.

Uncommon
- Retained root fragment
- Sensitivity from adjacent tooth.

Teeth and gums: loose teeth

Common
- Periodontal disease
- Trauma.

Uncommon
- Tumours/jaw cysts
- ORN/BRONJ.

Teeth and gums: miscellaneous related problems

Common
- Denture rubbing/ulceration
- Loose dentures
- Broken dentures/orthodontic appliance
- Denture candidiasis.

Uncommon
- Flabby ridge, denture hyperplasia, denture fibroma.

Useful questions and what to look for

Bleeding (non-extraction)

Ask about
- History of trauma or dental treatment
- Duration
- Generalized or discrete
- Swelling or other symptoms (pain/ulceration/blisters)
- Bleeding from other sites
- PMH/drug history
- Family history of bleeding disorders.

Look for
- Confirm site and degree
- Oral hygiene
- Associated structures, e.g. loose/painful teeth
- Bruising/petechiae, hepatosplenomegaly
- Signs of injury/infection/malignancy at site of bleeding.

Bleeding following dental extraction

Ask about
- How long after the extraction did the bleeding start
- History of bleeding disorders
- Anticoagulant medication.

Look for
- Signs of active bleeding from soft tissue and bone
- OPT to exclude retained root fragments
- Signs of local or systemic infection—inflamed gums, swelling, abscess, lymphadenopathy
- Signs of underlying bleeding disorder.

Change in colour

Ask about
- How has colour changed
- Smoking/sun exposure/diet/known precipitant
- Associated changes in lesion (growth, itching, bleeding, pain, etc.)
- Discrete or widespread
- Other sites on body.

Look for
- Single/multiple lesions
- Blanching or bleeding
- Possible melanoma.

Depapillation (loss of surface roughness)

Ask about
- How long
- Painful/painless
- Diet and nutritional status
- History of trauma, friction, and burns.

Look for
- Confirm depapillation
- Blood tests—haematinic screen: iron, folate, vitamin B12, magnesium, and zinc to rule out micronutrient deficiency
- Adjacent sharp or rough teeth causing trauma.

Difficulty swallowing (dysphagia)

(See also ➲ Chapter 8.)

Ask about
- Duration
- Progressively worsening
- Smoking/alcohol history
- Is it causing issues with aspiration or nutrition?
- Signs of chest infection
- Signs of reflux or vomiting indicating oesophageal obstruction
- PMH of diabetes, stroke, cancer
- Any paroxysmal nocturnal dyspnoea.

Look for
- Oral hygiene or signs of odontogenic infection, such as swelling, trismus, elevated tongue, and floor of mouth.
- Any ulcerations in the oral cavity, tongue, floor of mouth, or throat suggestive of a tumour
- Hoarse voice
- Signs of facial nerve or hypoglossal nerve palsy
- Signs of chest infection
- Wasting, cachexia, signs of nutritional deficiency.

Discoloured teeth

Ask about
- Single tooth or multiple teeth affected
- History of trauma to teeth
- History of foods causing staining—wine, soy sauce, tea/coffee, or smoking
- History of tetracycline antibiotics in childhood.

Look for
- Confirm whether single or multiple teeth affected
- Colour—black/grey, brown/yellow.

Exposed bone

Ask about
- History of recent extraction or trauma from denture
- History of radiation therapy to jaws
- History of bisphosphonate medication
- History of immunocompromise, diabetes, steroids, smoking
- Oral hygiene
- Severity of pain, or problems with malnutrition.

Look for
- Site, extent
- Signs of pathological fracture—check on OPT
- Signs of necrosis or infected bone—pus, swelling, or fistula
- Signs of oral cancer with induration, ulceration and lymphadenopathy.

Halitosis

Ask about
- How long
- Painful/painless
- Symptoms of chest/throat/sinus/dental infection
- Any gastric/oesophageal symptoms
- Tongue scrubbing and oral hygiene regimen.

Look for
- Confirm halitosis objectively
- Anaemia, signs of diabetic ketoacidosis, liver failure, lung abscess, or bowel obstruction
- Poor oral hygiene
- Dental infection
- Tonsillitis, sinusitis.

Injuries (dental—fractured, avulsed, loose)

Ask about
- Trauma history
- If avulsed tooth, time out of mouth
- Gradually loosening tooth/teeth
- Does the bite feel normal?

Look for
- Ensure all broken teeth are accounted for. Consider imaging.
- Single tooth affected, or segment of loose teeth suggesting alveolar bone fracture
- Signs of tooth root and jaw fracture on OPT and PA mandible
- Changes in bite (occlusion).

Injuries (oral)

Ask about
- When it occurred—date and specific time
- Mechanism of injury—high/low impact, likely cervical spine injury
- Loss of consciousness
- Progression of symptoms since time of injury
- Difficulty swallowing or stridor
- Numbness or weakness
- Change in bite
- Other injuries
- Clean or dirty injury and tetanus vaccination status.

Look for
- Other injuries—face and spine
- Lacerations—check intra- and extraorally. Document size, depth, and involvement of key structures, such as vermillion border. Note any gross tissue loss
- Mobility of jaw or teeth suggesting fracture
- Account for any missing or chipped teeth—CXR to exclude aspiration
- Floor of mouth swelling or sublingual haematoma suggesting potential for airway compromise.

Lumps

Ask about
- History trauma or dental treatment
- Cheek-biting habits
- Duration
- Generalized or discrete
- Painful/painless
- Is it growing?

Look for
- Confirm site and size
- Mobile or fixed
- Associated structures, e.g. loose/painful teeth
- Bony or soft tissue
- Lumps elsewhere
- Blanching or pulsation
- Are the lumps bilateral and part of normal anatomy?

Pain and numbness

Ask about
- History of facial trauma, surgery, or dental treatment
- Episodic or progressive
- Rapid onset or gradual
- Any improvement

- Exact site (perioral/dermatome)
- Associated masses or swelling
- Other neurological symptoms, e.g. dysarthria, limb weakness, hemiplegia, tetany
- Past history of surgery to head and neck with nerve damage or sacrifice
- Recent stress or viral infection.

Look for
- Confirm site and degree (unilateral vs bilateral, dermatomal or nerve distribution)
- Test cranial nerves (especially facial and trigeminal). Forehead sparing
- Associated structures, e.g. loose/painful teeth
- Parotid mass.

Painful extraction socket

Ask about
- Nature of extraction—simple or surgical
- Onset of pain
- Associated symptoms of dry socket—inflammation, bad taste
- Risk factors for dry socket—smoking, poor oral hygiene, contraceptive pill, past history of dry socket
- Symptoms of infection—fever, swelling, pus, lymphadenopathy
- Symptoms of nerve damage—numbness, tingling, sharp shooting or electric shock pain.

Look for
- Is the clot present or absent?
- Is the socket inflamed or pus present?
- Signs of food packing and poor oral hygiene
- OPT to exclude retained root fragments.

Swellings

Ask about
- Onset—acute or gradual/duration
- Localized or generalized
- Episodic or persistent
- Obvious triggers/allergies
- Trauma or lip biting history.

Look for
- Is the swelling soft tissue or bony?
- Painful, hot, or fluctuant
- Associated bleeding or ulceration
- Any lymphadenopathy
- Systemic features—hypotension, flushed, rash
- Dental pain or infection.

Toothache, dental pain, wisdom teeth

Ask about
- Pain duration, intensity, location, character, exacerbating and relieving features
- Symptoms of systemic infection
- Analgesia taken (can overdose with severe toothache)
- History of trauma to teeth.

Look for
- Confirm affected tooth/teeth with OPT and clinical examination
- Tongue mobility—able to swallow secretions
- Trismus
- Fever
- Swelling, lymphadenopathy and pus.

Ulceration and blistering

Ask about
- Duration
- Progressive or episodic
- Painful or painless—ability to maintain oral intake
- Solitary or multiple
- Risk factors (heavy smoker, sun exposure)
- Widespread mucocutaneous involvement
- Weight loss/fatigue
- Any new medications.

Look for
- Signs of malignancy—persistent ulcer with round rolled margins, induration
- Lymphadenopathy
- Iron/B12/folate deficiency
- Ill-fitting dentures or sharp teeth causing trauma.

Miscellaneous: denture/orthodontic appliance (braces)-related problems

Ask about
- Age of dentures
- Loose and rubbing
- Tight dentures
- Any pain, mobility, or problems with adjacent teeth and soft tissues.

Look for
- Signs of traumatic ulceration
- Signs of reactive hyperplasia of supporting soft tissues under denture base or flange
- If patient complains of tight dentures, check for signs of acromegaly and Paget's disease.

Examination of the mouth, lips, tongue, teeth, and gums

The extent to which the mouth and its associated structures will need to be examined will depend on the nature of the problem at hand and the degree of urgency it presents. Clearly a detailed head and neck examination will not be required in every patient (e.g. a patient with an obvious mucocoele of the lip), but then again, it is important not to jump to conclusions too early and miss something more important. Like skin lesions, many oral conditions are diagnosed to an extent by 'pattern recognition' and with experience, accurate 'spot diagnoses' become easier. However, for the novice it is best to start methodically and be thorough. It is important to have a system which ensures that all the hard and soft tissues are examined (including the cervical lymph nodes, jaw bones, and TMJ) and that any lesion that is encountered is also assessed carefully, noting its key features. A mirror, bright light, and tongue depressor are all required.

Start at one place (usually the inside of the lips) and slowly move clockwise (or anticlockwise) around the oral cavity, gently stretching the mucosa to look at its surface. Hand held dental mirrors, one in each hand, make excellent retractors that patients tolerate well. They can also be used to reflect light into any recesses. Work your way slowly to the back of the mouth, but be careful not to induce gagging. Use a mirror to gently retract the tongue to each side to look at its lateral surface and floor of the mouth. *Actively inspect key sites known to harbour oral cancer.* These include the posterior floor of the mouth, where it dips down to join the posterior lateral surface of the tongue—sometimes referred to as the 'coffin—corner' (so-called because advanced cancer here has a poor prognosis). Look carefully at the lips, tongue, buccal mucosae (and their recesses), floor of mouth (ask the patient to curl their tongue backwards), gingiva, teeth, palate, and tonsils. *Then palpate the tissues.* Deep tumours may not be obvious on inspection alone. This seems a lot, but with practice a thorough examination is possible within a very short period of time.

Airway assessment

Note the degree of any trismus and any problems with limited tongue movement or floor of mouth swelling. Check speech, breathing, and swallowing for signs of airway compromise. Look at the adequacy of the posterior airway space. If a general anaesthetic is indicated this information should be communicated to the anaesthetist. The patient may require a nasal tube. Occasionally, awake fibreoptic intubation with rapid sequence induction is required for difficult airways.

The oral mucosa and lips

Look at the colour of the oral mucosa. It is often described as salmon-pink. However, variations in pigmentation, vascularity, and keratinization are common. Pigmentation can be patchy. The amount of oral pigmentation a patient has is generally proportional to the amount of skin pigmentation they have. Increased pigmentation (e.g. Addison's disease) is usually accompanied by increased pigmentation in the skin of the head and neck. The buccal mucosa may sometimes have a milky-white appearance called leukoedema. This is normal and disappears when the cheek is stretched. Don't confuse this with candida. Ectopic sebaceous glands

(Fordyce spots) are common and appear as bilateral whitish-yellowish papules speckled on the surface of the buccal mucosa (and less commonly on the labial mucosa). A horizontal whitish ridge (the line alba) is also commonly seen running along the level of the teeth in the buccal mucosa. This is a benign keratosis secondary to chronic mild irritation from the teeth. The orifice of the parotid gland duct can be found as a small raised flap of mucosa opposite the first permanent molar tooth. Pressure on the parotid gland should cause a small amount of clear saliva to exude from the opening. Severe dryness or tackiness suggests xerostomia.

Evert the lips and look the labial mucosa. This is a site commonly affected by increased pigmentation. The surface is often slightly irregular due to the presence of minor salivary glands. These give a fine knobbly appearance to the labial mucosa. Those in the lower lip are often palpable. The mucosa otherwise should be smooth, soft, and well lubricated by the minor salivary glands. The lower lip is a common site for mucocoele and haemangioma. Actinic (sun) damage to the lips, especially the lower lip, is common in people who work outdoors. The exposed surfaces of the lips are dry, scaly and keratotic to varying degrees. *Note any non-healing lesions as these may be dysplastic/neoplastic.* Look at the corners of the mouth. Maceration and cracking (angular cheilitis) may be associated with several medical problems (nutritional deficiency, especially iron, folate and B vitamins, diabetes, and candida).

Saliva
Clear saliva should usually be seen coming from the parotid and submandibular ducts on massaging the glands. There should be no discomfort. Thicker mucus, or pus, indicate problems with drainage and infection. Look at the orifice of the duct for inflammation or a stone.

The tongue and floor of the mouth
The dorsal (upper) surface of the tongue is inspected by asking the patient to protrude the tongue. Surprisingly, some patients find it difficult to control movements of their tongue to command. If necessary, gently grip the tip in a piece of gauze. The dorsal surface should be uniformly covered by numerous short hair-like papillae and scattered mushroom-shaped fungiform papillae. Filiform papillae can become elongated (hairy tongue) and collect debris, resulting in halitosis. Food and drink dyes can result in a wide array of colouring. Atrophy of the dorsal surface can result from a variety of causes (nutritional deficiencies). If patchy this is sometimes referred to as a 'geographic tongue'. Further back, at the junction of the anterior two-thirds and posterior one-third of the tongue are the circumvallate papillae and lymphatic tissue. These are sometimes confused with 'growths' on the tongue. Fissures may be present but are generally of no clinical significance. The lateral borders of the tongue should be carefully examined by pushing the tongue laterally. The mucosa is smoother with no papillae. Posteriorly there are often irregular clumps of lymphoid tissue (lingual tonsil). The ventral (under) surface of the tongue seen by asking the patient curl the tip of the tongue backwards. The veins here can be very prominent. The lingual frenum is a membrane joining the tongue to the floor of the mouth. In some patients it can be short and extend to the tip of the tongue (tongue tie).

The floor of the mouth has similar appearances to the lateral surface of the tongue as one merges with the other. On palpation, symmetrical bony lumps may be felt on the inner (lingual) surface of the mandible. These are mandibular tori and are not significant. They are sometimes confused with tumours of the sublingual glands. The ostia of the submandibular glands are seen as two papillae either side of the lingual frenum in the midline. Look for clear saliva and stones. Examine it along its entire length, passing back towards the wisdom teeth area (coffin corner). *Both the ventrolateral surface of the tongue and the floor of the mouth are common sites for squamous cell carcinoma.*

The palate

The hard palate has a relatively thicker keratinized mucosa which is pale pink. Anteriorly it is covered by numerous fibrous ridges (rugae). The incisive papillae (lower end of the nasopalatine duct) is posterior to the maxillary incisor teeth. Occasionally a hard bony lump is seen in the centre of the hard palate—palatal torus. These are benign and do not require treatment if symptomless. They can be quite impressive. Don't confuse these with other lumps. Tori are bone hard. The soft palate is non-keratinized and salmon-pink in colour. Depress the posterior tongue and ask the patient to say 'Ahhh'. This may be difficult in some patients due to a pronounced gag reflex. The entire palate contains numerous minor salivary glands. These can develop into salivary gland neoplasms. Note any swellings and ulcers.

The tonsils

The tonsillar pillars are visualized by moving the tongue to each side The crypts are highly vascular and appear more erythematous than the surrounding tissues. There may be accumulations of food and debris, resulting in local irritation and halitosis. Accessory lymphoid tissue (adenoids) is common.

The teeth and gums

From an emergency department perspective, examination is relatively limited. Check for obvious signs of decay or trauma. Some decay between the teeth (interproximal) may not be obvious without the aid of radiographs. Bleeding or pus exuding around the necks of the teeth suggests a problem with the tooth or the jaw. If there is a copious amount of pus leaking there is probably a cyst or cavity somewhere nearby. Check for tenderness by lightly tapping each tooth in turn. Tenderness to percussion usually indicates root pathology, such as an abscess underneath the tooth. Teeth may also be mobile, but this may be longstanding.

Look at the gums (gingiva). This is best done with the mouth partially closed and the lips retracted. Do they look healthy (pale pink and tightly adherent), or diseased (swollen, friable, ulcerated, bleeding)? The commonest cause of inflammation is poor oral hygiene. The gingiva is frequently pigmented and is a common site involved in mucocutaneous diseases.

There are several ways to determine whether the tooth (i.e. its dental pulp) is alive, dead, or pulpitic (inflamed):

• Cold testing (cold spray of ethyl chloride): a freezing cold stimulus is applied to the teeth individually using a cotton bud. The patient is asked to indicate when they become aware of the coldness. A normal tooth should react quickly, and the cold sensation disappears within seconds. A tooth with a dead nerve (necrotic pulp) will not react at all, whereas a tooth with an inflamed pulp (pulpitis) will often produce an exaggerated reaction such as extreme sensitivity which lingers for minutes before subsiding to a dull throbbing pain.

- Electric pulp testing: using a specialized gadget, an increasing electric current is applied through the teeth individually, and a quantifiable reading recorded when the patient begins to experience tingling in the tooth. A vital tooth will produce a response with low levels of current, whereas non-vital teeth will not respond.
- FracFinder™: a hard plastic instrument is placed on each cusp of a sore tooth in turn and the patient instructed to bite on it. Pain on biting or release can indicate a hairline crack or fracture within the tooth.

Examining a patient with a history of oropharyngeal cancer

- Anatomy may be deranged, especially if the patient has undergone major resections (hemimaxillectomy/mandibulectomy) with free flap reconstruction.
- Radiation makes the tissues leathery and erythematous. This makes it difficult to differentiate induration and infection from radiation change.
- Any new lesions should be investigated (often biopsied). Keep a low threshold of suspicion for recurrence or a new cancer.

Investigations

Laboratory tests

FBC and CRP

An elevated WCC is seen in infections, typically with a corresponding neutrophilia. Anaemia can be associated with a number of oral symptoms. Thrombocytopenia may be a cause of post extraction bleeding. If platelets are <40, urgent haematology advice is necessary. In patients with bleeding gums whose FBC reveals a pancytopenia with blasts, leukaemia is the likely diagnosis, and urgent haematology referral is required. The CRP will typically be raised >100 for systemically unwell patients

U&Es, creatinine, and LFTs

In severe oral infections, patients experience dysphagia and may become dehydrated. These patients will look unwell and are unable to tolerate oral fluids. LFTs are required in bleeding patients with a history of alcoholic liver disease or viral hepatitis.

Coagulation screen

Derangements in coagulation may signify an underlying bleeding disorder, particularly in the setting of a patient with a bleeding extraction socket, where bleeding has persisted slowly for days. In warfarinized patients the international normalized ratio (INR) is a useful measure of whether the patient will require adjuvant haemostatic measures or vitamin K supplementation. If the INR is <3 the patient is unlikely to have significant complications.

Haematinic screen

Patients with recurrent aphthous ulceration, burning mouth, or atrophic glossitis should have a haematinic screen. Haemoglobin will give an indication of anaemia, and mean corpuscular volume will help to determine whether microcytic or macrocytic. Low iron and ferritin causes microcytic anaemia. Ferritin is also an acute phase marker, which can be falsely elevated in times of acute inflammation. It is therefore recommended to order CRP concurrently to exclude an erroneous normal/high ferritin result.

Low vitamin B12 and folate result in macrocytic anaemia.

Zinc and magnesium: if deficient, these can also contribute to soft tissue ulceration.

If corrected, these may result in resolution of some oral lesions.

Swabs

Microbiology swabs are useful to determine antibiotic sensitivities and direct treatment. If the patient has already been commenced on empirical antibiotics at the time the swab is taken, these should be documented on the pathology request. Virology swabs can be taken if primary herpetic stomatitis is suspected; the blisters can be swabbed and sent for virology. Swabs can take >48 hours for a result, so it may be better to commence aciclovir if the patient presents early. Fungal culturing is of little value in the acute setting because of the slow growth rate of the organism. *Candida* is also a normal commensal in around 90% of the normal population.

Plain films

OPT is an excellent starting point as it includes all the teeth on the one film. It is useful for characterizing tooth fractures, avulsions and subluxations. It will also detect gross caries, and associated periapical pathology, including cysts and abscesses. Interpretation usually requires experience, as anatomical radiolucencies such as maxillary sinuses, mental foramen, or submandibular depression can be mistaken for cysts or dental abscesses. OPTs can be difficult to interpret in the vicinity of the anterior teeth as there is superimposition from the vertebral column in this region. In children, an OPT can also help to determine the state of the unerupted developing permanent dentition. Other useful plain film dental X-rays include periapical films, which are X-rays of single teeth. These are most commonly taken in dental practice.

CT and MRI

These are useful in determining the spread of cancer. If the patient shows clinical signs of a deep fascial space infection, CT may be useful to determine the spread (Ludwig's angina or mediastinitis).

Ultrasound

This is excellent for characterizing whether there is a drainable collection in a soft tissue swelling. It is also useful to distinguish an enlarged lymph node from a salivary gland. It is sometimes possible to perform FNA at the same time.

ⓘ Injuries to the teeth

The most important thing to ascertain when a patient presents with loose or fractured teeth is whether there has been any other significant trauma involved. Assess the airway, C-spine, brain, eyes, and facial bone fractures as outlined elsewhere in this book.

ⓘ Fractured teeth

Fractured teeth are usually obvious. Any missing fragments which cannot be accounted for require a CXR and soft tissue view of the neck to ensure they are not in the throat or lung. Radiographic assessment, such as an OPT, or periapical view are important to define exactly which part of the tooth has fractured and what the treatment should be.

Crown fractures

These are either complicated (involve the pulp) or uncomplicated (do not involve the pulp). Uncomplicated fractures can be treated with a filling or crown. Complicated fractures will require either 'pulp capping' or root canal treatment before the tooth is restored.

Root fractures

These are divided into coronal, middle, or apical-thirds. They are diagnosed by X-ray. Typically coronal-third root fractures are very unstable, and often these teeth must be removed. Middle and apical-third fractures may recover with splinting. If a maxillofacial laboratory service is available, impressions can be taken and a clear plastic splint fitted to stabilize the teeth for at least 2 weeks. Alternatively, a semi-rigid splint with wire and composite resin can be applied. Patients require a soft diet for 2 weeks. Long-term follow-up (general dental practitioner) is required.

☼ Avulsed teeth

When a tooth has been completely avulsed from its socket, it should be immediately re-implanted at the scene. If this is not possible, the tooth should be transported in milk, or the patient's own saliva. It should never be handled by the root, and should not be washed, scrubbed, or brushed. There is a window of around 1 hour in which avulsed teeth can be successfully re-implanted. *Only permanent teeth are suitable for reimplantation.* Avulsed deciduous teeth are not re-implanted due to the risk of damage to the deeper unerupted adult tooth bud.

Under local anaesthetic, the tooth is placed back in its socket. If the clot does not dislodge from the socket, it may require gentle debridement to make space. Once re-implanted, the patient may need to bite down on a gauze swab to help seat the tooth, and X-rays can be taken to confirm tooth position. These patients require a semi-rigid splint for several weeks while the tooth reattaches. Root canal treatment is required later. Patients should be given antibiotics, chlorhexidine mouth rinse, and if required, tetanus prophylaxis. They should be advised to eat only a soft diet while the splint is in place. Long-term follow-up with a dentist is mandatory.

If the avulsed tooth has been out of the mouth for more than 1 hour, the tooth is unlikely to reattach. Maxillofacial opinion should be sought as sometime this may still be possible. If reimplantation is not possible, the patient will need still dental follow-up. *Incorrect management of the avulsed tooth is a source of litigation.*

ⓘ Loose teeth

Loose teeth following a trauma always require dental X-rays to ascertain whether there is a root fracture, or fracture of the alveolar, or even the jaw. If there is no sign of fracture, but the tooth appears to be loose or displaced, it is said to be subluxed.

If a crown-root fracture is present, the tooth should be treated as described earlier (see ➜ 'Fractured teeth', p. 413). If there are multiple adjacent, loose teeth, then it is likely that a fracture of the alveolar bone has occurred. This is often treated by constructing a splint to support all the teeth for up to 6 weeks, and advising the patient to have a pureed soft diet while the bone heals. If there has been a fracture of the jaw involving the tooth-bearing segments, it is likely that the patient will present with loose teeth on either side of the fracture line. Patients will require maxillofacial assessment.

Other causes of loose teeth

Patients complaining of gradually loosening crowns, intermittent bleeding from the teeth, or receding gums, over a period of months or years, are more likely to be suffering from periodontal disease. Cemented crowns can also loosen following trauma. These patients should be referred to their own dentist. Loose teeth may also be associated with a cyst or cancer. If a loose tooth is associated with soft tissue induration and ulceration, this may be indicative of a squamous cell carcinoma. These patients should be checked for lymphadenopathy and referred urgently to an appropriate specialty (maxillofacial/ENT etc.). An OPT is useful in the assessment of loose teeth as it will define changes in the supporting bone (such as erosion or cyst formation). Large well-defined radiolucencies involving tooth roots are likely to represent radicular cysts, odontogenic keratocysts, or ameloblastoma, the management of which is typically surgical. ORN and BRONJ can present with mobile, painful teeth, exposed bone, and ulceration. These require careful assessment and urgent referral.

ⓘ Tooth damage from general anaesthesia

Trauma to the anterior teeth can occur during laryngoscopy and intubation. It is more likely if the patient has crowns, decay, or periodontal disease. Patients are usually warned of this risk during anaesthetic consultation, and due care is taken during instrumentation. If a tooth has fractured during intubation, the broken segment should be retained. The patient will require dental assessment to see whether the broken part can be re-bonded. It is not always possible to save the tooth, especially if the tooth was grossly decayed, or already loose from pre-existing periodontal disease. If any broken or avulsed teeth cannot be accounted for, the patient will require imaging to exclude aspiration.

ⓘ Soft tissue injuries

ⓘ Lip lacerations

Lip lacerations are a common presentation to the emergency department following facial trauma. Lips have an abundant vascular supply and there may be seemingly dramatic bleeding and swelling, which usually looks more severe than it really is. Bleeding is easily controlled with pressure, and wounds should be closed with sutures where practicable. Swelling can be minimized with ice. Lip lacerations tend present following trauma, or lip-biting following seizures or dental local anaesthetic. *It is important to ascertain from the history whether there is a likelihood of a retained foreign body, such as tooth fragments, gravel, or glass.*

Assessment

External lacerations tend to be self-evident. The internal surfaces of the lips should be inspected to check for intraoral lacerations and damage to the teeth. Gently feel for possible retained foreign bodies within the substance of the lip. Consider soft tissues X-rays. Assess the following:

- Does the laceration cross the vermillion border? If so, consider specialist referral for primary closure (although this is not mandatory if you can clearly see the border). If you suture the lip yourself, it is make sure you re-oppose the wound margins anatomically to prevent a step in the vermillion.
- Is the laceration 'through-and-through'? That is, is there an obvious hole extending from the external lip through to the inside of the mouth? If so, consider referral for a layered closure.
- Wound depth. If the wound is >0.5 cm deep it is likely to involve deeper tissues such as muscle. Deep lacerations have a tendency to gape, and should be closed layers. Glue and steri-strips are not appropriate for deep wounds.
- Is the wound clean or dirty? This will dictate whether extensive debridement is required prior to wound closure. It will also influence whether antibiotics and tetanus prophylaxis should be given.
- Is there any frank tissue loss? If so, refer for assessment.

Repair of lacerations

If the laceration is deep, gaping, through-and-through, or involves vermillion border, it should be closed primarily. If the wound is contaminated, it should be thoroughly debrided prior to closure. For dirty wounds and animal bites, antibiotics and tetanus prophylaxis should be considered. Local anaesthetic is often sufficient for wound closure. If the patient is uncooperative, such as a young child, consider sedation or a short general anaesthetic. It is safe to use adrenaline (epinephrine)-containing local anaesthetics in the oral cavity and face, due to the abundant blood supply. Their vasoconstrictive effects also aid in haemostasis.

Options for wound closure include steri-strips, glue, and sutures. Steri-strips have very limited application in lip lacerations, and will not adequately close a gaping wound, particularly when the patient speaks or smiles. Glue is not suitable for intraoral wounds, and will not satisfactorily close a deep or gaping wound. Sutures are required in most cases. For lip lacerations a layered closure involves deep slowly-resorbing sutures (such as 3/0 or 4/0 plain Vicryl®) to muscle layers, with inter-rupted sutures for skin or mucosa. Intraoral lacerations are typically repaired with fast-resorbing sutures (such as 4/0 Vicryl® Rapide). If in doubt, specialist referral is recommended.

Afterwards, patients should be given suitable oral analgesia, chlorhex-idine mouthwash, and antibiotics (as required). Sutures are usually removed 5–7 days later.

ⓘ Intraoral lacerations

Intraoral lacerations are usually self-evident. Blood in the mouth mixes with saliva and bleeding seems more extensive than it really is. If it is not possible to see where the blood is coming from, the patient should be instructed to rinse their mouth out. Remember that blood in the mouth is not always from an oral source. Other causes such as epistaxis, hae-moptysis, and haematemesis should be considered. Again, it is important to assess the location, size, and depth of the wound, noting whether they are gaping, or contaminated. Involvement of key structures, such as submandibular ducts in the floor of mouth, or parotid ducts inside the cheeks adjacent to the upper second molar, will determine whether specialist referral is required for assessment and repair. Not all intraoral lacerations need repair. The tongue heals extremely well without sutur-ing, although this may still be desirable. Treatment involves symptom-atic relief, including analgesia, together with chlorhexidine or salt water mouth rinse to prevent wound contamination. If the laceration is large, deep, gaping, or involving important structures, it may require repair, either under local or general anaesthetic.

Be careful with penetrating soft palate injuries in children. The typical his-tory is a fall while running with a pencil or pen in the mouth. Although the palatal wound itself is usually small, carotid injury and delayed onset of stroke have been reported.

ⓘ Bleeding (non-traumatic)

In the absence of trauma, oral bleeding is typically mild, and most likely to be coming from the gums (gingivae). *It is important not to miss rare but serious causes, such as oral and haematological malignancy.*

ⓘ Gingivitis

The most common cause of oral bleeding is that of gingivitis. It pres-ents with diffusely inflamed gums, which bleed on tooth brushing and is usually associated with poor oral hygiene and periodontal disease. It can be amplified in pregnancy, as hormonal changes can cause an exag-gerated inflammatory response to plaque. Gingivitis is a clinical diag-nosis. Treatment is coordinated through a dentist or periodontist, and involves intensive cleaning, oral hygiene instruction and chlorhexidine mouth rinse.

ⓘ Infections

Dental or oral infections can also present with discrete areas of intraoral bleeding due to inflammation. There is also swelling, pain, and (if systemi-cally ill), pyrexia. Treatment may include surgical drainage and antibiotics.

① Oral cancer

Oral cancer, usually squamous cell carcinoma, tends to present as indu-rated painless ulceration with associated necrosis. The most commonly involved sites include the ventrolateral surface of the tongue, floor of mouth, retromolar region, and alveolus. Due to the fragility of the affected mucosa, these lesions tend to bleed easily on being touched. Biopsy is necessary to confirm diagnosis. Treatment will depend on the type, site, and extent of the cancer, but may include any combination of surgery, radiotherapy, chemotherapy, or palliation.

① Anticoagulation (aspirin, clopidogrel, warfarin)

Quickly elicit whether the patient is taking any anticoagulant medica-tions. Overdose or dietary/drug interactions, can result in spontaneous bleeding. Coagulation studies are useful in patients who are anticoagu-lated. In warfarinized patients with elevated INR, discuss management with haematology. Don't just give vitamin K.

Control of bleeding may be possible with local measures, such as Surgicel® and biting on a gauze pack soaked in tranexamic acid. It is usu-ally safe to perform dental extractions on patients taking anticoagulation without having to alter or withhold the drug, so long as extra haemo-static measures are employed.

① Haematological disease (thrombocytopenia, haemophilia, leukaemia)

The patient with oral bleeding from an unknown source should be ques-tioned regarding unintentional weight loss, malaise, and night sweats. If a haematological malignancy is suspected, look for clinical signs of anae-mia, lymphadenopathy, and hepatosplenomegaly. In cases of idiopathic thrombocytopenic purpura, the skin should be inspected looking for purple bruises (purpura). If a coagulopathy is suspected, the patient should have FBC, LFTs and a coagulation screen. In males where haemo-philia is suspected, testing of factor VIII and IX levels will help.

Other causes

See also ➔ 'Ulceration and blistering', pp. 418–24.

Management of oral bleeding

This is surprisingly straightforward in most cases and can usually be con-trolled with pressure, and the use of tranexamic acid mouthwash if nec-essary. Tranexamic acid acts an antifibrinolytic. It inhibits activation of plasminogen to plasmin, and thereby prevents premature clot degradation. Desmopressin (DDAVP®) may be useful in patients with von Willebrand disease, haemophilia, or thrombocytopenia. Thrombocytopenia is also treated by steroids, and platelet transfusion if necessary. Haemophilia may require factor replacement. Leukaemia may require treatment with che-motherapy, radiotherapy, and possible bone marrow transplant. *All man-agement of bleeding patients with anticoagulation or haematological disease should be coordinated via liaison with specialist haematologists.*

① Ulceration and blistering

While lip and mouth ulcers are usually benign, it is important not to over-look oral cancer. The duration of ulceration can be of help in arriving at a differential diagnosis. For example traumatic, aphthous, and herpetic ulcers typically resolve spontaneously within a few weeks. In contrast, malignancy tends to present as a progressive, non-healing ulcer, which is relatively painless in many cases. For lesions extending beyond the oral cavity into other mucocutaneous sites, conditions such as pemphigoid, pemphigus, and SJS should be considered.

① Traumatic ulcers and burns

Patients with traumatic ulcers or burns from hot food or drinks will usu-ally have a clear history of this. Ulcers commonly occur in areas of the mouth which can be bitten, namely the lips, cheeks (buccal mucosa), and tongue, while burns are more common on the palate and tongue. Both are often painful. Ulcers and burns can also present as blisters, with a sloughy white surface membrane, which sheds to reveal an erythema-tous or bleeding base. These lesions tend to look inflamed around the periphery.

Ulcers caused by repeated trauma (such as a sharp broken tooth, or denture flange) can be difficult to distinguish from an oral cancer. Malignancies however, tend to have a firmer, indurated consistency, with round rolled margins. An important differentiating factor is chronicity—traumatic ulcers and burns tend to heal spontaneously within 2 weeks, so long as the cause of the trauma has been removed. In contrast, malig-nancy tends to be more progressive and persistent. If in doubt, clini-cal photographs and biopsy by a specialist will assist in giving a clearer diagnostic picture.

Management

Treatment of traumatic ulcers and burns is symptomatic. Patients can use simple oral analgesia. If necessary, topical local anaesthetic gels and mouth rinses can be prescribed. Patients should have a bland diet, avoiding irritant flavours (such as salt, vinegar, citrus, and chilli). Very hot food and drinks should be avoided. Antibacterial chlorhexidine mouth rinse may help in preventing bacterial superinfection. Patients should be reviewed by a dentist or maxillofacial surgeon to ensure the lesion has resolved. *All non-healing ulcers need urgent referral.*

① Herpetic infection (primary herpetic stomatitis, cold sores)

Widespread oral ulceration and blistering is commonly due to herpetic viral infection. This may be primary herpetiform stomatitis, or second-ary cold sores. Primary HSV typically presents in children and teenagers as painful widespread oral mucosal blisters. Patients may also experi-ence malaise, fever, and lymphadenopathy. Eating and drinking may be restricted by pain. In contrast, secondary HSV (cold sores) present as more localized vesicular swellings, typically periorally, with a character-istic prodrome of tingling and pain. These swellings are *highly contagious*, and can be triggered by stress or immunocompromise. Herpetic infection is often diagnosed clinically, but can be confirmed with viral swab.

Shingles (herpes zoster virus) can involve the oral cavity. Usually it is confined to one side (dermatomal distribution), whereas HSV is more widespread.

HSV and herpes zoster virus infection may respond to aciclovir if treatment is initiated promptly at the onset of symptoms. Otherwise treatment is symptomatic, involving analgesia, hydration, and rest. Rarely, hospital admission is required for severe eruptions where pain prohibits any oral intake. In these instances, patients may benefit from systemic analgesia and IV hydration.

⚙️ Stevens–Johnson syndrome

Where lesions are extensive and acute, SJS should be considered (Figure 13.1). Also known as toxic epidermal necrolysis, SJS presents as widespread mucosal and skin ulcers, resulting from a delayed hypersensitivity reaction with separation of the epidermis from the dermis and subsequent epidermal necrolysis. SJS occurs typically in response to medications (in particular antibiotics) and following some infections (including HSV, influenza, and mumps). SJS is a medical emergency with a high mortality, often due to secondary wound infection. Patients are often managed conservatively, with all non-essential medication stopped. Patients with severe oral ulceration require IV hydration and nutritional support. Analgesic mouth rinse and wound dressings may aid in supportive therapy. Treatment with corticosteroids is controversial. If there is ocular involvement, refer also to ophthalmology. SJS frequently causes scar tissue inside the eyelids and a host of other ocular problems.

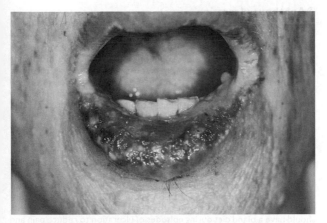

Figure 13.1 Stevens–Johnson syndrome.

✿ Mucous membrane pemphigoid, pemphigus vulgaris

If widespread blistering and ulceration occurs without an obvious cause consider uncommon causes such as pemphigus vulgaris and mucous membrane pemphigus.

Pemphigus vulgaris is an autoimmune mediated mucocutaneous disease which results in intra-epidermal blistering. It is known to affect the oral mucosa prior to other cutaneous sites. It can produce painful blisters which inhibit oral intake. Diagnosis is via biopsy—fresh specimens are preferred as they better permit immunofluorescence. Once confirmed, referral for ophthalmic assessment is prudent, as vesicular lesions are known to affect the corneal surfaces of the eyes, potentially threatening vision.

Mucous membrane pemphigoid is another form of autoimmune blistering disease restricted to mucosal surfaces, particularly gingivae, sinuses and genitourinary tract. It is heralded clinically by a positive Nikolsky's sign—that is rubbing a non-affected site will create a bulla, due to reduced intraepithelial adhesion. Formal diagnosis is made via biopsy with immunofluorescence.

Management

Prompt treatment of pemphigus is essential to prevent sepsis from infection of the blisters once they have burst. Treatment typically involves high-dose oral prednisolone as a first-line drug. Antibiotics should be prescribed for any wound infection, and analgesia titrated according to need. Admission may be warranted for severe vesiculobullous disease preventing oral intake, or with established infection.

In contrast, management of mucous membrane pemphigoid tends to be more localized than for pemphigus, and involves soft diet, oral hygiene, and topical steroids.

⑦ Aphthous ulceration

Patients presenting with episodic oral ulcers may be suffering from aphthous ulceration. Aphthous ulcers are non-contagious, painful ulcers which predominately affect the labial and buccal mucosa, lateral tongue and floor of mouth. They most commonly affect teenagers and young adults, and tend to spontaneously resolve within 2 weeks of onset. Although the exact cause of aphthous ulceration is unknown, several factors are postulated to contribute, including haematinic deficiency (vitamin B12, folate, and iron), immunocompromise, and stress. Ulcers are typically erythematous macules, with intensely red halos of inflammation surrounding them. The surface may be covered by a yellow-grey fibrinous slough.

While the diagnosis of aphthous ulceration is often clinical, ulcers should be followed up to ensure they resolve. In resistant cases blood tests are employed to exclude a haematinic deficiency.

The treatment of aphthous ulceration is typically symptomatic, as for traumatic ulcers and burns. In addition, vitamin B12, folate, and iron supplementation as required may help to prevent episodes of ulcer recurrence. Patients should have a bland diet during episodes of ulceration to reduce pain and irritation. Topical steroids may help. Severe episodes of painful ulceration precluding oral intake may require admission for IV hydration and systemic steroids, although this is rare.

ⓘ Oral/lip cancer

Oral/lip cancer typically presents as a non-healing ulcer, with raised rolled edges. The patient may have a history of risk factors, including smoking, alcohol, and sun exposure. Any ulcer which is progressively enlarging, and persists for >2 weeks, should be referred for urgent biopsy to exclude dysplasia or malignancy. Patients with suspected cancer should also be checked for signs of cervical lymphadenopathy, weight loss, and chest involvement.

Clinical features of a malignant ulcer include:
- Firm
- Fixed
- Indurated
- Non-healing ulcers
- Often painless
- Friable
- Round/rolled/heaped margins.

While oral squamous cell carcinomas can occur anywhere in the mouth, the most common locations are the floor of mouth and posterolateral tongue. Other less common types of cancer include salivary gland malignancy (consider this in any palatal swelling or non-healing ulcer) and lymphoma. See Figures 13.2 and 13.3.

Malignant melanoma is rare. Management involves further imaging to determine whether there is regional lymph node involvement or distant spread. Following discussion at a head and neck multidisciplinary team meeting, treatment may be active or palliative, comprising surgery, chemotherapy, and radiation.

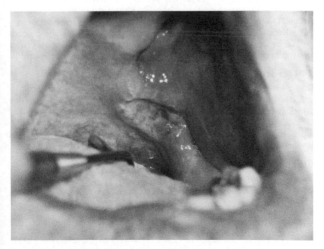

Figure 13.2 Example of oral cancer (1).

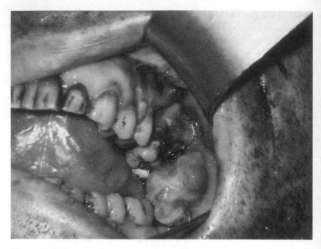

Figure 13.3 Example of oral cancer (2).

① Kaposi's sarcoma

Kaposi's sarcoma is rare, often presenting in HIV-positive patients, as a clinical manifestation of AIDS. It is an angiosarcoma caused by human herpesvirus 8 (HHV8). It typically presents as a violaceous (dark red, blue, or black) macule on the palate which then ulcerates and becomes painful. Diagnosis is via biopsy of the lesion, which tends to be highly vascular. Kaposi's sarcoma cannot be cured, but it may regress and be controlled by use of HAART (highly active anti-retroviral therapy). Other treatment options include cryotherapy, radiation, and chemotherapy.

⑦ Necrotizing sialometaplasia

This is a benign ulcerative lesion found mostly on the posterior hard palate. It is due to necrosis of the minor salivary glands sometimes following an injury (such as palatal infiltrations of local anaesthetic or trauma during intubation). It can also arise spontaneously. Necrotizing sialometaplasia is more common in smokers. It may be confused with malignancy as it shares common features. Biopsy is necessary in most cases to be sure.

① Syphilitic lesions

Syphilis, although uncommon, can present with a characteristic triad of oral lesions

- Primary syphilis—chancre
- Secondary syphilis—condyloma lata
- Tertiary syphilis—gumma.

Primary syphilitic chancres are typically painless, firm ulcers, which present approximately 1 month after oral sexual contact with an infected individual. Chancres are infectious, caused by *Treponema pallidum*. They typically heal spontaneously after several weeks. If syphilis is untreated, it will progress to the secondary stage.

Secondary syphilis presents approximately 3 months after initial infection as a non-itchy rash which can involve the whole body, even the palms and soles. On mucosal surfaces including the oral cavity, the lesions present as infectious wart-like projections, called condyloma lata. Patients may also complain of malaise, fever, and sore throat at this time. These symptoms tend to self-resolve within 1 month of occurring.

Tertiary syphilis presents years after initial infection, and can present as a gumma—an exophytic round soft tissue swelling which can involve the skin, bone, or internal organs. Intraorally, the palate is the most common site of involvement. Tertiary syphilis can also affect the brain (neurosyphilis), with seizures, paresis, or dementia. Tertiary syphilis is not infectious.

Syphilis is diagnosed with serology, or dark field microscopy of a biopsy to identify the characteristic causative spirochete, *Treponema pallidum*. Treatment is with a single injection of penicillin. Once syphilis advances to the tertiary stage, the damage is generally irreversible.

⑦ Angina bullosa haemorrhagica

This is characterized by the sudden appearance of one or more blood blisters within the oral cavity. The cause is unknown. Blisters may occur following mild trauma but usually rupture quickly and heal without scarring. Generally the condition is not serious. Blisters usually affect the palate or oropharynx. Diagnosis is based on exclusion of other conditions and the history of blood as the blister (hence the name).

⑦ Angular cheilitis

Cracked painful fissures at the corners of the mouth (commissures) are termed angular cheilitis. This may signify a nutritional deficiency, such as iron, vitamin B12, or folate. It is also seen in denture-wearers with prominent perioral wrinkles that collect salvia, allowing opportunistic candidal infection in the moist tissue folds. Angular cheilitis can be diagnosed clinically, Exclude deficiencies of iron, vitamin B12 and folate. Construction of new dentures with increased vertical dimension should open the facial height, thereby reducing perioral wrinkling to prevent pooling of moist saliva in these regions.

① Drug induced

Chemotherapy (and radiotherapy) can produce widespread painful ulceration. Nicorandil (used to manage angina) can result in large solitary oral ulceration which may resemble major aphthous ulcers or squamous cell carcinoma. The ulcers may cause severe symptoms, including weight loss from pain and dysphagia. They usually resolve completely on cessation of the drug.

⑦ Erosive lichen planus

This is a chronic painful condition affecting mucosal surfaces, mainly the mouth (oral lichen planus) and the genitals (vulval or penile lichen planus). Ulceration commonly occurs in the mouth and gums. It is sometimes associated with classical cutaneous lichen planus or other forms of mucosal lichen planus.

Management
The management of erosive lichen planus can be very challenging. Topical and systemic treatment may be required. Topical steroids generally applied daily are the mainstay of treatment in most patients. Systemic steroids such as prednisone may be prescribed for severe cases.

⑦ Behçet's disease
This is a rare immune-mediated vasculitis that often presents with recurrent oral aphthous ulcers, genital ulcers, and uveitis. It can also involve the GI tract, pulmonary, musculoskeletal, cardiovascular, and nervous systems. Treatment includes steroids, but patients should be referred to a specialist.

Summary of systemic causes of oral ulceration
- Bacterial infections—TB, secondary syphilis
- Behçet's disease
- Candidia
- Chemotherapeutic agents
- Chronic renal failure
- Crohn's disease
- Dermatitis herpetiformis lichen planus
- Epidermolysis bullosa
- Haematological disease—vitamin B12, folate, and iron deficiencies
- Kawasaki disease
- Linear immunoglobulin A disease
- Nicorandil
- Reiter's syndrome
- SJS, SLE
- Strachan's syndrome
- Sweet's disease
- Viral infections—HSV, herpes zoster virus, coxsackievirus, Epstein–Barr virus, hand, foot, and mouth disease, HIV infection
- Wegener's granulomatosis.

Swellings

Diffuse oral swelling can have many causes. Some of them can progress rapidly. Life-threatening causes of swelling, such as anaphylaxis and Ludwig's angina, must not be overlooked.

Swelling is fairly self-evident and can be diffuse or relatively localized. It can also be acute or chronic. Diffuse swelling is more likely to be related to a systemic cause such as anaphylaxis, whereas localized swelling is more likely with an abscess, or following trauma. It is important to identify the chronicity of the swelling, and to determine whether it primarily involves the soft tissues or the underlying bones.

Patients presenting with swelling of the lips should always be checked for swelling intraorally, notably the tongue and airway. If advanced, oral swelling (particularly in the floor of mouth), can cause problems with swallowing, speech, or even breathing. In severe infection, such as

Ludwig's angina, potentially life-threatening swelling can occur rapidly over a few hours.

If the onset of the swelling has been more gradual, soft tissue conditions such as haemangioma, lymphangioma, orofacial granulomatosis, and amyloidosis could be considered. If the swelling appears to be due to underlying bony distension, it may signify a bony disease, such as ossifying fibroma, fibrous dysplasia, or Paget's disease. *The recent onset of pain and increased growth in any swelling suggests the possibility of infection or malignancy.*

ⓘ Traumatic swelling

Localized lip and oral swelling is very common following an acute trauma, in which case there is usually a clear history of injury. If there is a wound, consider the possibility of a foreign body.

ⓘ Sublingual haematoma

Sublingual haematoma is usually secondary to trauma or dental treatment, and may resemble a large, firm bruise in the floor of the mouth, with distension of the sublingual tissues and tongue displacement. Patients may experience problems with moving the tongue, speaking, and swallowing. Massive sublingual haematoma is often a sign of significant trauma, and patients should be assessed for a mandibular fracture. *Beware of patients taking anticoagulants as the swelling may continue to grow.* Occasionally CT is required.

ⓘ Infections/abscesses

See also ➲ Chapter 11 and ➲ Chapter 12.

Clinical features

Patients most commonly present with a focal infection (abscess). Occasionally, a cellulitis may develop, resulting in more diffuse swelling, redness and pain. Abscesses and cellulitis are associated with acute onset of swelling, typically occurring 24–48 hours prior to presentation. They tend to be painful, warm, and fluctuant to touch. Most intraoral infections arise from an infected tooth. Other causes include an infected fracture (or its fixation plate) and osteomyelitis. An OPT should be taken to check the status of the teeth and bones. Bloods including FBC and CRP will aide in determining whether the patient is systemically unwell. Some patients with a lip or facial abscess may have a history of skin infection, dental pain, or recent facial/tongue piercing, which helps with diagnosis. If an oral, facial, dental, or lip abscess is suspected, maxillofacial referral may be required.

Management

Abscesses should be treated by incision and drainage, either in an inpatient or outpatient setting, depending on the site/size of the abscess, patient cooperation, and whether they are systemically unwell. Antibiotics are commonly given, but it is important to remember that antibiotics alone are never a substitute for surgical incision and drainage of pus.

☼ Ludwig's angina

Patients with deep-seated facial or dental infections may present with rapidly progressive swelling within the mouth and neck. Examination of the floor of mouth is essential to check for impending airway compromise. *If the floor of the mouth is elevated, tense, with restricted tongue movements, and inability to swallow saliva, the patient requires urgent intubation and surgical decompression.* Even if there is no demonstrable collection of pus, cellulitic swelling still benefits from incision and drainage, to reduce bacterial load and inflammatory tissue oedema. *Ludwig's angina is life-threatening, and occurs when fascial space infections track down into the neck and mediastinum.* Patients will be systemically unwell, febrile, with an accompanying leucocytosis and elevated CRP. CT scanning of the neck and chest may demonstrate fascial space collections along with mediastinitis, but this is a very late and imminently life-threatening sign.

☼ Anaphylaxis

This acute life-threatening condition results from immunoglobulin E-mediated massive degranulation of mast cells in response to an allergen, commonly food, latex, or medication. Anaphylaxis may present with diffuse swelling of the lips, tongue, and face (angio-oedema), and can threaten the airway. It may or may not present with a rash. Established anaphylactic shock is characterized by hypotension, tachycardia, and warm peripheries. The allergen must be removed, and the patient treated with oxygen, adrenaline (epinephrine), and antihistamines as appropriate (refer to local guidelines) Facial swelling tends to resolve spontaneously as the anaphylaxis settles.

☼ Hereditary angio-oedema

Hereditary angio-oedema results from a deficiency of C1 esterase inhibitor in the complement cascade. This can result in increased vascular permeability and subsequent tissue oedema. It causes episodic swelling of the face, hands, feet, airway, and GI tract. Episodes may be triggered by stress, surgery, and dental treatment. Diagnosis is made by blood test via liaison with haematology. Prior to surgical or dental treatment, C1-inhibitor concentrate, or fresh frozen plasma can be given prophylactically. Treatment of emerging oedema is the same as for anaphylaxis.

⑦ Haemangioma/lymphangioma

Haemangioma and lymphangioma represent benign lymphovascular malformations with proliferation of lymphatic or vascular capillaries in a localized area. This results in a localized swelling, which may be blue or purplish in colour. The most common oral sites include the lips, buccal mucosa, and tongue. Haemangioma may be congenital and typically enlarge with age. If bitten or traumatized, they may bleed.

Treatment of haemangioma depends on the size of the lesion. If small (<1 cm), many can be successfully excised. If larger, options such as cryotherapy or sclerotherapy or embolization may be considered. In children, until recently the mainstay of treatment was oral corticosteroid therapy. Propranolol has been shown to reduced severe haemangioma in infants. Other treatments include interferon or vincristine.

⑦ Orofacial granulomatosis

Orofacial granulomatosis (OFG) comprises gradual, painless, persistent enlargement of the lips and perioral tissues, which typically presents in adolescence. The lips often feel firm and rubbery. Diagnosis is made by biopsy. OFG may be linked to other granulomatous conditions, including Crohn's disease. Patients should be questioned regarding GI symptoms, and referred for gastroenterology assessment if necessary. Treatment of OFG tends to be conservative, involving dietary restriction (avoiding cinnamon and benzoate preservatives). Occasionally, intra-lesion steroids or tissue debulking can be performed for massive and persistent lip swelling.

⑦ Amyloidosis

Amyloidosis produces gradual oral swelling, which can be either localized or generalized. The localized form predominates and most commonly involves the tongue. Systemic amyloidosis involves the kidneys and heart, and can initially present with fatigue and weight loss, progressing to proteinuria and signs of congestive cardiac failure. Oral amyloidosis tends to resemble benign soft nodules with overlying mucosal discolouration, which may be yellow, purple, and blue. The diagnosis can only be made by biopsy. Once diagnosed, treatment is targeted to the organs involved (e.g. diuretics and dialysis), while surgery and laser excision may help to minimize localized symptoms, including dysphagia.

⑦ Dermal fillers (side effects)

Dermal fillers come in many forms, from resorbable to permanent, and are now commonly undertaken by the cosmetic industry. The face (especially the perioral region) is a commonly injected site. Each kind of dermal filler has its own side effects and these may occur at different times. The most common side effects include:

- Bruising and bleeding
- Itching
- Skin discolouration
- Viral/bacterial infection
- Redness and swelling at the region of injection
- Allergic reactions
- Lumps under the skin
- Skin ulceration in the injected site.

Most of these are uncommon. Allergic reactions are rare. Refer back to the practitioner that placed the filler.

⑦ Fibrous dysplasia

This typically presents in teenagers as a progressive bony expansion. In most cases a single bone is involved (monostotic), and the skull and jaws are commonly implicated. The patient may present with physical bony deformity or, in some cases, painful bony expansion. The exact cause of fibrous dysplasia is unknown, but it is not a neoplasm. Diagnosis is usually made formally by CT and bone biopsy. Bone pain can be treated symptomatically, and in extreme cases, surgical debulking may be required.

⑦ Paget's disease

This is a metabolic bone disorder which typically presents from middle age with progressive bony deformity. Paget's disease involves the skull, spine, pelvis, and femur. Patients may present with bone pain, pathological fractures, increasing bony deformity, or mention that previously well-fitting dentures (or hats) now seem too tight. Occasionally Paget's disease of the skull can cause deafness due to excess ossification in the petrous temporal bone surrounding the inner ear. Diagnosis is typically made via blood tests, which show an elevated alkaline phosphatase. Plain film skeletal survey X-rays may show a cotton-wool appearance, resembling multiple sclerotic bony patches in the skull. Treatment is often under the care of endocrinologists, and bisphosphonate medication may be required, together with vitamin D supplementation. For pathological facial fractures or significant deformity of the jaws, referral may be required.

Pain and numbness in the mouth

Changes in sensation involving the lips, mouth, or tongue can usually be diagnosed by a thorough history and anatomical knowledge of the sensory nerve supply to the oral cavity.

① Trigeminal neuralgia

(See also ➲ Chapter 12.) Trigeminal neuralgia can present with pain within the mouth. This is episodic, sharp, lancinating, or shock-like localized to one or more divisions of the trigeminal nerve. It typically begins around the age of 50, and shooting pain can be triggered by tooth brushing, shaving, or chewing. If pain becomes bilateral, systemic disease should be suspected, such as MS, and the patient referred to a neurologist for testing. The diagnosis of trigeminal neuralgia is typically clinical, based on presentation and anatomical distribution of symptoms. In an emergency setting, a local anaesthetic block will settle severe trigeminal neuralgic pain. For longer-term control, patients may find relief from gabapentin, carbamazepine, or amitriptyline.

⑦ Burning mouth syndrome

Burning mouth syndrome is common. It refers to a burning, scalding, tingly pain inside the mouth, which predominantly affects the tongue, and occurs in the absence of another medical or dental cause. Paraesthesia and xerostomia (dry mouth) may also be present. Patients may experience temporary relief while eating, and occasionally benefit from topical local analgesia. Antidepressants and neuropathic pain agents are commonly prescribed. Cognitive behavioural therapy may also be beneficial in sufferers.

⑦ Reflux oesophagitis

Patients with a history of burning pain extending from the epigastric region may be suffering from reflux oesophagitis. They may have accompanying halitosis, indigestion, or episodes of acid reflux or vomiting. Patients may require medical management with proton pump inhibitors and antacids as required. Spicy food and alcohol intake should be reduced, and patients should be tested for *Helicobacter pylori*.

① Perioral tingling of hypocalcaemia

One of the earliest signs of hypocalcaemia is perioral tingling. Severe hypocalcaemia can then progress on to tetany, and potentially arrhythmias. Causes of hypocalcaemia can include hypoparathyroidism, chronic renal failure and vitamin D deficiency. Patients may demonstrate a positive Chvostek's sign, whereby tapping on the cheek elicits facial spasms. Diagnosis can be confirmed with blood tests, showing low ionized calcium. Calcium can be replaced either orally or intravenously, with vitamin D supplementation. Refer urgently to a physician.

① Multiple sclerosis

MS can cause diverse symptoms throughout the body, including the head and neck. In particular, it may result in hypoaesthesia or neuropathic pain. MS can also cause muscle cramps, weakness, unusual fatigability, and movement difficulties, together with dysphagia or dysarthria, visual problems (diplopia and nystagmus), and bladder/bowel incontinence. Initially MS may present as episodic attacks, which become progressively worse as demyelination continues. Diagnosis may require MRI scanning, neurology referral, and nerve conduction studies. Treatment may involve a combination of medication, such as interferon, methotrexate and steroids, together with physiotherapy.

① Tumours

Malignancy and large lesions may cause oral and facial paraesthesia by compressing or eroding nerves. In these cases, patients usually report a worsening progressive numbness or pain (dysaesthesia). There may be a neoplastic mass evident clinically, on palpation or imaging. Diagnosis is confirmed by biopsy and CT or MRI imaging.

① Hypoglossal nerve lesion (motor weakness)

In patients with tongue weakness, hypoglossal nerve lesions should be considered. Typically, when asked to protrude the tongue, it will deviate towards the affected side. There may or may not be accompanying fasciculation or wasting of the tongue. Patients with a weak tongue may also experience slurring of speech and swallowing difficulties. Since pathology can occur in the brainstem, at the hypoglossal nucleus, or in the nerve itself, an MRI of the skull and neck is required for formal diagnosis. Treatment is dependent on the cause of the problem.

Toothaches and the wisdom teeth

① Dental pain

Patients will commonly present to the emergency department or their general practitioner with dental pain, without first having seen a dentist. For non-dentally trained healthcare providers, dental pain can be a daunting topic. Table 13.1 summarizes different types of tooth pain, and differences in symptomatology, examination, and X-ray findings, and outlines treatment. Often treatment is required in dental practice.

Table 13.1 Classification of dental pain

Condition	Presentation, pain descriptors, clinical and radiographic findings, treatment
Pulpitis	Presentation is typically severe pain.
	Pain described as constant, intense, 10/10, throbbing, interrupting sleep, worse with hot and cold, little relief from simple analgesia. Usually localized to the offending tooth, sometimes pain can be vague, and only localized one side. Pain does not cross the midline.
	Clinically and radiographically the offending tooth will show deep caries or dental restoration involving the pulp. If periapical pathology is present, the condition had likely progressed on to an abscess.
	Treatment is extraction of the offending tooth, or extirpation of the pulpitic nerve, with later root canal treatment. Patients will often require opiate analgesia.
Dental or periodontal abscess	Presentation is one of pain, local or facial swelling, pus, halitosis, and tender or mobile tooth. Deep-seated abscesses may also present with fever, trismus, dysphagia, or stridor, which constitutes a medical emergency.
	Pain is severe, constant, throbbing, worse when biting on the abscessed tooth. Little relief from simple analgesia.
	Clinically the patient may have trismus, fluctuant facial swelling, mobile tooth which is tender to percussion. Pus may be visible extruding from the gingivae around the tooth. OPT will often reveal a grossly decayed tooth with underlying periapical radiolucency and bone loss.
	Treatment involves extraction of the affected tooth and incision and drainage of associated abscess. Patients may also require admission and IV antibiotics.
Recent dental treatment	Presentation is typically within days of dental treatment, such as a deep filling. The patient may complain of toothache, worse with hot and cold foods, but often not constant or severe enough to disturb sleep. If the filling is slightly high, the patient may complain of deranged occlusion or tenderness to biting.
	A peri-apical X-ray will typically show a restoration in the symptomatic tooth, which may be close to the pulp.
	Patients should be prescribed suitable analgesia, and referred back to their dentist for adjustment of the filling. While minor nerve irritation will spontaneously settle over 2–4 weeks, if it persists, the filling may need to be removed and a sedative dressing placed in the tooth. If the filling has been particularly deep the nerve requires extirpation and later endodontic treatment.

Table 13.1 (Contd.)

Condition	Presentation, pain descriptors, clinical and radiographic findings, treatment
Dentine hypersensitivity	Presentation is typically of short, sharp pain to cold food and drinks. Pain resolves in seconds. It may involve a single tooth, or, if erosion or abrasion, multiple teeth. Examination usually reveals teeth with exposed dentine, typically following a filling, chipped tooth, or long-term toothbrush abrasion or acid erosion. Dentine lies just below the protective tooth enamel, and contains tubules with nerve endings which can be sensitive to cold temperature in particular. X-rays are not usually required. Treatment is via the patient's dentist, and may require chemical desensitizing agents, such as concentrated fluoride gel application, or physical barriers such as varnish or fillings. In the interim, the patient should be advised to topically apply desensitizing toothpaste to the affected area and to avoid cold food triggers.
Cracked tooth	Cracked teeth are usually heavily restored, and are more likely to be molars, which take the brunt of chewing and grinding forces. Cracks are often hairline, and rarely visible on X-rays. Patients with a hairline crack in a tooth often complain of short, sharp pain on biting and pain to cold. The teeth should be examined with a FracFinder™, to elicit which cusp or cusps are fractured. X-rays should be taken to exclude abscess formation. Treatment is via dental practice. The tooth may be reduced from occlusion, and in some cases the filling removed to explore for a crack. If a crack is found, the tooth may be stabilized by orthodontic band or crown. Occasionally cracks can propagate right through the crown of the tooth, into the root structure. These teeth are not restorable and extraction will be required.
Referred pain—sinusitis	Patients with sinusitis often present with pain affecting the upper molars, which may be unilateral or bilateral. The pain is often constant, dull, and throbbing, and can be confused with pulpits, resulting in unnecessary dental extractions or endodontics. The main distinguishing feature of sinusitic pain is that it worsens with postural change. For instance, it may become extreme a few minutes after the patient lies down, or sits up. The patient may report a recent cold, or nasal congestion or discharge. OPT will show both the sinuses and teeth and may assist in diagnosis. Acute sinusitis is treated with antibiotics, and the patient may benefit from steam inhalation. ENT evaluation for culture, antibiotics, and possible washout.

In an emergency department setting, patients can be issued appropriate analgesia, and antibiotics. It is worth noting that some dental pain can be severe, and it is possible for patients to unintentionally overdose, particularly on paracetamol-containing preparations. Any patient with a suspicion of liver injury will require urgent LFTs and paracetamol levels, with treatment of overdose as per departmental protocol. Diffuse jaw pain can also be referred pain from myocardial ischaemia.

⑦ Wisdom teeth

Patients can present with painful wisdom teeth for a multitude of reasons. These include eruption pain, pericoronitis, dental caries, pulpitis, and infected (dentigerous) cysts. Wisdom teeth typically erupt between the ages of 18 and 22, provided there is sufficient space. This may be accompanied by some teething pain, which may require paracetamol and chlorhexidine mouth rinse.

⑦ Pericoronitis

If there is insufficient space for complete eruption of the tooth, it is said to be impacted. Sometimes impacted teeth only have space to erupt partially and part of the tooth remains covered by a flap of gum, called an operculum. This can trap food debris and bacteria, causing infection—pericoronitis. Pericoronitis is more common with lower wisdom teeth and presents with pain, swelling, trismus, and pus extruding from around the tooth. OPT confirms chronic pericoronitis with bone loss around the crown of the impacted tooth. Treatment requires irrigation and antibiotics to settle the condition, with eventual extraction of the tooth, ideally when the acute episode has settled. Wisdom tooth removal carries risks of infection and nerve damage, with the possibility of numbness to the lower lip, chin, and tongue on the affected side.

Other problems

Wisdom teeth with caries or pulpitis will tend to present with the same symptoms as for other dental toothache (see Table 13.1). Treatment typically requires extraction of the tooth. It is not practical to perform endodontic treatment in wisdom teeth, which tend to have curved roots and variable anatomy.

Unerupted wisdom teeth remain covered by dental follicle, which can gradually expand, forming a dentigerous cyst. Over many years, these cysts can slowly enlarge, weakening the jaw, and are at risk of infecting. An OPT is useful in patients with wisdom tooth pain to exclude cyst formation, which appears as a well-defined radiolucency involving an unerupted wisdom tooth. Cysts require careful removal. Infected cysts may present with pus extruding from the site, and are typically accompanied by high WCC and CRP. Antibiotics are usually required in addition to surgical enucleation of infected cysts. The offending wisdom tooth is always removed along with the cyst.

The extracted tooth: socket problems

① Bleeding socket

- Bleeding which commences approximately *2 hours following an extraction* may relate to reflex vasodilation. Standard dental local anaesthetic contains the vasoconstrictor adrenaline and a rebound bleed can occur as the drug off. In most cases local pressure by biting on a gauze pack for 20 minutes will stem the bleeding. Additional measures such as exploration and the use of Surgicel®, sutures or bone wax may occasionally be required.

- Bleeding within the *first 24 hours* is often a sign that the blood clot has been disturbed, often by the patient sucking or poking the socket, or by premature rinsing or spitting. The mouth should be gently cleansed with saline or damp gauze to remove any blood, and the patient asked to bite on a gauze pack for 20–30 minutes. The pack should be changed and the procedure repeated. This usually stops the bleeding. The patient must be advised to be careful not to disturb the socket in the ensuing 24 hours.

- Bleeding which does not commence until the *second or third postoperative day* may be a sign of infection. The patient may have accompanying pain, pus, and erythema of the gums around the extraction socket. In severe infections there is lymphadenopathy and trismus. An X-ray should be taken to exclude retained roots in the socket, and the socket explored and debrided under local or general anaesthesia as appropriate. The patient should be given chlorhexidine mouth rinse, antibiotics if appropriate, and advised not to smoke. Any bleeding will settle as the infection resolves.

- Slow bleeding which *continues over many days* following the original extraction may be a sign of an underlying clotting or haematological disorder. The patient should be given a gauze pack soaked in tranexamic acid to help stabilize any clot and stem the bleeding. Bloods such as FBC, LFTs, and a coagulation screen should be taken and the patient urgently sent for further haematological assessment.

Always consider the possibility of a retained root in any socket which fails to heal uneventfully.

① Painful socket and dry socket

(See also ➲ 'Exposed bone', pp. 434–6.) A painful extraction socket can have many causes, ranging from normal postoperative pain, to infection or iatrogenic nerve injury. Often the history regarding the onset, nature, and duration of pain can help in diagnosing the likely cause:

- Patients who have undergone surgical removal involving the raising of a mucoperiosteal flap and bone removal are likely to have moderate to strong postoperative pain, which is worse over the first 3 postoperative days. These patients will often complain of intense, aching or throbbing pain from the bone of the socket, which may prevent sleep. X-rays may be useful to exclude any retained root fragments in the socket. The socket should be checked to ensure it is not inflamed and the clot is still present. Treatment of postoperative pain may involve regular simple analgesia (such as codeine or tramadol). Ice packs and soft diet may also provide symptomatic relief. Patients should be reassured that pain is likely to spontaneously regress with healing.

- In those patients who had minimal pain initially, but who then develop worsening symptoms after the first 2–3 days, alveolar osteitis (dry socket), retained roots, or infection should be considered. An X-ray should be taken to check for residual root fragments. Patients with a deeper seated postoperative abscess or cellulitis may present with fever, swelling, lymphadenopathy, trismus, suppuration, and halitosis. WCC and CRP are often high. If the patient appears systemically unwell, they may require hospital admission for IV antibiotics and debridement of the socket.
- If the patient reports a shooting or electric-type sensation running along the lower lip or tongue, this suggests iatrogenic nerve injury. This is more likely following removal of impacted lower wisdom teeth, the roots of which can lie in close proximity to the inferior alveolar nerve. Wisdom tooth removal carries approximately 1% risk of damage to the nerve. Occasionally patients can develop dysaesthesia. In many cases no intervention is required and the nerve recovers slowly over the ensuing months. However, in a handful of cases, there may be lingual nerve compression from tight sutures, a haematoma causing inferior alveolar nerve compression, or frank nerve transection. In these cases early surgical intervention may be indicated. In an emergency department setting, dental local anaesthetic blocks should relieve neuropathic pain. Patients may experience relief from amitriptyline or gabapentin.
- Patients experiencing short, sharp pain from teeth adjacent to extraction sockets are likely to have dentine sensitivity, especially if the pain is triggered by eating cold or icy food. Adjacent teeth can be checked by their own dentist to ensure there are no cracks or mobility, and X-ray can be taken to check the integrity of the roots. Typically dentine hypersensitivity will reduce over time, but the use of sensitive toothpaste, or application of concentrated fluoride gels should help.

Always consider the possibility of a retained root in any socket which fails to heal uneventfully.

Exposed bone

(See also ➲ Chapter 12.)

ⓘ Alveolar osteitis (dry socket)

Dry socket is the most common cause of exposed bone in the oral cavity. It typically occurs at least 48–72 hours following dental extraction. While the exact pathogenesis is not known, patients are found to have a bare bony socket, with premature loss or dissolution of the protective blood clot. Alveolar osteitis is more likely in smokers, diabetics, immunocompromised patients, females taking the contraceptive pill, and patients with poor oral hygiene. It is more common following removal of impacted lower wisdom teeth. It is less common in simple extractions, and extractions where the socket has been closed primarily with sutures.

Clinical features

Alveolar osteitis typically presents as severe pain, which begins on the second or third postoperative day. The pain is intense, throbbing, and constant. Examination reveals an open empty socket, with no residual clot. There may be erythema in the surrounding gingivae, but there is not usually pus, swelling, or fever. There may also be halitosis or a foul taste in the mouth. Although dry socket is typically a clinical diagnosis, OPT may be useful to exclude any retained root fragments or foreign bodies within the socket.

Management

Treatment is directed at symptomatic relief, and involves gently irrigating and packing the socket with a sedative dressing (Alvogyl®). Patients should be prescribed appropriate analgesia, and chlorhexidine mouth rinse. Provision of a small, curved-tipped syringe may facilitate oral hygiene. Routine prescription of antibiotics is controversial. Dry socket can take 2–4 weeks to resolve.

① Osteomyelitis

Unlike dry socket, which presents days following dental extraction, osteomyelitis tends to present in the ensuing weeks or months. It represents bone marrow inflammation, and most commonly occurs secondary to odontogenic infection or jaw fracture. Acute osteomyelitis of the jaw tends to present as dull, severe throbbing pain, with swelling, redness, and lymphadenopathy. In advanced cases, patients may present with trismus or dysphagia. Adjacent teeth may appear loosened or tender to percussion. In chronic osteomyelitis, patients may present with persistent fistulas. Osteomyelitis more commonly affects the mandible than maxilla, due to its poorer blood supply. Patients most at risk include diabetics, immunocompromised, elderly, and smokers.

OPT may show a mixture of bony destruction (radiolucency) and healing (sclerosis), and may also indicate a cause, such as a fracture, or infected tooth. Treatment requires antibiotics and debridement as outlined in the chapter on the lower jaw.

① Osteoradionecrosis

ORN occurs in bone following radiotherapy, notably the mandible. Radiotherapy impairs the ability of tissues to heal and can result in large necrotic areas of exposed bone. This can be painful, suppurative, and lead to long term fistula formation, ongoing bony destruction, and pathologic jaw fracture. Although ORN can develop spontaneously, it is much more likely following a dental extraction in previously irradiated bone, particularly when the total radiation dose exceeds 60 Gy.

Although diagnosis and treatment of ORN is similar to that of osteomyelitis, ORN may sometimes also be treated with hyperbaric oxygen therapy. In advanced cases, surgical resection and reconstruction is required.

ORN prevention is important. All patients requiring head and neck irradiation should undergo pre-treatment dental assessment, with removal of any dubious teeth prior to commencing radiotherapy.

ⓘ Bisphosphonate-related osteonecrosis of the jaws

BRONJ is exposed necrotic bone found in a subset of patients with bisphosphonate exposure. Bisphosphonates are commonly prescribed for osteoporosis, multiple myeloma, and painful bony metastases. It can be given in an oral or IV form, with the latter being much more potent. Bisphosphonates bind irreversibly to bone, inhibiting osteoclasts and bone remodelling. Although BRONJ can occur spontaneously, it is much more likely following direct trauma to the bone, such as dental extraction. The risk of BRONJ is said to be moderate to high in patients with a history of oral bisphosphonates for 5 or more years, or any IV bisphosphonates. Surgical removal of impacted teeth and full dental clearances pose a higher level of risk than simple extractions.

BRONJ presents with pain, suppuration, halitosis, and fistulae. The extent of osteonecrosis is often delineated on OPT. Treatment is conservative wherever possible, and may include analgesia, chlorhexidine mouth rinse and antibiotics. If the area of necrotic bone becomes extensive, radical resection and reconstruction may be required.

BRONJ is a significant problem, and prescribers of bisphosphonates are urged to send patients for dental assessment and extractions prior to commencing the drug.

ⓘ Oral cancer with bony invasion

Exposed bone in the jaw can be a sign of malignancy. While primary bone tumours (such as osteosarcoma) and metastases from breast, lung, and renal cell carcinoma can occur, the most common form of oral cancer affecting bone is primary squamous cell carcinoma with local bony invasion. In these cases, patients may present with exposed necrotic bone, surrounded by soft tissue ulceration, induration, and erythema. *Sometimes, symptoms can mimic a dental infection, and include painful and loose teeth.*

Denture and orthodontic appliance-related problems

For the vast majority of denture problems, patients should be redirected to their local dentist for assessment and further treatment.

ⓘ Denture rubbing/ulceration

In the case of new dentures, or loose old dentures, the prosthesis may rub against the adjacent soft tissues, causing painful ulceration. This is usually obvious on clinical examination. Patients should be advised not to wear the denture and may benefit from topical lignocaine gel to affected areas. The patient should see their dentist for denture evaluation and adjustment. Ulcers typically resolve within 2 weeks following removal of the traumatic stimulus. *Any ulcer which fails to heal requires a biopsy to exclude malignancy.*

ⓘ Loose or broken dentures

Dentures typically tend to loosen with age, due to resorption and remodelling of the supporting bone. Patients with severely loose or broken dentures should not wear them, and instead see their dentist for repair or relining of the prosthesis.

⑦ Denture stomatitis

Patients with denture stomatitis present with persisting redness of the tissues underneath the denture, most commonly the palate. It is often seen in patients who do not remove their dentures at night, or who do not clean them adequately. Although harmless, denture stomatitis often represents candidal infection. Diagnosis is often a clinical one, but swabs can be taken to confirm the presence of candidal hyphae if desired. Treatment tends to involve a combination of antimicrobials, such as nystatin or miconazole, together with educating the patient on removing the denture at night, and cleaning it with dilute Milton's solution.

⑦ Soft tissue changes: denture hyperplasia, flabby ridge, denture fibroma

Patients with long-standing, ill-fitting dentures may develop firm fibrous soft tissue protuberances underneath the denture base or flanges. These can be in the form of generalized tissue thickening (denture hyperplasia), or discrete pedunculated soft tissue masses (denture fibroma). In the region of the edentulous alveolus, the term flabby ridge is used to describe thickened and mobile tissue. These are the oral equivalent to corns or calluses if poorly fitting shoes are worn. The thickened tissues are typically non-inflamed and have no sinister signs. Treatment involves surgical resection of the offending tissue, and relining or remaking the dentures to ensure a snug fit.

⑦ Dentures too tight

It is very unusual for patients to present with dentures which become tighter over time, particularly to the point where they can no longer be worn. This should arouse suspicion of conditions such as acromegaly, or Paget's disease.

⑦ Orthodontic appliances ('braces')

Orthodontic appliances are commonly used in the UK to 'straighten' teeth. There are many reasons why they are used and these are not only cosmetic in nature. Appliances can be removable or fixed. Problems include:
- Pain and sensitivity—usually after recent adjustment
- Staining/demineralization of the teeth
- Gingivitis
- Bad breath
- Broken/loose appliance.

All of these should be referred back to the orthodontist. Broken appliance may lacerate the soft tissues, which should be managed first. Don't try and remove these, unless they are very loose. Make a note of how many brackets have been removed. If there has been significant trauma or a history of loss of consciousness consider the possibility of foreign body aspiration.

Index